THE CLIMACTERIC
IN PERSPECTIVE

THE CLIMACTERIC
IN PERSPECTIVE

Proceedings of the Fourth International Congress
on the Menopause, held at Lake Buena Vista, Florida,
October 28–November 2, 1984

Edited by
M. Notelovitz and P. van Keep

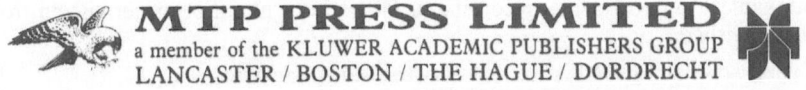
MTP PRESS LIMITED
a member of the KLUWER ACADEMIC PUBLISHERS GROUP
LANCASTER / BOSTON / THE HAGUE / DORDRECHT

Published in UK and Europe by
MTP Press Limited
Falcon House
Lancaster, England

British Library Cataloguing in Publication Data
International Congress on the Menopause
 (4th: 1984: Lake Buena Vista, Fla)
 The climacteric in perspective:
 proceedings of the Fourth International
 Congress on the Menopause, held at Lake
 Buena Vista, Florida, October 28–
 November 2, 1984
 1. Menopause
 I. Title   II. Notelovitz, M.
 III. Keep, Pieter A. van
 612'.665   RG186

 ISBN-13:978-94-010-8339-3   e-ISBN-13:978-94-009-4145-8
 DOI: 10.1007/978-94-009-4145-8

Published in the USA by
MTP Press
A division of Kluwer Boston Inc
190 Old Derby Street
Hingham, MA 02043, USA
Library of Congress Cataloging in Publication Data
International Congress on the Menopause (4th: 1984:
 Lake Buena Vista, Fla.)
 The climacteric in perspective.

 Includes index.
 1. Menopause—Congresses.   I. Notelovitz, Morris.
II. Keep, Pieter A. van.   III. Title. [DNLM:
1. Menopause—congresses. W3 IN667 4th 1984c/
WP 580 I61 1984c]
RG186.I57 1986   612'.665   86-668
ISBN-13:978-94-010-8339-3

Typeset by Blackpool Typesetting Services Ltd., Blackpool.

Contents

List of Contributors   ix

Preface   xvii
M. Notelovitz and P. A. Van Keep

1   Keynote address: menopause and the developing world   1
    Egon Diczfalusy

Section 1: Climacteric medicine and science: a societal need

2   Climacteric medicine and science: a societal need   19
    M. Notelovitz

3   Medicine and science – the role of the basic scientist   23
    R. J. B. King

4   Nutritional needs of climacteric women   27
    E. B. Feldman

5   Exercise and the postmenopausal woman   41
    B. L. Drinkwater

6   Health needs of climacteric women   51
    B. G. Wren

7   Health status and health care utilization by menopausal   59
    women
    S. M. McKinlay and J. B. McKinlay

Section 2: Osteoporosis

8   Pathogenesis of postmenopausal osteoporosis   79
    R. Lindsay, D. M. Hart, H. Abdalla and D. Dempster

9   Etiology of postmenopausal osteoporosis   87
    J. C. Stevenson

10 Bone mineral assessment: a practical guide for primary 95
    care physicians
    B. Ettinger, H. K. Genant and C. Cann

11 Prophylactic treatment for age-related bone loss in   105
    women
    C. Christiansen

Section 3: Climacteric in the cultural context

12 The climacteric syndrome: historical perspectives   121
    J. Wilbush

13 The climacteric in different cultural contexts   131
    P. A. van Keep and T. Abe

14 Climacteric expressions in a crosscultural study   139
    Y. Beyene

15 Climacteric in a Newfoundland fishing village   149
    D. L. Davis

16 A survey of perimenopausal symptoms in Nigeria   161
    O. Bajulaiye and P. M. Sarrel

17 The cultural climacteric in crosscultural perspective   177
    B. M. du Toit

Section 4: How do hormones work?

18 Presentation of estrogens to target tissues   193
    V. H. T. James, R. C. Bonney and M. J. Reed

19 Recent progress in the study of the mechanism of   203
    action of progesterone
    F. Logeat, R. Pamphile, M. Applanat, M. T. Vu Hai and
    E. Milgrom

20 Ovarian hormone action in the brain: implications for   207
    the menopause
    B. S. McEwen

Section 5: Hot flashes

21 An animal model for pharmacologic evaluation of the   213
   menopausal hot flush
   J. W. Simpkins and M. J. Katovich

22 Vascular responses in menopausal flushers   253
   J. Ginsburg and B. O'Reilly

23 Description of the hot flash: sensations, meaning and   259
   change in frequency across time
   A. M. Voda, B. M. Feldman and E. Gronseth

24 Therapy for hot flushes   271
   D. W. Sturdee

Workshops

1 The breast   285
  R. D. Gambrell

2 The aging male   295
  A. Vermeulen

3 Lifestyles; coping with life events and stress at the   299
  climacteric
  L. Severne

4 Genital tract and other target tissues   315
  S. Campbell

5 Hormones and metabolism   321
  G. Samsioe

6 Technology and techniques   329
  W. Utian

7 Sexuality in the climacteric   337
  L. Dennerstein

8 Nutrition   343
  L. Reimer

9   Self-help groups at middle age   361
    R. Schmid-Heinisch

10 Contraception in the premenopause   367
    H.-D. Taubert

11 Progestins   381
    R. Sitruk-Ware

13 Pharmacology of estrogens   393
    T. E. Shellenberger

14 Anthropology   411
    P. Kaufert

15 Joint and musculoskeletal problems   419
    J. Dequeker

16 Psychoneuroendocrinology   429
    L. Speroff

Other scientific contributions

    Special lectures   439

    Short communications   443

    Poster session   449

    Index   457

List of Contributors

H. Abdalla
Menopausal Clinic,
Stobhill Hospital,
Glasgow G21 3UW, UK

T. Abe
Department of Obstetrics/
  Gynecology,
Tohoku University School of
  Medicine,
1–1 Seiryo-Machi,
Sendai 980, Japan

M. Applanat
Laboratoire d' Hormonologie,
INSERM U.135,
Hôpital de Bicêtre,
78 rue du Général Leclerc,
94275 Le Kremlin-Bicêtre Cédex,
France

A. J. M. Audebert
40 Cours de Verdun,
33000 Bordeaux, France

G. Backmann
Department of Obstetrics/
  Gynecology,
UMDNS Rutgers Medical Center,
Academic Health Science Center,
CN19, New Brunswick, NJ 08903,
USA

S. W. Ballinger
University of Sydney,
Faculty of Medicine,
Department of Behavioural Sciences,
Blackburn Building,
Sydney, NSW 2006, Australia

A. Basdevant
Service du Professor Guy Grand,
Hotel Dieu, 1 Clinique Medicale,
Place du Parvis Notre Dame,
Paris, France

C. S. Berkun
University of Maine at Orono,
Department of Sociology and Social
  Work,
221 East Annex,
Orono, ME 04469, USA

Y. Beyene
Medical Anthropology Program,
University of California,
San Francisco,
Center for Social and Behavioral
  Science,
1350 Seventh Avenue, CSBS-317,
San Francisco, CA 94143, USA

K. I. Bland
Department of Surgery,
J-286 JHMHC,
University of Florida College of
  Medicine,
Gainesville, FL 32610, USA

R. C. Bonney
Department of Chemical Pathology,
St Mary's Hospital Medical School,
London W2 1PG, UK

E. Brecher
Yelping Hill,
West Cornwall, CT 06796,
USA

M. Breckwoldt
Universitaets-Frauenklinik,
Hugstetter Strasse 55,
D-7800 Freiburg, West Germany

M. Brincat
Dulwich Hospital,
Menopause Clinic,
East Dulwich Grove,
London SE22 8PT, UK

J. Brown
Clinical Dietician,
Center for Climacteric Studies,
Gainesville, FL 32601, USA

J. Buchanan
Department of Radiology,
Methodist Evangelical Hospital,
315 East Broadway,
Louisville, KY 40201, USA

S. Campbell
Department of Obstetrics &
 Gynaecology,
King's College School of Medicine
 and Dentistry,
Denmark Hill,
London SE5 8RX, UK

C. E. Cann
Department of Radiology,
University of California,
San Francisco, CA 94143, USA

L. Cardozo
Menopause Clinic,
Dulwich Hospital,
East Dulwich Grove,
London SE22, UK

C. H. Chesnut, III
Division of Nuclear Medicine RC-70,
University of Washington,
Seattle, WA 98195, USA

C. Christiansen
Department of Clinical Chemistry,
Glostrup Hospital,
University of Copenhagen,
Norde Ringvej,
DK-2600 Glostrup, Denmark

E. Connell
3159 Marne Drive, NW,
Atlanta, GA 30305, USA

J. Davidson
Physiology Department,
Stanford University,
Stanford, CA 94305, USA

D. L. Davis
Department of Social Behavior,
University of South Dakota,
414 East Clark Street,
Vermillion, SD 57069, USA

D. Dempster
Regional Bone Center,
Helen Hayes Hospital,
Route 9W, West Haverstraw,
NY 10993, USA

L. Dennerstein
University of Melbourne,
Department of Psychiatry,
Austin Hospital,
Heidelberg, Victoria 3084, Australia

J. Dequeker
University of Leuven,
Rheumatology Unit,
UZ Pellenberg,
B-3041 Pellenberg, Belgium

J. O. Deslypere
Academic Hospital,
Department of Endocrinology,
De Pintelaan 185,
B-9000 Gent, Belgium

E. Diczfalusy
Reproductive Endocrinology
 Research Unit,
Karolinska Institutet,
Box 60500,
S-104 01 Stockholm, Sweden

B. L. Drinkwater
Department of Medicine,
Pacific Medical Center,
1200 12th Ave S,
Seattle, WA 98144, USA

B. Dusterberg
Schering Berlin,
Pharmakokinetik,
Muellerstrasse 170-178,
1000 Berlin 65, West Germany

B. Du Toit
University of Florida,
Department of Anthropology,
350 GPA,
Gainesville, FL 326110, USA

L. Ellenbogen
Lederle Laboratories,
Pearl River, NY 10965, USA

B. Ettinger
Department of Medicine,
The Kaiser Permanente Medical
  Center,
2200 Farrell Street,
San Francisco, CA 94115, USA

M. Featherstone
Teeside Polytechnic,
Department of Administration and
  Social Studies,
Middlesbrough,
Cleveland TS1 3BA, UK

B. M. Feldman
School of Nursing,
University of Minnesota,
5–140 Unit F,
308 Harvard Street,
Minneapolis,
MN 55455, USA

E. B. Feldman
Medical College of Georgia,
Department of Medicine,
Section of Nutrition,
Augusta, GA 30912, USA

J. Fishman
The Rockefeller University,
1230 York Avenue,
New York, NY 10021, USA

M. Flint
Klinik Raden Saleh,
Department of Obstetrics and
  Gynaecology,
School of Medicine,
University of Indonesia,
Jalan Radeh Saleh 49,
PO Box 3180,
Jakarta, Indonesia

P. Fottrell
University College,
Galway, Ireland

C. Gallagher
Section of Endocrinology and
  Metabolism,
Creighton University School of
  Medicine,
Omaha, NB 68131, USA

R. D. Gambrell
Department of Endocrinology,
Medical College of Georgia,
Augusta, GA 30912, USA

H. K. Genant
Department of Radiology,
University of California,
San Francisco, CA 94143, USA

J. Ginsburg
Academic Department of Medicine,
Royal Free Hospital,
Pond Street,
Hampstead,
London NW3 2QC, UK

R. Good
The University of Texas Medical
  Branch,
1.200 Graves Building D-29,
Department of Psychiatry and
  Behavioral Sciences,
Galveston, TX 77550, USA

R. Goswamy
King's College Hospital Medical
  School,
Denmark Hill,
London SE5 8RX, UK

R. Greeenblatt
Medical College of Georgia,
Department of Endocrinology,
Augusta, GA 30192, USA

J. G. Greene
Department of Clinical Psychology,
Gartnavel Royal Hospital,
Lansdowne Clinic,
3 Whittinghame Gardens,
Great Western Road,
Glasgow G12 0AA, UK

E. Gronsett
College of Nursing,
Arizona State University,
Tempe, AZ 85287, USA

D. Hart
Menopausal Clinic,
Stobhill General Hospital,
Glasgow G21 3UW, UK

M. Hepworth
King's College University,
University of Aberdeen,
Aberdeen, UK

A. Holte
Institute of Behavioral Sciences in
  Medicine,
University of Oslo,
PB 1111 Blindern,
Oslo 3, Norway

V. H. T. James
Department of Chemical Pathology,
St Mary's Hospital Medical School,
University of London,
Paddington,
London W2, UK

C. Johnston
Division of Endocrinology and
  Metabolism,
Indiana University School of
  Medicine,
Emerson Hall 421,
545 Barnhill Drive,
Indianapolis, IN 46223, USA

M. J. Katovich
Department of Pharmacodynamics,
College of Pharmacy,
University of Florida,
Gainesville, FL 32610, USA

P. Kaufert
Department of Social and Preventive
  Medicine,
University of Manitoba,
750 Bannatyne, Winnepeg R3E OW3,
Canada

J. B. King
Imperial Cancer Research Fund
  Laboratories,
Department of Hormone
  Biochemistry,
PO Box 123,
Lincoln's Inn Fields,
London WC2A 3PX, UK

C. Kitchens
College of Medicine,
University of Florida,
The J Hillis Miller Health Center,
Gainesville, FL 32610, USA

C. Lauritzen
Universitaet Frauenklinik,
Prittwitzstrasse 43,
D-7900 Ulm, West Germany

R. Lindsay
Regional Bone Center,
Helen Hayes Hospital,
Route 9W,
West Haverstraw, NY 10993, USA

R. Lobo
Section of Reproductive
  Endocrinology and Infertility,
University of South Carolina Medical
  Center,
1240 Mission Road, Room 1M2,
Los Angeles, CA, USA

M. Lock
McGill University,
Dept of Humanities and Social
  Studies,
3655 Drummond Street,
Montreal, PQ H3G 1Y6, Canada

F. Logeat
Laboratoire d'Hormonologie,
INSERM U.135,
Hôpital de Bicêtre,
78 rue du Général Leclerc,
94275 Le Kremlin-Bicêtre Cédex,
France

C. Longcope
University of Massachusetts,
Department of Obstetrics/
  Gynecology,
Worcester, MA 01605, USA

K. Macpherson
University of South Maine, School of
  Nursing,
96 Falmouth Street,
Portland, ME 04103, USA

R. B. Mazess
Department of Medical Physics,
1530 Medical Sciences Center,
1300 University Avenue,
Madison, W1 53706, USA

B. S. McEwen
Laboratory of Neuroendocrinology,
Rockefeller University,
1230 York Avenue,
New York, NY 10021–6399, USA

J. McKinlay
American Institutes for Research in
  The Behavioral Sciences,
22 Hilliard Street,
Cambridge, MA 02138, USA

S. McKinlay
American Institutes for Research in
  The Behavioral Sciences,
22 Hilliard Street,
Cambridge, MA 02138, USA

J. Mehta
Department of Medicine,
University of Florida,
J-277 JHMHC,
Gainesville, FL 32610, USA

G. B. Melis
Department of Obstetrics/
  Gynaecology,
University of Pisa,
Via Roma,
56100 Pisa, Italy

E. Milgrom
Laboratoire d'Hormonologie,
INSERM U.135,
Hôpital de Bicêtre,
78 rue du Général Leclerc,
94275 Le Kremlin-Bicêtre Cédex,
France

G. Myrberg
Hagvagen 45,
S-149 OD Upplans Vasby,
Sweden

C. Nagant De Deuxchaisnes
Louvain University in Brussels,
Department of Internal Medicine,
St Luc University Hospital,
B-1200 Brussels, Belgium

M. Notelovitz
The Center for Climacteric Studies
  Inc,
901 NW 8th Avenue,
Gainesville, FL 32601, USA

E. Olbrich
Universitât Erlangen-Nurnberg,
Institut für Psychologie,
Hindenburgstrasse 14/11,
D-8520 Erlangen, West Germany

B. O'Reilly
Academic Department of Medicine,
Royal Free Hospital,
Pond Street,
London NW3 2QG, UK

R. Pamphile
Laboratoire d'Hormonologie,
INSERM U.135,
Hôpital de Bicêtre,
78 rue de Général Leclerc,
94275 Le Kremlin-Bicêtre Cédex,
France

R. Recker
Section of Endocrinology and
    Metabolism,
Creighton University,
601 North 30th Street,
Omaha, NE 68131, USA

C. Rector
CLOUT Coordinator,
Center for Climacteric Studies,
901 NW 8th Avenue Suite B-1,
Gainesville, FL 32601, USA

M. J. Reed
Department of Chemical Pathology,
St Mary's Hospital Medical School,
London W2 1PG, UK

L. Reimer
Halifax Hospital Medical Center,
PQ Box 1990,
Daytona Beach, FL 32015, USA

J. Resnick
Psychological and Vocational
    Counselling Center,
University of Florida,
311 Little Hall,
Gainesville, FL 3611, USA

R. Rivlin
Memorial Sloan Kettering Cancer
    Center,
1275 York Avenue,
New York, NY 10032, USA

G. Samsioe
Department of Obstetrics/
    Gynaecology,
Sahlgrenska University Hospital,
S-41345 Göteborg, Sweden

P. Sarrel
Yale University Health Services,
17 Hillhouse Avenue,
New Haven, CT 06520, USA

I. Schiff
Department of Obstetrics/
    Gynecology,
Boston Hospital for Women,
221 Longwood Avenue,
Boston, MA 02115, USA

R. Schmid-Heinisch
International Health Foundation,
Berliner Allee 56,
D-4000 Dusseldorf 1, West Germany

J. Semmens
Medical University of South Carolina,
Department of Obstetrics/
    Gynecology,
80 Barre Street,
Charleston, SC 29425, USA

E. Severne
International Health Foundation,
Naamestraat 43,
B-1000 Brussels, Belgium

T. Shellenberger
Pharmacopathics Res. Labs., Inc.,
9705 N Washinton Blvd,
Laurel, MD 20707, USA

N. Siddle
King's College Hospital,
Medical School,
Denmark Hill,
London SE5 8RX, UK

G. Silfverstolpe
Department of Obstetrics/
    Gynaecology,
Sahlgrenska University Hospital,
S-413 45 Göteborg, Sweden

J. Simpkins
Department of Pharmacodynamics,
College of Pharmacy,
University of Florida,
Box J-4 JHMHC,
Gainesville, FL 32610, USA

S. Sipinen
Steroid Research Laboratory,
Department Medical Chemistry,
University of Helsinki,
Siltavuoienpenger 10,
SF-00170 Helsinki 17, Finland

R. Sitruk-Ware
Hôpital Necker,
Gynecologie Medicale,
149 Rue de Sevres,
75730 Paris,
Cédex 15, France

L. Speroff
2105 Adelbert Road,
Cleveland, OH 44106, USA

J. C. Stevenson
Endocrine Unit,
Royal Postgraduate Medical School,
Hammersmith Hospital,
Ducane Road,
London W12 0HS, UK

J. Studd
120 Harley Street,
London W1, UK

P. Stumpf
Department of Obstetrics/
  Gynecology,
Pennsylvania State University,
College of Medicine,
Room C-310 Hershey Medical
  Center,
Hershey, PA 17033, USA

D. W. Sturdee
Department of Obstetrics and
  Gynaecology,
Solihull Hospital,
Lode Lane,
Solihull,
West Midlands B91 2JL, UK

H. -D. Taubert
Division of Gynecological
  Endocrinology,
J W Goethe University,
Theodor-Stern-Kai 7,
D-6000 Frankfurt Main, West Germany

J. H. H. Thijssen
Academisch Ziekenhuis Utrecht,
Universit Eitskliniek voor in Wendige
  Geneeskunde,
Catharijnesingel 101,
3511 GV Utrecht, The Netherlands

V. Upton
Wyeth International Ltd,
Box 8616,
Philadelphia, PA 19101, USA

W. Utian
Reproductive Biology,
Mount Sinai Medical Center,
University Circle,
Cleveland, OH 44116, USA

P. van Keep
International Menopause Society,
8 Avenue Don Bosco,
1150 Brussels, Belgium

A. Vermeulen
Department of Endocrinology,
Academic Hospital,
University of Ghent,
De Pintelaan 185,
B-9000 Ghent, Belgium

A. Voda
The University of Utah,
College of Nursing,
25 South Medical Drive,
Salt Lake City, UT 84112, USA

B. V. Schoultz
Department of Obstetrics/
  Gynaecology,
University Hospital,
S-901 85 Umea, Sweden

H. Vorherr
Department of Obstetrics and
  Gynecology,
The University of New Mexico,
School of Medicine,
2211 Lomas Blvd NE,
Alberquerque, NM 87131, USA

M. T. Vu Hai
Laboratoire d'Hormonologie,
INSERM U.135,
Hôpital de Bicêtre,
78 rue du Général Leclerc,
94275 Le Kremlin-Bicêtre Cédex,
France

P. Wagner
University of Florida,
Human Nutrition,
3014 McCarty Hall,
Gainesville, FL 32611, USA

M. Whitehead
Department of Obstetrics/
  Gynaecology,
King's College Hospital,
Denmark Hill,
London SE5 8RX, UK

J. Wilbush
Apt.36, 11112 129th Street,
Edmonton, T5M 0Y5,
Alberta, Canada

H. Wotiz
Department of Biochemistry,
Boston University School of
  Medicine,
80 East Concord Street,
Boston, MA 02118, USA

B. G. Wren
Menopause Clinic,
Royal Hospital for Women,
Paddington, NSW 2021, Australia

S. Zeisel
Boston University School of
  Medicine,
33 Conant Road,
Weston, MA 02193, USA

L. Zichella
Università di Roma,
Policlinico Umberto 1,
IV Patologia Obstetrica-Gynecologia,
00161 Roma, Italy

Preface

The Fourth International Congress on the Menopause was held in Lake Buena Vista, Florida, USA in October – November 1984. It was different from the previous meetings held under the auspices of the International Menopause Society in three respects: the duration of the Congress was extended to five days, plenary sessions were held on each day, and the scope of the subject matter was expanded to provide a total or holistic overview of the subject – hence the theme for the Congress 'Climacteric Medicine and Science: A Societal need.'

In recent years there has been an increased interest in the menopause and middle year aging by scientists and clinicians in fields as diverse as anthropology, urodynamics, nutrition and exercise physiology, while 'newer' issues in clinical medicine, such as osteoporosis prevention and management, attracted specialists in nuclear immaging techniques and internal medicine. Over 120 invited speakers plus numerous contributors to the free communication, special lectures and the poster sessions provided a virtual cornucopia of information on the menopause, that has indeed brought a newer perspective to a subject previously the domain of a single specialty, the gynecologist, and dominated by a single therapy, estrogen replacement.

The organizers were fortunate in being able to attract experts from many parts of the world, all of whom were experienced practitioners in their respective fields, and who were able to share their knowledge with 700 participants from 23 countries in a relaxed environment conducive to postgraduate learning. This information has been summarized by the contents in this volume. The first five sessions are devoted to papers presented at the plenary sessions; this is followed by the summaries of the various workshops and a listing of the free communications and poster presentations.

The detailed papers and workshop reports provide a reference text while an excellent overview of ongoing research (and the researchers involved) can be gleaned from the listed presentations.

A great deal of behind the scenes activity goes into the planning of a meeting: sincere thanks are extended to the program committee, R. Don Gambrell, Wulf Utian, Malcolm Whitehead, Jos Thijsen, and

Vivian James and to the local organizers, staff members of the Center for Climacteric Studies. Although it is an invidious task to select special names for mention, there are three non-Center volunteers whose help was critical to the financial and organizational success of the Congress, Dorma Stanley, Monique Boulet and Beryl Notelovitz.

Finally, a word of thanks to the pharmaceutical industry. Through their generous support, we were able to attract the experts, and stage innovative and educational events such as the cheese and wine poster sessions, an osteoporosis workshop geared to the needs of the clinician and a luncheon seminar exploring alternatives to estrogen replacement therapy.

The quality of the data presented endorsed the hope expressed in the official welcome namely '... that when you return to your respective countries and homes, you will be much richer from the intellectual and social experiences of your visit to Florida and participation in the Fourth International Congress on the Menopause.' We hope you agree after reading this book.

Morris Notelovitz, M.D., Ph.D.
Pieter van Keep, M.D.

Chapter 1

Keynote address: menopause and the developing world

Egon Diczfalusy

> And he that will not apply new remedies must expect new evils; for
> time is the greatest innovator.
>
> (Sir Francis Bacon, *Essayes*, XXIV, 1625)

I would like to start this keynote address by quoting Macbeth: 'If you can
look into the seeds of time and say which grain will grow and which will
not, then speak to me . . .' (Macbeth I, iii); and I wish to speak to you
about a very special grain, ourselves, which will not only grow too
rapidly, but which may grow in such a way that it may cause global
problems, unless new remedies are applied. And new remedies are
urgently needed, since the extent and especially the rate of change around
us is almost overwhelming; indeed, the changes are so rapid that our
perception of these changes seems to lag more and more behind. This is
my main concern and the reason for selecting the well-known quotation
from Sir Francis Bacon as the motto of this address.

BACKGROUND

Various lines of evidence indicate that human settlements existed in
Africa at least a million years ago. However, it took mankind a very long
time to reach the first billion, which happened around the year 1850
(Table 1.1). Then – as indicated by the data of Table 1.1 – growth started
to accelerate; the next billion was reached within 80 years, in 1930; the
third in some 30 years' time, in 1961; and the fourth in only 15 years' time,
in 1976. In this way my own generation in our lifetime has witnessed a

Table 1.1 World population growth during the past two centuries

Year	Billions
1850	1
1930	2
1961	3
1976	4
1987	5

doubling of the world population from 2 to 4 billion. We have seen the birth of another world of 2 billion human beings, equal in numbers, demands, hopes and aspirations . . . and it looks now virtually certain that we will reach the fifth billion within 11 years, some time in 1987. And beyond 1987? What can we expect? The 1982 year's low, medium and high projections of the United Nations Population Division[1] are presented in Table 1.2; according to the most likely medium variant projection, the global population is expected to reach 6.1 billion in the year 2000 and 8.2 billion in 2025. It is estimated by the United Nations that in the years 2000 and 2025, 4.8 and 6.8 billion human beings, respectively, will live in countries which are presently classified as developing ones.

Table 1.2 World population projections of the United Nations Population Division from 1982[1] (millions)

Year	Projection		
	Low	Medium	High
1974	–	3994	–
1984	–	4763	–
2000	5899	6127	6367
2025	7278	8177	9185

Furthermore, according to R. M. Salas, the Executive Director of the United Nations Fund for Population Activities (UNFPA), the United Nations estimate that the world population will continue to grow for another 110 years; according to the medium variant projection, it is expected to stabilize at 10.5 billion by the end of the 21st century. Ninety-five per cent of this future growth of global population will occur in the developing countries of the world[2].

These data can be put into stronger focus by comparing and complementing them with the detailed population projections recently prepared by the World Bank, using available data from 126 member states[3]. By allowing for a number of assumptions, certain global projections can be made[4], like those presented in Table 1.3. These figures are similar to those shown in Table 1.2 and indicate a significant shift that will take place in

Table 1.3 World population projections based on the 1984 World Bank estimates[4] (millions)

Year	World	Developing countries
1980	4435	3298
2000	6147	4884
2025	8298	6941
2050	9780	8400
2100	10 870	9463

the distribution of the future populations between developing and developed countries; it can be seen from the data of Table 1.3 that, whereas in 1980 approximately 26% of mankind was living in the developed, industrialized part of the world, only 13% is expected to do so by the end of the next century, when as much as 87% of the global population will live in developing countries.

Indeed, as stated by A. W. Clausen, the President of the World Bank, in the 1984 World Development Report: 'Population growth does not provide the drama of financial crisis or political upheaval, but as this Report shows, its significance for shaping the world of our children and grandchildren is at least as great'[3]. The complex and interrelated consequences of rapid population growth on the future standard of living and quality of life were succinctly summarized by Mrs Gertrud Sigurdsen, Minister of Health of Sweden, at the United Nations Population Conference in Mexico City: 'Population growth will result in major strains on the already limited availability of food, clean water, shelter, energy, education, health services and job opportunities. It will also speed up desertification, deforestation and soil erosion'[5].

The present extent of these changes has been assessed in detail by the various Specialized Agencies of the United Nations. Thus, the United Nations Environmental Programme (UNEP) reports that in 1981–82 some 1.7 billion human beings lacked safe drinking water and 1.2 billion lacked any form of sanitation[6], and the recent Stockholm Conference devoted to the Year of the Forest (1983) described the other environmental effects of population growth in a rather dramatic way: '*this day* world population has increased by 175 000 persons. *This day* an additional 160 square kilometers have been turned into deserts. *This day* fully 300 square kilometers of tropical forests have been cut down.' Indeed, the UNEP considers that as much as 35% of Earth's land area is at risk from desertification[6]. Furthermore, the International Labour Office (ILO) estimates that: 'Between 1980 and 2000 employment must be found for 700 million new entrants into the labour force, approximately twice the number of the 1960–80 period. Moreover, a back-log of unemployed or seriously under-employed workers need jobs. This group constitutes one-third of the existing labour force of 1200 million'[7]. I hope that these few

Table 1.4 Urban population as percentage of total in selected countries[3]

Country	Population in 1982 (millions)	Percentage of urban population	
		1960	1982
Bangladesh	93	5	12
Brazil	127	45	69
China	1008	18	21
India	717	18	24
Indonesia	153	15	22
Mexico	73	51	68
Nigeria	91	13	21
Pakistan	87	22	29
United States	232	70	78
USSR	270	49	63

examples sufficiently emphasize the importance of the interrelationships between population, environment, resources and development.

Population growth will also be accompanied by increasingly rapid urbanization, predominantly in the developing world. Some of the past changes are indicated in Table 1.4; the rate of change will increase dramatically during the coming years. Thus, whereas in 1974 the number of cities with 4 million or more inhabitants was only 28, and 15 of these were situated in developing countries, the United Nations estimates that by the year 2000 there will be 66 such cities (50 of these in the developing world), and by 2025 their number is projected to increase to 135, out of which as many as 114 are expected to be in developing countries[1]. Expressed in percentages, this would mean that by the year 2025 almost two-thirds of the global population will live in large metropolis, and 58% of the population of developing countries. The impact of this on the provision of health services and sanitation hardly needs any comments.

Pari passu with these changes, the 21st century will also witness a rather dramatic increase in life expectancy at birth, and the marked differences in this respect which exist today will gradually disappear, as illustrated by the data of Table 1.5[1]. Indeed, the United Nations medium projections foresee such a major increase in this respect that it is believed that by 2025

Table 1.5 Life expectancy at birth (years); figures based on the medium projections of the United Nations Population Division[1]

Year	World	Developing countries
1974	55.4	52.7
1984	58.9	56.6
2000	63.5	61.8
2025	70.0	68.9

the global life expectancy at birth will be as high as 70 years[1]. The projections also indicate that the difference between developing and developed countries will gradually diminish, to such an extent that by the year 2025 the average life expectancy at birth in the developing world will be around 69 years. This rate of change becomes very impressive when compared to the 1960 and 1982 estimates of life expectancy at birth. Table 1.6 illustrates the changes that occurred in 10 selected countries, representing roughly two-thirds of the global population. It can be seen from the data of Table 1.6 that during the past 22 years life expectancy at birth for Chinese women increased from 41 to 69 years[3].

Table 1.6 Life expectancy at birth (years) in selected countries[3]

| | | Life expectancy at birth | | | |
| | | 1960 | | 1982 | |
Country	Population in 1982 (millions)	Males	Females	Males	Females
Bangladesh	93	45	42	48	49
Brazil	127	53	57	62	66
China	1008	41	41	65	69
India	717	43	42	55	54
Indonesia	153	40	42	52	55
Mexico	73	55	59	64	68
Nigeria	91	37	40	48	52
Pakistan	87	44	42	51	49
United States	232	67	73	71	78
USSR	270	65	72	65	74

It is easy to see that the rapidly increasing life expectancy at birth will in its turn significantly alter the dependency ratio and the age structure; as shown in Table 1.7, the Vienna International Plan of Action on Aging (1982) estimates that in developing countries the number of persons aged 60 and over will double between 1975 and 2025. It can also be seen from the data of Table 1.7 that by 2025 as much as 23% of the population of developed countries will consist of persons aged 60 and over[8]. Indeed, as shown in Table 1.8, as late as in 1950, the number of persons aged 60 and over did not exceed 200 million; 40% of these persons lived in developing

Table 1.7 Projected age structure as percentage of population[8]

| | Developed countries Age group | | Developing countries Age group | |
Year	<15	>60	<15	>60
1975	25	15	41	6
2000	21	18	33	7
2025	20	23	26	12

Table 1.8 Projected population size of persons aged 60 and over[8]

Year	World (millions)	Developing countries (millions)
1950	200	80
1975	350	178
2000	590	355
2025	1100	792

countries. According to the figures published by the United Nations World Assembly on Aging[8], the number of aged persons is expected to increase to 1100 million within the next 40 years, and by 2025 more than 70% of them will live in developing countries.

With the background information presented in Tables 1.1–1.8, we can now address the subject proper: menopause and the developing world.

MENOPAUSE IN THE 21st CENTURY

It follows from the estimates of life expectancy at birth that the number of women aged 60 and over will exceed that of men in the corresponding age group in most parts of the world. According to the figures of the Vienna International Plan of Action on Aging[8], the present sex ratio, i.e. the number of males per 100 females in industrialized countries, is around 75 for age group 60–69, and approximately 50 for those aged 80 and over. Furthermore, from the country-by-country data reported in the latest edition (1983) of the *World Health Statistics*[9], it is possible to estimate the number of women approaching, or reaching, menopause by calculating the world population of women aged 45 and over. These figures are presented in Table 1.9. It can be seen from these data that by year 2000, in some 15 years time from now, there will be more than 700 million in this category, and two-thirds of them in the developing world. Furthermore, it can be calculated from the data of Table 1.9 that by 2000 almost 24% of the global population will consist of women aged 45 and over,

Table 1.9 The world population of women aged 45 and over (in millions)[9]

Region	Year 1960	1980	2000
Developed countries	155	204	251
Developing countries	175	274	468
Total	330	478	719

and that – as far as the developed countries are concerned – almost 39% of their population will be made up by this category.

However, even in the developing world, by the year 2000 the percentage of such persons will approach 20%. Hence, it is naive to think – what I frequently hear from developing country administrators – that the menopause as a problem mainly concerns the well-to-do Western societies. Within 15 years it will be a major problem also in the developing world, and by the middle of the 21st century it may, or may not, develop into a problem of overwhelming proportions in several developing countries which lack a suitable medical infrastructure. I say it may, or may not, since 'there are virtually no data on the age distribution of the menopause and no information on its sociocultural significance in the developing countries', as was stated by a WHO Scientific Group just a few years ago[10].

In the discussion that follows, the WHO definitions will be used: *menopause* being the permanent cessation of menstruation resulting from loss of ovarian follicular activity, *perimenopause* (climacteric) is the period immediately prior to the menopause and at least the first year after it, and *postmenopause* is the period dating from the menopause, which can only be assessed in retrospect[10]. In my own view the definition of the perimenopause is probably outdated by now, since a considerable body of evidence indicates that it is a considerably longer period than indicated above.

Many factors influence the *age at menopause*, such as important ethnic differences, secular trends, age at menarche, marital status, parity, occupation, smoking habits, altitude, socioeconomic conditions and perhaps also contraceptive use[10]. The above data are, however, mainly based on observations made in developed countries, and little, if any, information is available on the age distribution, sociocultural significance and prevalence of various symptoms and major disorders in developing countries. This lack of information makes it very difficult to adequately assess the health- and social-service needs of these countries today, and especially tomorrow. Indeed, very little is known of the perception of developing country women of lack of menstruation, childlessness, the attitude of husbands, the social status and extent of economic deprivation of such women, or the alternative roles they may play and the medical services available to them[10]. Similarly, information is extremely scanty about the perimenopausal symptoms, their prevalence in various developing country settings, their sociocultural impact, and last, but not least, the optimal hormonal therapy needed, which is also a controversial subject in the developed world. Hence, information is urgently needed on the prevalence and sociocultural impact of the various vasomotor and psychological symptoms, sexual decline, vaginal dryness, dyspareunia, insomnia, urinary problems, skin changes and bleeding disturbances.

OSTEOPOROSIS

Among the major *disorders*, it will be extremely important to find out the prevalence of *osteoporosis* in various developing countries, in view of the rapid change in lifestyle and the equally rapid increase in life expectancy at birth. Of course, osteoporosis is a monumental problem in the developed world, since it is established that, by the age of 80, some 25% of Western women have sustained one or more fractures of the proximal femur, vertebrae, or distal radius[10]. In the United States osteoporosis is affecting as many as 15–20 million individuals, and about 1.3 million fractures attributable to osteoporosis occur annually in people aged 45 and over[11]. In fact, the cost of osteoporosis in the United States has been estimated at US \$3.8 billion annually. Among those who live to be 90, 32% of women and 17% of men will suffer a hip fracture, mostly due to osteoporosis. Most patients fail to recover normal activity, and mortality within 1 year approaches 20%[11].

Why do people develop osteoporosis? Epidemiological studies point to a number of risk factors – but again, only in Western populations. The *established risk factors* include age, sex, race, body weight-for-height, menopause, estrogen- and calcium deficiency, lack of exercise, immobilization and prolonged bed rest. The risk increases with age and is higher in women than in men, and in whites than in blacks[11]. The estimates are based on data obtained in the United States; no information is available as far as developing countries are concerned.

Among *possible risk factors*, hereditary factors; smoking; various dietary factors, such as alcohol, vitamins A and C, magnesium and protein are under consideration. Again, no data are available from developing countries.

There has been a significant improvement in our diagnostic possibilities to ascertain accelerated bone loss, with methods ranging from simple spine radiography, radiogrammetry, photodensitometry, estimation of Singh index, photon absorptiometry, neutron activation techniques, Compton scattering, improved tomography to classical histomorphometry[11]. However, there still are many unsolved problems with regard to suitable methodology to assess bone loss during relatively short periods of time, especially in epidemiological studies to be conducted in developing countries.

It is established that in Western women, four factors are of cardinal importance for the reduction of the *rate of bone loss*: estrogen, calcium, vitamin D and exercise[10, 11]. It is also agreed that adequate nutrition should include a daily dose of 1500 mg elemental calcium in the absence, and 1000 mg in the presence, of estrogen substitution therapy[11]; however, opinions greatly differ as to what dose, and particularly what type, of estrogen will provide an optimal substitution. A number of other agents are also under study[11]; they include sodium fluoride, calcitriol, calcitonin, anabolic steroids, large doses of progesterone, thiazides, bisphosphonates and parathyroid preparations (such as the 1–34 fragment). The relative merits of these therapies remain to be ascertained.

However, the overwhelming problem is that we do not have any effective agent which could accelerate bone formation and replace bone that is lost. All the presently available therapeutic regimens can do is to reduce the rate of bone loss.

Why is it so important to establish whether or not osteoporosis is a major risk factor in Oriental or Indian women? Is it not possible to simply extrapolate the data obtained in Western women? Certainly not. It is known that genetic heterogeneity is frequently associated with *metabolic heterogeneity*, as indicated in the examples shown in Tables 1.10–1.12,

Table 1.10 Poor metabolizers* of debrisoquine in various populations[12]

Population	Percentage
Saudi Arabians	1
Egyptians	1
Ghanaians	5
Canadians	6
Nigerians	8
Britishers	9
Orientals	32

*Defined as a urinary drug/metabolite ratio of 12.6 or above

which have been adapted from the classical paper of Kalow[12]. The data of Table 1.10 indicate population differences with respect to the metabolism of debrisoquine; it is obvious that Egyptians metabolize the drug far better than Orientals. The data of Table 1.11 indicate major differences in the percentage distribution of slow acetylators of isoniazid; the difference between Caucasians and Chinese or Japanese is impressive. The data

Table 1.11 Percentage distribution of slow acetylators of isoniazid in various populations[12]

Population	Slow acetylator	Fast acetylator	
		Heterozygotes	Homozygotes
South Indians	59	36	5
Caucasians	59	36	5
Negroes	55	38	7
Chinese	22	50	28
Japanese	12	45	43
Eskimos	10	44	46

Table 1.12 Percentage distribution of alcohol dehydrogenase variants in liver specimens from various populations[12]

Country of origin	'Usual'	'Atypical'	
		Heterozygotes	Homozygotes
Switzerland	82	18	0
Germany	93	7	0
England	93	7	0
Japan	13	44	43
China	11	44	45
India	100	0	0

of Table 1.12 indicate the percentage distribution of alcohol dehydro-genase variants in liver specimens; again, the difference between European and Chinese or Japanese findings is striking.

Hence, an over-all assessment of the *research priorities* with regard to osteoporosis strongly suggests that it will be important to study possible demographic differences, the influence of nutritional factors and the effect of socioeconomic conditions. It will also be of crucial importance to develop safe, simple, reliable and inexpensive diagnostic procedures and preventive measures. Last, but not least, a major effort is required to find a drug which will not only diminish the rate of bone loss, but which will accelerate bone formation.

CARDIOVASCULAR DISEASE

The second disorder of major importance is atherosclerotic cardio-vascular disease. It is established that cessation of ovarian function is associated with a significantly increased risk of morbidity and mortality from such diseases[10], as is indicated in Table 1.13. This table was com-piled on the basis of the data of the latest edition of the *World Health Statistics*[9]. The point is that the data indicate major differences not only between developing and developed countries, but also among various Western countries. The fact that senility without psychosis was indicated

Table 1.13 Selected causes of death for women aged 65 and over in various countries[9]

Cause of death	WHO classification	USA	UK	France	Japan	Thailand
Diseases of circulatory system	(25–30)	63	55	47	53	7.1
Malignant neoplasms	(08–14)	17	17	16	16	1.1
Senility without psychosis	(465)	0.1	0.4	3.4	7.6	67
Atherosclerosis	(300)	2.6	2.0	0.7	1.1	0.0
Number >65 who died		641 163	240 188	220 551	252 158	40 149

Figures indicate percentage of women who died that year at the age of 65 and over

Table 1.14 Selected causes of death for women aged 65 and over in various countries[9]

Cause of death	WHO classification	USA	UK	France	Japan	Thailand
Breast cancer	(113)	2.6	2.9	2.2	0.5	0.1
Uterine and cervical cancer	(120 + 122)	1.0	0.8	1.1	1.1	0.2
Myocardial infarction	(270)	16	16	7.2	4.0	0.2
Other ischemic heart disease	(279)	18	8.4	2.2	3.8	0.1
Cerebrovascular disease	(29)	14	16	17	27	1.6
Number >65 who died		641 163	240 188	220 551	252 158	40 149

Figures indicate percentage of women who died that year at the age of 65 and over

as the predominant cause of death in Thailand most probably indicates flaws in the diagnosis and data collection, and reflects the fact that the diagnosis was not based on autopsy findings.

However, whereas it is relatively easy to criticize and dismiss the relevance of the Thai data shown in Table 1.13, it is more difficult to neglect the significance of the differences shown in Table 1.14. Indeed, the data strongly suggest that significant differences exist in the frequency of myocardial infarction and of other ischemic heart diseases as causes of death for women in the United States, compared to the figures reported not only from Japan, but also from France. Therefore, a detailed study of the various risk factors involved appears to represent a very high priority. Also, as rightly emphasized by the WHO Scientific Group[10], because of the overwhelming size of the underlying risk, in-depth epidemiological studies on the effect of possible preventive agents, such as estrogens with or without added progestins should be undertaken in various populations with the highest possible priority.

MUSCULOSKELETAL DISORDERS

The third group of major disorders is represented by the various forms of rheumatic and degenerative musculoskeletal disorders. Here again, the same considerations apply as in the case of osteoporosis and cardiovascular disease; we have to find out the prevalence in different populations, including a large variety of developing countries; we have to ascertain whether or not estrogen administration is protective, and if so, what type of estrogen should be given in what dose. Last, but not least, the relative risks and benefits of such therapy must be carefully evaluated. What are those risks? The risks under discussion include endometrial and breast cancer, hypertension, cardiovascular complications, gall-bladder disease and urinary tract stones (the last-mentioned in connection with high calcium doses).

RISKS OF SUBSTITUTION THERAPY

The 'estrogen risk' can be brought into focus by relating the established
and/or probable risk factors for endometrial and breast cancer, as shown
in Table 1.15. As indicated by the data in this table, there is indeed a
strong association between exogenous estrogens and risk of endometrial
cancer[13]. This poses an 'estrogen dilemma', shown in Fig. 1.1. What this
figure intends to illustrate is that inadequate estrogen therapy will increase
the risk of osteoporosis but decrease the risk of endometrial hyperplasia
and endometrial cancer, whereas excessive estrogen therapy may diminish

Table 1.15 Risk factors for endometrial cancer and their relation to breast cancer[13]

	Relative strength of association	
Risk factor	*Endometrial cancer*	*Breast cancer*
Late menopause	+	+
Estrogen-secreting hormones	+ +	×
Polycystic ovary/anovulatory cycles	+ +	+
Obesity	+	±
Nulliparity	+	+
Low parity	+	±
Menstrual irregularity	+	−
Exogenous estrogens	+ +	+

+ +: strong; +: moderate; ±: probable; ×:insufficient data

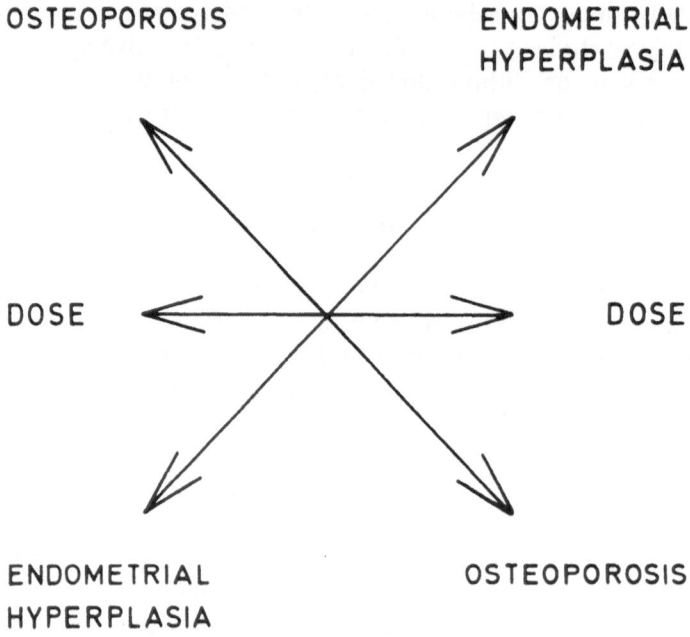

Figure 1.1 A simplistic view of the estrogen dilemma; how much is too much?

the risk of osteoporosis but increase the frequency of endometrial hyperplasia. However, while this seems to be true, it may be worth remembering that endometrial cancer is relatively infrequent; osteoporosis is not.

EPILOGUE

The United Nations Vienna International Plan of Action on Aging[8] states with emphasis that 'diseases do not need to be essential components of aging', and then it predicts that 'It is expected that, as men and women live to increasingly greater ages, major disabilities will largely be compressed into a narrow range just prior to death.' This sounds reassuring. It is clear, however, that if we really wish to achieve this objective for the benefit of the women of this world, a number of urgent tasks will be confronting us, mainly, but not entirely, in the developing world. First of all, we have to establish the age distribution and sociocultural significance of the menopause and the prevalence of the various symptoms and disorders which to a large extent will determine the health and social service needs of individual developing countries in this area. Major progress must also be made in the fields of diagnosis, prevention and cure of osteoporosis and atherosclerotic vascular disease, and – at the same time – we have to eliminate, as far as possible, the risks associated with preventive hormonal therapy. Also, the prevention of senility will acquire greater and greater importance *pari passu* with the unprecedented global increase in life expectancy at birth. Since all this will prove to be exceedingly expensive, and since tomorrow, like today, the setting of national priorities in different countries may, or may not, reflect the primary needs of a rapidly aging population, I strongly believe that there is also a clear need to establish an international code of ethics for the protection of the elderly within the framework of the United Nations and to impress the member states to ratify it rapidly.

The very expensive national and international measures required to foot the above bill raise, of course, the perennial question as to where to find the funds needed. Like so many of my fellow scientists, I also lack any 'great ideas' for a breakthrough to provide the necessary money. However, I cannot resist the temptation to record here the global expenditures on arms and health, as reported by the UNEP in 1984. According to this publication, in 1978 the military expenditures of developed countries amounted to US$ 345 billion, and those of the developing countries to 102 billion. The pooled health expenditures of developed countries during the same year amounted to US$ 213 billion, whereas all developing countries together spent only US$ 22 billion for health services[6]. Hence, in 1978 the developing world spent almost five times as much money on armaments as on health services. Furthermore, the above figures seem to suggest that in 1978 global expenditures on armaments were somewhat less than half a trillion dollars. A more recent figure published by the Stockholm International Peace Research Institute (SIPRI) in its 1984 *Yearbook* indicates that the world military expenditure in the year 1983 (expressed in constant price figures at 1980 prices and exchange rates) amounted to US$ 637 billion, which comes pretty close to US$ 1 trillion at current prices and exchange rates[14]. This raises the question, how much money really is US$ 1 trillion? If we divided this figure by 5 billion (the expected global population in the year 1987), this mathematical exercise would yield US$ 200, a sum which in another world could have been spent to improve the life condition of every single human being living on this Earth today. So much money is US$ 1 trillion.

A. L. Mackay quotes Meister Eckhart (1260–1327) as having said more than 600 years ago that 'the greatest power available to man is *not to use it*'[15]. As I view it, Meister Eckhart (like many of us on other occasions) was wrong, since the greatest power available to man is *to use it* in order to improve the human condition. I therefore prefer to close this address with a quotation from William Faulkner: 'I decline to accept the end of man . . . I believe that man will not merely endure: he will prevail . . .'.

REFERENCES

1. United Nations Population Division (1984). World Population Prospects: Estimates and Projections as Assessed in 1982, to be issued as a United Nations Publication; data reproduced in the Review and Appraisal of the World Population Plan of Action; Report of the Secretary General, United Nations International Conference on Population, Mexico City, August 1984; E/Conf. 76/4 Corr. 1.26, July, pp. 29–30
2. Salas, R. M. (1984). Population: The Mexico Conference and the Future. Opening Address for the International Conference on Population, Mexico City, 6 August. UNFPA/ICP/84/E/2500
3. *World Development Report* (1984). Published for the World Bank by Oxford University Press
4. The World Bank (1984). 1984 Estimates and Projections; cf. McNamara, R. S. (1984) *The Population Problem: time bomb or myth*. Washington, DC. 1 July
5. Delegation of Sweden to the United Nations International Conference on Population, Mexico City, August 1984. Statement by Ms Gertrud Sigurdsen, Minister of Health
6. United Nations Environment Programme (UNEP), Nairobi (1984). The State of the Environment 1984: The Environment and the Dialogue between and among developed and developing countries, UNEP, Nairobi, Kenya
7. International Labour Office (ILO), Geneva (1984). *Population, Development, Family Welfare. The ILO's contribution*, p. 55
8. United Nations World Assembly on Aging, Vienna (1982). The Vienna International Plan of Action on Aging, 192, paras 9 and 11. Cf. Swedish Ministry for Foreign Affairs (1983): *Förenta Nationernas åldrandekonferens i Wien 26 juli–6 augusti 1982*. Norstedts Tryckeri, Stockholm
9. World Health Organization (1983). *World Health Statistics Annual*, Geneva
10. World Health Organization (1981). *Research on the menopause*. Techn. Rep. Ser. 670, Geneva
11. National Institutes of Health (1984). *Osteoporosis*. Consensus Development Conference Statement, vol. 5, no. 3 (US Government Printing Office: 1984-421-132:4652)
12. Kalow, W. (1982). Ethnic differences in drug metabolism. *Clin. Pharmacokinet.*, 7, 373–400 (ADIS Press Australasia Pty Ltd)

13. Thomas, D. B. (1984). Do hormones cause breast cancer? *Cancer*, **53**, 595–604
14. Stockholm International Peace Research Institute (SIPRI) (1984). Armaments and Disarmament. *SIPRI Yearbook*. (London: Taylor and Francis)
15. Mackay, A. L. (1977). *Scientific Quotations: the harvest of a quiet eye*, p. 50. (New York: Crane, Russak & Co.)

Section 1

Climacteric medicine and science: a societal need

Chapter 2

Climacteric medicine and science: a societal need

M. Notelovitz

The climacteric is a natural and inevitable event. All women will experience this period of change just as they did puberty. The reproductive senescence of the climacteric is a mirror image to the maturation associated with puberty and parallels the cessation of menstruation (menopause) with its onset (menarche). The menopause is thus a single event which lasts approximately 4–5 days, whereas the climacteric spans a 30-year continuum between age 35 and 65 years. Many of the changes which occur are remote from the reproductive tract; in addition pathology, associated with aging *per se*, imposes additional clinical realities creating a spectrum of conditions far removed from the traditional view of the menopause: amenorrhea and its associated 'badge' – the hot flash.

Why choose the age range 35–65? The first recognizable features of failing steroidogenesis occur at this time with shortening of the menstrual cycle and subtle yet measurable decrements in plasma estradiol, and elevated levels of FSH. In addition, bone mass maturity is reached at this time – a little recognized clinical feature that can have a significant impact on later life and well-being. The distinguishing biologic features at the opposite end of the spectrum are less clear-cut: here traditional (yet arbitrary) definitions are applied to age 65 as being the onset of the geriatric years and so serves as the dividing line between the middle and older years.

The needs of women vary during the climacteric. Latent changes in the early phase have the potential for significant morbidity in the later years; by early recognition and prevention, conditions such as osteoporosis and atherogenic cardiovascular disease may be ameliorated or even prevented.

It is for this reason that the theme for the Congress – Climacteric Medicine and Science: A Societal Need – has been chosen. By recognizing the needs of the total woman, the expertise of the primary care physician (gynecologist or family practitioner) is complemented by the skills and talents of nutritionists, exercise physiologists, psychologists and social counsellors. Traditional health care specialists, in turn, need to work with the basic and social scientist.

THE CLIMACTERIC

THREE DECADES OF HEALTH NEEDS

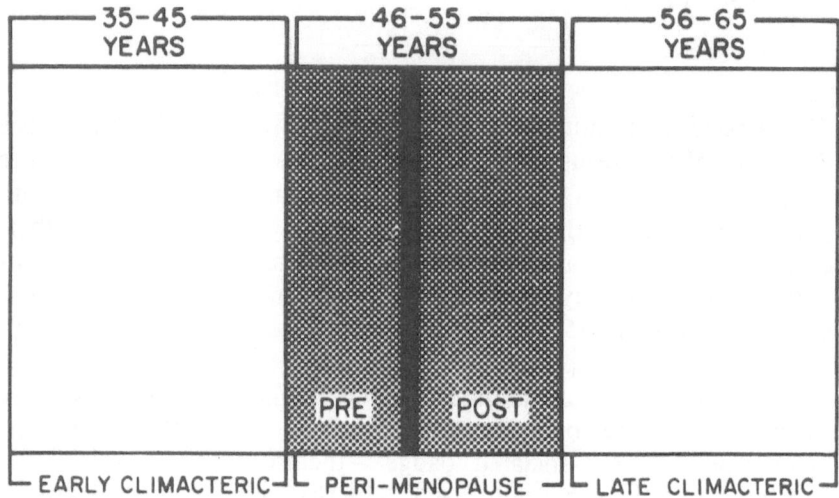

Figure 2.1

As a clinician involved with the care of women during their middle years, I have arbitrarily subdivided the climacteric into three decades: the early and late climacteric, separated by the perimenopause (Fig. 2.1). The early climacteric (when symptomatic) presents in women between the age of 35 and 45 years with gynecologic problems associated with abnormal steroidogenesis: dysfunctional uterine bleeding and the premenstrual syndrome. A need that has been neglected for many years – safe and effective contraception – is yet another common clinical requirement of early climacteric women. The perimenopausal period – premenopause (age 45–50) and the postmenopause (50–55) – is when the traditional signs and symptoms of 'the menopause' occur and hormonal therapy is often needed. As more experience is gained it is increasingly recognized that menstruating premenopausal women may exhibit 'classic' menopausal symptoms which are responsive to estrogen and/or progestins. On the other hand, why do only a minority of postmenopausal women develop significant symptoms. An important question that still needs to be answered is: Who needs to be treated with hormone replacement therapy? During the late climacteric (age 55–65), signs of osteoporosis and atherogenic cardiovascular disease frequently present as the overt feature of earlier asymptomatic change. These diseases are due as much to lifestyle (diet and activity) and social habits (smoking and alcohol) as they are to a loss of hormonal function. Hence the need for physicians to be as comfortable with exercise prescription and nutritional advice as they are with hormone usage. Finally, the age-related consequences of non-menopause-related conditions – cancer of breast, colon and lung; hypertension; diabetes etc. – need to be considered and measures taken to ensure their early recognition, treatment and prevention or cure.

The development of new technology aids in this process. Densitometers are now available for the early detection of osteoporosis; stress and treadmill tests can be used to determine cardiorespiratory fitness; mammography is used for breast cancer detection; urodynamics to determine the cause for urinary incontinence; while biofeedback technology may aid in stress management. The use of this and other technology is additive and should not replace the skills and clinical judgment of the clinician.

Climacteric medicine is a discipline waiting to be born. In short, it may be defined as preventive medicine for women (and men) in their middle years, and has as its basic premise consideration of the individual as a whole, with the objective of achieving a healthy mind in a healthy body in a healthy environment. As such, it may be regarded as a national insurance policy. A healthy middle-age population will be a productive population; by preventing or ameliorating chronic illnesses much of the need for and cost of long-term geriatric care can be avoided. We have noted the benefit of preventive medicine in obstetrics and dentistry. Why should the climacteric be any different?

It is in this context that climacteric medicine has emerged as a science and has become a societal need.

Chapter 3

Medicine and science:
the role of the basic scientist

R. J. B. King

Basic and medical scientists interact in several ways to the benefit of both scientists and patients. In this chapter two examples will be used to illustrate the various components of that interaction.

Most scientific discoveries are the result of one of two processes: logical thought and experimentation is the commonly perceived method of progress but frequently serendipity is a major factor.

SERENDIPITY

Many examples can be cited of chance observations in one field being translated into major advances in a different area of scholarship. This is sometimes ascribed to luck but in most cases reflects the scientific insight of the person(s) proposing the altered use of an observation. A classical example from the scientific/medical area is the development of medical X-ray techniques from physical studies of uranium by Curie and Bequerel. As a more recent example, I shall use current work of Taylor-Papadimitriou and her colleagues. They have been characterizing the membranes of normal and neoplastic human mammary epithelial cells with the main objective of learning more about the biochemical changes accompanying carcinogenesis. As a consequence of these studies, they are now pursuing a very different goal, the detection of ovarian tumors in patients by non-invasive means. Data relating to this work can be found in references 1–4.

At the cellular level, cancer is characterized by unregulated growth in which cells do not respond to inhibitory signals in their environment such as contact with other cells, basement membranes or growth factors and nutrients in plasma. This altered perception of the environment has focused attention on the cell membrane as the interface between the inside and outside of the cell. Dr Taylor-Papadimitriou has been using monoclonal antibodies to probe the components of the membrane. To obtain such antibodies, antigens must first be obtained which can then be used to immunize mice. Given that antibodies are often species-specific, it was desirable to use human material, which can often be a major difficulty for the scientist. Normal human breast tissue is only rarely available in the quantities required, so alternative sources had to be used. Ceriani had pointed the way out of this dilemma by using delipid-ated cream from human milk[4]. When milk is secreted by mammary epithelium, the fat droplets are surrounded by regions of the apical cell membrane which, after purification, can be used to immunize mice. Alternatively, milk also contains a small number of intact mammary epithelial cells which, after amplification in culture, can be used as the immunogen. Both methods were used.

Two antibodies were obtained which, as part of the essential scientific work, had to be characterized. This was mainly done by histochemical monitoring of their ability to recognize antigens in tissue sections from different sources. As expected, the antibodies reacted with lactating mammary gland and, interestingly, with some but not all breast tumors. The surprise came when ovary was examined; the antibody stained neo-plastic but not normal epithelial membranes. It is this observation that opened the collaboration with the medical scientists.

The antibody can be labeled with radioactive iodine and injected into the blood stream. As the antigen is exposed on the cell surface it can interact with the labeled antibody. By the choice of an appropriate iodine isotope [^{123}I] and conditions, the antibody bound to ovarian carcinoma can be detected by means of external scintigraphy with a gamma camera.

The validity of this research as an aid in the detection and diagnosis of ovarian cancer is being assessed but it does illustrate important features that are relevant to the topic of this talk. Firstly, for basic scientists to contribute to medical science they must have the appropriate materials with which to work; blood and urine present less of a problem than tissue samples. In the example quoted, ingenuity overcame that difficulty. Probably the most common source of human material is surgical speci-mens; although by their very nature, caution has to be used in applying such data to normal processes. Secondly, the interaction between scientist and physician can occur at many levels. In this example, human milk was obtained from an obstetrician whilst gynecologists, oncologists and nuclear medical physicists were approached for the tumor localization work.

LOGIC

To illustrate this approach I will use the collaborative research of Dr Whitehead and myself. Data referred to in the text can be found in references 5-7. In this example the reverse situation occurred to that described for the breast/ovary - the clinician approached the basic scientist with a well-defined problem. The problem arose from the cancer scare associated with the use of unopposed estrogen for treating the climacteric. It had been realized that a progestin should be included in the treatment schedule but virtually no information was available as to type, dose or duration of progestin therapy. Controlled trials on the relationship of cancer incidence to all the possible hormone combinations were impossible. However, animal studies had provided insights into the way in which estrogens and progestins exert their effects on the uterus, and it was also known that much of this information was relevant to human premenopausal endometrium. Furthermore, women attending the menopause clinics at King's College Hospital and the Chelsea Hospital for Women in London routinely had a dilation and curettage in order to monitor the histological status of the endometrium; part of this tissue was available for biochemical analysis. The choice of parameters to be analysed was based on knowledge derived from premenopausal endometria and included estrogen- and progestin-sensitive reactions such as receptor quantities, enzyme activities and [^{3}H]thymidine labeling as an index of cell multiplication. These were all logical candidates especially when coupled with the morphological data generated from the other part of each sample. However, they also highlight a basic dilemma often facing a laboratory scientist in this situation: just because we have a method of measuring something, it does not follow that it is relevant to the clinical question being asked. Thus, there is no doubting that cell multiplication is an important component in tumor production but many other processes are also involved and we cannot unequivocally equate inhibition of DNA synthesis in normal cells with cancer prevention. Likewise, the ability of progestins to induce certain enzymes gives us indications of potencies at the end organ for that particular biochemical pathway; these may be relevant to progestin effects on cancer prevention but we have no direct proof to that effect. In other words, we could only measure events that were our best guess at being relevant given our paucity of data as to how hormones alter the risk of developing endometrial cancer. We measured as many parameters as possible with the tissue available and it turned out that they all gave the same answers. The answers were that one needed a minimum of 6 days progestin to counteract the estrogen and that substantially lower doses of compounds such as norethindrone (norethisterone) and norgestrel could be used than was originally recommended. They further pointed the way to potentially the most effective form of therapy: continuous combined estrogen plus progestin. Preliminary trials indicate that endometrium can rarely be obtained from such patients, suggesting that they have an atrophic endometrium.

I now feel that the ball is firmly back in the court of the physician. The biochemical analyses have shown how to protect the endometrium; it is now up to the physician together with his/her patient to decide whether the regime we have evolved corrects the presenting symptoms and does not generate other side-effects.

CONCLUSIONS

Medical science requires a symbiotic relationship between basic science and the physician so that clinical problems can be identified and the powerful techniques of modern biology applied to answering those problems. I see the symbiosis as being a partnership of equals, with the patient being the overall beneficiary.

REFERENCES

1. Epenetos, A. A., Mather, S., Granowska, M., Nimmon, C. C., Hawkins, L. R., Britton, K. E., Shepherd, J., Taylor-Papadimitriou, J., Durbin, H., Malpas, J. S. and Bodmer, W. F. (1982). Targeting of iodine-123-labelled tumour-associated monoclonal antibodies to ovarian, breast, and gastrointestinal tumours. *Lancet*, **2** (8306), 999–1004
2. Burchell, J., Taylor-Papadimitriou, J., Granowska, M. and Britton, K. (1984). Monoclonal antibodies for successful tumour imaging. *Behring Inst. Mitt.*, **74**, 87–93
3. Wilkinson, M. J. S., Howell, A., Harris, M., Taylor-Papadimitriou, J., Swindell, R. and Sellwood, R. A. (1984). The prognostic significance of two epithelial membrane antigens expressed by human mammary carcinomas. *Int. J. Cancer*, **33**(3), 299–304
4. Ceriani, R. L., Thompson, K., Peterson, A. and Abraham, S. (1983). Surface differentiation antigens of human mammary epithelial cells carried on the human milk fat globule. *Proc. Natl. Acad. Sci. (Wash.)*, **12**(2), 143–54
5. King, R. J. B. and Whitehead, M. I. (1983). Estrogen and progestin effects on epithelium and stroma from pre- and postmenopausal endometria: application to clinical studies of the climacteric syndrome. In Jasonni, V. M., Nenci, I. and Flamigni, C. (eds.) *Steroids and Endometrial Cancer*. pp. 105–15. (New York: Raven Press) (*Progress in Cancer Research and Therapy*, vol. 25)
6. Whitehead, M., Lane, G., Siddle, N., Townsend, P. and King, R. (1983). Avoidance of endometrial hyperstimulation in estrogen-treated postmenopausal women. *Sem. Reprod. Endocrinol.*, **1**(1), 41–53
7. Whitehead, M. I., Siddle, N. C., Townsend, P. T., Lane, G. and King, R. J. B. (1983). The use of progestins and progesterone in the treatment of climacteric and postmenopausal symptoms. In Bardin, C. W., Milgrom, E. and Mauvais-Jarvis, P. (eds.) *Progesterone and Progestins*. pp. 277–94. (New York: Raven Press)

Chapter 4

Nutritional needs of climacteric women

E. B. Feldman

The nutritional needs of climacteric women can be described in three parts: (1) a characterization of the status of middle-aged women; (2) a prediction of what the future may hold for these women considering the prevention of important disorders and pathology; and (3) promotion of good health into the later years with prolongation of life of high quality. These needs are addressed in three sections: nutritional excesses, nutritional deficiencies and nutritional factors in health promotion.

NUTRITIONAL EXCESSES

In our affluent society we are faced primarily by the consequences of overnutrition. The principal offender is calories. We also consume a diet high in fat, principally saturated fat, and also high in cholesterol. Consumption of sodium chloride is also high. The American diet contains about 40% of calories from fat, 20% as sugar, 500–700 mg of cholesterol, and 8–10 g of salt. Of the fat calories, about 15% are derived from saturated fat, 9% from polyunsaturated fat and the remainder from monounsaturated fat[1].

Excessive intake of calories results in a population in which 24% of adult women are obese[2]. The peak incidence is in middle age with obesity more prevalent in black women than in white women. There are multiple determinants of obesity[3]. Fundamentally, there is an excess of intake of calories in the diet versus the expenditure of energy. As seen in Fig. 4.1 a study in males, the decline in energy expenditure from age 30 to 80 is due mainly to a decrease in expenditure for activity of about 400 calories,

27

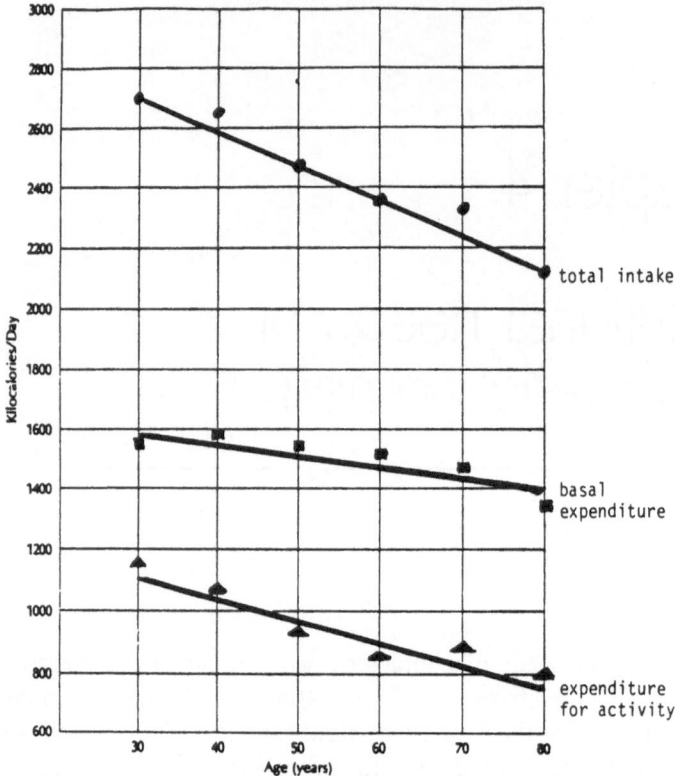

Figure 4.1 In a classic study of energy intake and expenditure in aging, R. B. McGandy *et al.* found that average daily calorie intake decreased about 600 kcal per day from age 30 to age 80 in men of high socioeconomic status. A third of the decline could be correlated with reduced basal metabolism; two-thirds with reduced physical activity. ● —— Total intake; ■ —— basal expenditure; ▲ —— expenditure for activity. (Adapted from Munro, H. N. (1982) Nutritional requirements in the elderly. *Hospital Practice*, August, p. 149)

or one-third. The decline in basal energy expenditure from age 30 to 80 is only about 200 calories, or about one-eighth. Unless the calorie intake declines proportionally, a total of about 600 calories, there will be an inevitable weight gain. The decline in basal energy expenditure of 2% per decade is probably inexorable and is related to the change in body composition relating primarily to the loss of cell mass and increase in body fat (Fig. 4.2). Thus, in providing for calorie needs with aging, calorie intake should be adjusted downward to prevent excess weight gain, starting at the age of 50[4]. For those who remain active, the reduction of caloric intake should be less. Food consumption should be adjusted to prevent overweight or underweight. The recommended decline in energy consumption is about 5% per decade between 40 and 60 years of age and 10% per decade after the age of 60. The specific recommendation for women is to reduce calories from about 2300 calories per day in the third decade to about 2200 calories in the fifth decade, 1800 calories in the

28

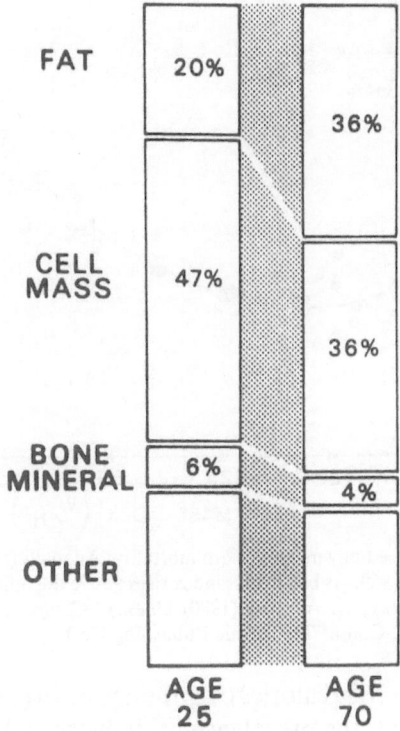

Figure 4.2 Idealized representation of the age-related change of body composition of male subjects. Young females (age 25) have nearly twice as much body fat as do males but show a smaller increase of fat (and loss of cell mass) with age than do males. From Gregerman, R. I. and Bierman, E. I. (1981) in Williams, R. H. (ed.) *Textbook of Endocrinology*, 6th edn., p. 1200. (Philadelphia: W. B. Saunders)

Table 4.1 Mean normal values, effects of age

	Age (years)		
	20–44	*45–59*	*60–74*
Blood pressure (mmHg)			
♀	118/75	135/84	151/86
♂	125/81	137/88	145/86
Age (years)	20–49	50–75	76+
Energy needs (kcal)			
♀	2100	1800	1600
♂	2900	2400	2050
Plasma cholesterol (mg/dl)			
♀	182	227	225
♂	192	212	205
Plasma triglycerides (mg/dl)			
♀	85	120	130
♂	127	143	130

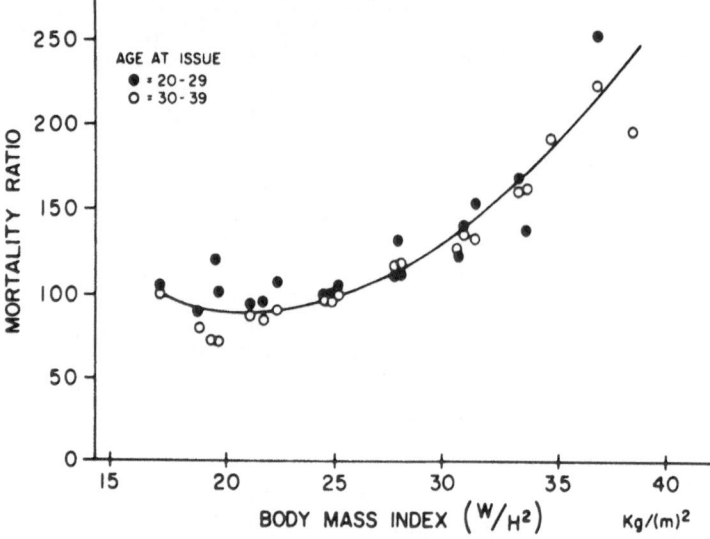

Figure 4.3 Relation of the body mass index to mortality. Adapted from data in the Build and Blood Pressure Study of 1959. As body mass index rises above the normal (25), the excess mortality increases. From Bray, G. A. (ed.) (1980) *Obesity: Comparative Methods of Weight Control.* p. 4. (Westport, Conn.: Technomic Publishing Co.)

seventh decade, and 1600 calories over the age of 70 (Table 4.1). As weight increases above ideal, the prevalence of diabetes and hypertension, and overall mortality, increase significantly (Fig. 4.3).

The changes in plasma lipids with age are shown in Table 4.2. In women plasma cholesterol levels increase after puberty until the fifth decade.

Table 4.2 Average levels of circulating lipids*

Age	White males Total C	LDL C	HDL C	TG	White females Total C	LDL C	HDL C	TG
15–19	152	93	46	68	157	93	51	64
20–24	159	101	45	78	165	102	51	80
25–29	176	116	44	88	178	108	55	76
30–34	190	124	45	102	178	109	55	73
35–39	195	131	43	109	186	116	53	83
40–44	204	135	43	123	193	122	56	68
45–49	210	141	45	119	204	127	58	94
50–54	211	143	44	128	214	134	62	103
55–59	214	145	46	117	229	145	60	111
60–64	215	143	49	111	226	149	61	105
65–69	213	146	49	108	233	151	62	118
70 +	214	142	48	115	226	147	60	110

*50th percentile
C = cholesterol; LDL = low-density lipoprotein; HDL = high-density lipoprotein; TG = triglyceride
Adapted from Lipid Research Clinics Prevalence Study

Plasma cholesterol levels in women are generally lower than those of men until the middle or later years[5]. About two-thirds of the plasma cholesterol is transported as low-density lipoprotein, LDL. LDL cholesterol levels parallel levels of total cholesterol. Levels of high-density lipoprotein, HDL, cholesterol are 9–17 mg/dl higher in women (Table 4.2). Cholesterol levels in postmenopausal women exceed those in males. Circulating triglyceride levels increase by 50–75% with age (Table 4.2). The levels of total cholesterol and LDL cholesterol increase with high intake of saturated fatty acids, cholesterol and with excess calories in the obese. Triglyceride levels are influenced by calories, fat, carbohydrate and alcohol. The diet associated with the development of atherosclerosis contains about 200 mg cholesterol/1000 kcal and is high in fat.

Blood pressure also increases with age (Table 4.1). Blood pressure is higher in blacks than in whites. Middle-aged and elderly black women have the highest prevalence of hypertension, with rates exceeding 50%. The incidence of hypertension rises steeply in young black women over the age of 30 and in middle-aged white women over the age of 50[5]. A reduction in elevated blood pressure, averaging about 8 mmHg, can be achieved with sodium restriction. For salt-sensitive people it has been suggested that salt intake be limited to less than 3 g/day or about 40% of the usual intake in the American diet. Other nutritional factors implicated in the etiology of hypertension[6] include a decrease in the relative amount of potassium. Increasing potassium intake can partially negate the blood pressure increment produced by sodium. Recently calcium deficiency has been advocated as an important factor in some groups with hypertension, and may explain the association of hypertension with soft water. Increase in calcium intake in some experimental models is associated with blood pressure lowering. The role of calcium deficiency in the etiology of osteopenia is discussed later.

Dietary fat may play a role specifically in the pathogenesis of obesity as well as in the etiology of hyperlipidemia and atherosclerosis and hypertension. Polyunsaturated fats in the diet have a blood pressure lowering effect, and essential fatty acid deficiency can raise blood pressure in experimental animals. Blood pressure is proportional to weight gain and a reduction to ideal body weight lowers blood pressure and decreases the risk of coronary heart disease and mortality from cardiovascular disease[7].

The non-insulin-dependent, more common type of diabetes mellitus affects a greater proportion of the population in the middle and later years in contrast to youth, and is especially prevalent in the obese. Thus, curtailment of calories will have a beneficial effect in the prevention of diabetes, especially in those with genetic predisposition. Since the diabetic is also predisposed to premature and severe atherosclerosis, control not only of the calorie level but the fat level of the diet is warranted.

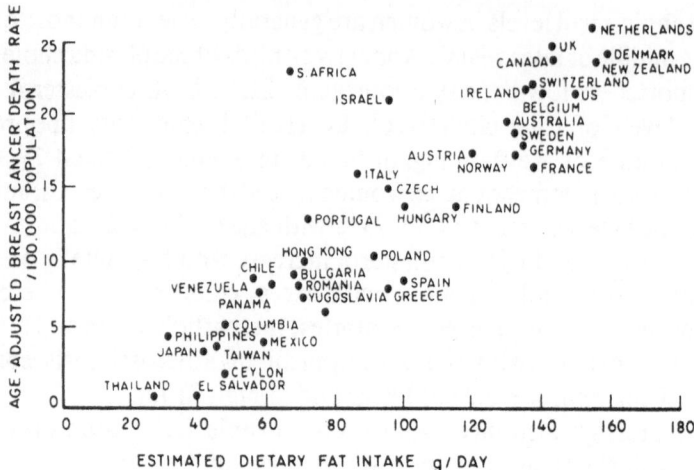

Figure 4.4 Correlation between per capita consumption of dietary fat and age-adjusted mortality from breast cancer. From Wynder, E. L., Chan, P. C., Cohen, L. A., MacCornack, F. and Hill, P. (1976). Etiology and prevention of breast cancer. In Grundmann, E. and Peck, L. (eds.) *Cancer Campaign, Early Diagnosis of Breast Cancer*, vol. 1, p. 12. (New York: Gustav Fischer)

The high fat/high calorie diet also has been implicated in the etiology of some types of cancer (Fig. 4.4). Particularly relevant to climacteric women are cancer of the endometrium and cancer of the breast. Both the fat level and type of fat have been related in epidemiologic studies of the various forms of cancer[9]. Calorie excess or obesity are associated with increased incidence of cancer of the uterus, gall bladder, kidney, stomach, colon and breast. Women more than 40% over ideal body weight have a 55% greater risk of cancer than subjects of normal weight. The strongest association of calorie excess is with endometrial cancer. The changes that produce the high-calorie diet may be an increase in the ratio of fat to carbohydrate or a decrease in the concentration of fiber. The latter will be discussed under the heading of deficiencies. Excessive fat intake increases the chance of developing cancer of the breast; this applies to excessive intake of either saturated or unsaturated fat from plant or animal sources. The amount of fat consumed might be decreased to 30% of total calories in order to prevent cancer. This can be achieved by moderating the consumption of fats, oils and foods rich in fat – this is also an effective way to reduce total calories and maintain ideal body weight. Dietary fat may act as a promoter of colon cancer which also may be related to high levels of cholesterol in the diet. These diets may increase excretion of bile acids and neutral sterols and alter intestinal bacterial flora to modify these sterols, transforming them to potential carcinogens.

Hormonal mechanisms have been suggested to be responsible for the effect of increased levels of dietary fat to influence the rate of breast cancer, specifically increased levels of estrogens. Estrogen synthesis and reabsorption may be increased by dietary fat. Fat also may affect breast cancer risk by altering prolactin secretion. Interaction between poly-unsaturated fats and antioxidants also may be related to increased risk of breast and other cancers. Prospective studies of diet and cancer in women are needed to characterize the relation between fat intake and breast cancer and address specifically the effect of various types of fat. Currently a trial of a low-fat diet as an intervention study is under way both in women at high risk of developing breast cancer and as adjuvant to chemotherapy of women with stage two breast cancer. Of all the dietary components that have been studied in relation to cancer, the evidence is most suggestive of a relationship between fat intake and the occurrence of cancer[10].

NUTRITIONAL DEFICIENCIES

Fiber

Too little fiber in the diet (less than 30 g/day) may relate to the patho-genesis of colon cancer. High fiber consumption, that is of various types of whole grains, fruits, and vegetables, may have a protective effect against colon cancer possibly diluting potential carcinogens and speeding their transit route through the colon. Fiber may also have a favorable or anti-cancer effect on bacterial flora. Even if fiber does not protect against cancer, the high-fiber diet of fruits, vegetables and whole grains should provide a wholesome substitute for fatty foods, thereby decreasing fat and calorie intake. The average American diet contains about 20 g of dietary fiber. Increasing dietary fiber intake to 30 g or more is associated with a lower prevalence of diverticular disease and is beneficial in the treatment of constipation. Cereal fiber in particular should be increased in terms of increasing fecal weight. In practice, consumption of fruit and vegetables as well as cereals should be encouraged. The high-fiber diet has also been used in the management of obesity, hyperlipidemia and diabetes[11, 12]. For the latter disorder, the use of legumes is particularly recommended (beans, peas, lentils). Oat bran and some soluble carbo-hydrates such as gums and pectins may lower levels of blood sugar and plasma cholesterol. In some of these diets, fiber is increased to 40–45 g daily. At that high fiber intake adverse effects include abdominal fullness, flatulence, and diarrhea.

For some, the high-fiber diet is a vegetarian diet. The combination of the increase in fiber and a decrease in meat intake may have beneficial effects on blood lipids and also on blood pressure. The vegetarian diet can be nutritionally adequate provided attention is paid to meals contain-ing complementary proteins that will provide all of the essential amino acids[1]. The high carotene content of some vegetables, as well as some unknown factor in cruciferous vegetables, may have protective effects against cancer[10].

Another nutrient in inadequate supply for middle-aged and older women is calcium[4]. Calcium is necessary for bone mineralization and skeletal growth and maintenance. Almost all the body calcium is located in teeth and bones. The calcium intake in the United States is provided mainly from milk and cheese. Vitamin D is required for calcium absorption. Vegetable calcium is less available than animal sources. Excessive intakes of phosphorus may lead to increased bone resorption and increased calcium loss. High dietary intake of protein may also tend to increase calcium excretion and bone resorption. Calcium absorption decreases with advancing age[13].

With all these threats to adequate calcium balance, it is important that dietary intake of calcium be ample throughout life to avoid depletion. In order to meet the other constraints of the diet which have been described earlier – e.g. calories, fat, fiber – it may be that for women, especially older or smaller women, adequate amounts of calcium can only be provided by the use of supplements. Osteopenia, a reduction in bone mass, whether due to decreased bone formation or increased resorption, may result from inadequate calcium intake. Calcium intake affects the bone mass achieved. Middle-aged and elderly individuals may require additional dietary calcium to maintain positive calcium balance in the face of decreased absorption, etc. Bone loss with osteoporosis also coincides with reduction of physical activity in later years[14]. Median calcium intake in women is estimated as ranging from about 700 mg/day in late adolescence to less than 500 mg/day in the elderly. These amounts do not meet the recommended dietary allowance for calcium, 800 mg/day[4].

Bone loss begins earlier in women than in men, age 40 vs. 50, and also occurs at an accelerated rate in women compared to men (8% vs. 3% per decade). This bone demineralization may be corrected in part by increasing calcium intake to 1.2–1.5 g/day and also by getting 1 hour of endurance, aerobic exercise 3–4 times per week. It is estimated that one-third of postmenopausal women have osteoporosis, and that one in five women suffers a hip or vertebral compression fracture. Up to the age of 80 women are affected four times more often than men. Blacks are less susceptible to osteoporosis than are whites; the reason is unknown. The decrease in estrogen activity in the menopause contributes to bone demineralization. While calcium supplements may not remineralize the bone, fracture frequency can decrease and the process of bone demineralization can be arrested. A high level of calcium intake can reduce bone resorbing activity and thereby have a prophylactic effect on bone loss. The calcium supplement can be taken in the form of calcium carbonate, calcium lactate or other salts in tablet or liquid form[14].

An important contributor to nutrient deficiencies in the middle and later years are the effects of medications taken for various ailments; thus diet/nutrient interactions may occur. Medications used in the treatment of hypertension, heart disease, peripheral vascular disease, pulmonary disease, Parkinson's disease, diabetes mellitus, arthritis, or cancer carry the risk of nutritional depletion, especially of minerals, or diet-related side-effects[13]. Good advice is to read labels, ask the physician or the pharmacist, and report medicines taken. Restricted diets in themselves may cause nutrient deficiencies. Thus, when calories are decreased to less than 1300 per day, a multi-vitamin supplement should be prescribed, probably also one that contains iron[14]. (Calcium supplementation has already been addressed.)

NUTRITIONAL FACTORS IN HEALTH PROMOTION

For the relatively sedentary climacteric women, in order to promote health and avoid consuming excess calories, nutrition needs may need to be provided by supplementing with pharmacologic preparations of vitamins or minerals to meet the RDA. Since body size and aging are inevitable and inexorable, perhaps only the level of activity is truly amenable to significant change. Thus exercise and an increased level of daily activity are to be recommended. The goal should continue to be a body weight close to ideal. Ideal body weight for women assumes a weight of 100 lb at 60 inches of height with an additional 5 lb per inch of height over 60. Weight can be adjusted upwards or downwards by 10% for large or small body frame respectively[15].

Prior to embarking on a program of regular exercise, the middle-aged woman should have a physical examination expecially with regard to cardiovascular status. There are numerous opportunities these days to engage in safe and beneficial forms of exercise. These will strengthen not only muscles but bone. Attention must be paid to avoiding injury and not to stress excessively cardiovascular parameters. If nothing else, women can be encouraged to walk rather than ride in automobiles. Bicycle riding is a form of locomotion that provides exercise. Unfortunately for our mechanized society, where the automobile is a fact of life on the road, it may be safer to ride an exercise bicycle at home. Even standing rather than sitting will increase caloric expenditure. It is not too late for middle-aged women to begin an exercise program that they can carry out into the later years. Of course, the woman who has been active in recreational sports should be encouraged to continue these activities. There are no special dietary requirements for sports activity or athletics other than a nutritionally balanced diet. All participants, especially those in warm climates, should maintain a good state of hydration.

It is particularly important for women not to succumb to the lure of dietary fads and nutrition quackery[16, 17]. Some dietary fads are good nutritional practices but unfortunately this is not always so. Thus, a vegetarian diet may be a healthful diet provided attention is paid to protein and vitamin content. There are no new vitamins other than the 13 that had been discovered by 1948. There is no benefit for a human being to ingest vitamins that have been found to be essential for rats. Similarly the requirements for vitamins is for microscopic amounts, measured in milligrams or even micrograms or nanograms. Increase in vitamin intake to megadoses (ten times or more the recommended dietary allowance) is wasteful, expensive and may be hazardous. In general the principle that if a little is good, a lot is better, is not advisable in terms of good nutrition. Vitamin E heads the list of vitamins touted to prevent or cure everything from acne to underarm odor, including prevention of senility and atherosclerosis, promotion of sexual potency and restoration of physical charm, especially to the skin.

Other unsubstantiated recommendations for vitamins include ribo-flavin to prevent or treat cataracts or glaucoma; vitamin C to prevent colds; megadoses of niacin and other B vitamins to prevent or cure schizophrenia and induce optimal health. Some non-vitamin myths about food are that specific combinations of foods cure disease, that special foods increase vigor, that elimination of foods achieves health and that 'natural' foods are better and prevent disease. There are no special nutrients needed to cope with the strains of everyday modern life. The potential for harm from large doses of vitamins A and D is well established and becoming increasingly visible from water-soluble vitamins as well. Unfortunately in many instances of vitamin toxicity, the vitamin has been prescribed by a physician.

Weight-reducing diets are the most popular of fad diets[16, 17]. Popular weight-loss diets are usually unbalanced in that they may be low or high carbohydrate, a protein-sparing modified fast, of one component primarily (fruit) or contain additives that 'keep you from getting fat'. Since carbohydrate retains salt and water, there is fluid loss when carbohydrate foods are restricted. This, however, does not represent loss of adipose tissue. Such diets produce a diuresis and may cause fatigue due to associated electrolyte loss. A high-protein diet may be bad for patients with some impairment of renal function. High-fat diets induce ketosis and promote hyperlipidemia. The protein-sparing modified fast is a modification of a starvation regimen and should be used only under strict medical supervision and where significant weight loss (greater than 20 lb) is required[3]. Starvation regimens use up the lean body mass and are not to be recommended for persons in the older age groups. Sudden arrhythmias and cardiomyopathy may result on this regimen. Fad diets may work because they temporarily relieve the dieter's choices and substitute what is generally few calories than the usual intake.

It is suggested that consumers shop carefully for correct nutrition information and not obtain this primarily from popular magazines, particularly those written for women. The nutrition information in the majority of these magazines is inconsistent or unreliable. Reliable sources of nutrition information are published by scientifically reputable organizations, are written by nutrition professionals, or are derived from legitimate government agencies. Checking with a knowledgable physician or registered dietition may help to distinguish nutrition reality from myths. Only registered dietitians or trained nutrition health professionals have nutrition training or credentials. Unorthodox tools of nutritional assessment should be avoided, including at the present time hair analysis, body chemistry balancing, saliva testing, etc. Not only are these worthless; they are expensive.

A major problem with all of these activities is that they deflect people from seeking assistance that will be helpful and safe rather than worthless and hazardous. Unfortunately nutrition is neither a panacea nor a fountain of youth.

Another factor to be considered is the increase in alcoholism among women, and particularly in middle-aged and older women[18]. Alcoholism is the leading cause of nutritional deficiencies in the United States. Deficiencies in B vitamins, particularly thiamin and folic acid, are found primarily in alcoholics. If alcoholism is combined with a poor dietary intake, such as might occur in the depressed, older patient, then serious nutritional problems can develop in which the fundamental cause may be unsuspected. Alcohol also contributes empty calories and may play an important role in the development of obesity. Alcohol intake can worsen high blood pressure. Chronic alcohol consumption may damage the liver, heart, brain and bone marrow.

CURRENT RECOMMENDATIONS

Although there is not a national policy on nutrition, governmental agencies in the past few years have issued a series of recommendations concerning diet, health and disease. The first of these was the dietary goals issued in 1977 (Table 4.3) based on concerns that overnutrition is related to coronary heart disease, obesity, cancer and stroke. The goals[19] stipulated that Americans should eat less food; less fat, particularly saturated fat; less cholesterol; less sugar; less salt; and increase consumption of fruits, vegetables, grain products and unsaturated oils. The goals were followed by the dietary guidelines first published in 1980 by the Departments of Agriculture and Health and Human Services (Table 4.3). The guidelines[20] were more modest, using the term 'too much' rather than providing specific amounts of saturated or polyunsaturated fat, cholesterol, sugar, sodium, or complex carbohydrate. In addition the guidelines introduce the concept of variety of foods and concern with alcohol intake.

The Food and Nutrition Board of the National Academy of Sciences recommended in 1980[21] that healthy Americans eat a variety of food, adjust their energy intake, and if the requirement is low, reduce consumption of alcohol, sugars and fats and use salt in moderation. Their publication did not recommend reduction of cholesterol and saturated fat intakes for the average person. They also did not specify eating foods with 'adequate starch and fiber'.

Table 4.3

Dietary goals	Dietary guidelines
1. Reduce overall fat consumption to about 30% of energy intake.	1. Eat a variety of foods.
2. Reduce saturated fat consumption to about 10% of total energy; polyunsaturated and monosaturated fat should account for about 10% each.	2. Maintain desirable weight. 3. Avoid too much fat, saturated fat and cholesterol.
3. Reduce cholesterol consumption to about 300 mg per day.	4. Eat foods with adequate starch and fiber.
4. Limit the intake of sodium by reducing salt to about 5 g per day.	5. Avoid too much sugar. 6. Avoid too much sodium.
5. Increase the consumption of complex carbohydrates and 'naturally occurring' sugars to about 48% of energy intake.	7. If you drink alcohol, do so in moderation.
6. Reduce the consumption of refined and processed sugars to account for about 10% of total energy intake.	
7. To avoid overweight, consume only as much energy (calories) as is expended. If overweight, decrease energy intake and increase energy expenditure.	

In my opinion the dietary guidelines are reasonable in suggesting moderation with an emphasis on maintaining desirable body weight and consuming a variety of foods. Until we know the implications of dietary excesses of fat, saturated fat, cholesterol, sugar or sodium, common sense should also pervade. The toxic and adverse effects of alcohol are well known.

Interim guidelines in 1982 provided recommendations aimed at cancer prevention[10]. These guidelines also include reducing intake of saturated and unsaturated fat, including fruits, vegetables and whole grain cereal products in the diet, minimizing consumption of foods preserved by salt curing or smoking, minimize contamination of foods with carcinogens from any source, identify mutagens in food and remove or minimize their concentration, and consume alcoholic beverages only in moderation. These items are not too dissimilar from the dietary guidelines with specific attention to carcinogens and mutagens.

SUMMARY AND CONCLUSIONS

Middle-aged women are afflicted with obesity resulting from a diet high in calories, fat, cholesterol and sodium. The tendency to obesity increases with advancing age due to a decline in energy expenditure. To improve health, fewer calories should be ingested and activity increased.

Hyperlipidemia and atherosclerosis also increase with age and may respond to a diet limited in fat, saturated fat, and cholesterol, achieved by increasing intake of complex carbohydrates. This diet may also protect against some forms of cancer (breast, endometrium, colon).

The increase in hypertension also can be modified by achieving ideal body weight and decreasing salt intake.

Calcium intake should be optimized throughout adult life. To improve bone mineralization women susceptible to osteoporosis should take calcium supplements and engage in an exercise program.

Women should beware of myths, fads and quackery relating to vitamins, weight reduction, longevity and seek reliable, scientific sources of nutrition information.

To promote health and prevent disease women also should eat a variety of foods and use alcohol, if at all, only in moderation.

Acknowledgement

This work was supported in part by National Institutes of Health Grant AM 30865.

REFERENCES

1. Feldman, E. B. (1985). The normal healthy diet. In *Essentials of Clinical Nutrition*. (Philadelphia: F. A. Davis) (In press)
2. Bray, G. A. (1983). Obesity. In Schneider, H. A., Anderson, C. E. and Coursin, D. B. (eds.) *Nutritional Support of Medical Practice*, 2nd edn. pp. 466-90. (Philadelphia: Harper & Row)
3. Feldman, E. B. (1985). Obesity, anorexia and bulimia. In *Essentials of Clinical Nutrition*. (Philadelphia: F. A. Davis) (In press)
4. Food and Nutrition Board, National Academy of Sciences, National Research Council (1980). *Recommended Dietary Allowance*, ed. 9. (Washington, DC: National Academy of Sciences)
5. Feldman, E. B. (1985). Nutritional factors in cardiovascular disease. In *Nutrition in the Middle and Later Years*. pp. 107-26. (Boston: John Wright-PSG)
6. Feldman, E. B. (1983). Diet and plasma lipids and lipoproteins. In Feldman, E. B. (ed.) *Nutrition and Heart Disease, Vol. 6: Contemporary Issues in Clinical Nutrition*. pp. 45-58. (New York: Churchill Livingstone)
7. Teague, R. J. (1983). Obesity and heart disease. In Feldman, E. B. (ed.) *Nutrition and Heart Disease, Vol. 6: Contemporary Issues in Clinical Nutrition*. pp. 125-44. (New York: Churchill Livingstone)
8. Bernstein, R. S. (1983). Evaluation and treatment of obesity. In Feldman, E. B. (ed.) *Nutrition in the Middle and Later Years*. pp. 71-92. (Boston: John Wright-PSG)
9. Feldman, E. B. (1985). *Diet and Cancer*. (Midpoint: Counseling Women through the Menopause (In press)

10. National Research Council (1982). *Diet, Nutrition and Cancer*. (Washington, DC: National Academy Press)
11. Kuske, T. T. (1983). Carbohydrate, fiber and heart disease. In Feldman, E. B. (ed.) *Nutrition and Heart Disease, Vol. 6: Contemporary Issues in Clinical Nutrition*. pp. 111–24. (New York: Churchill Livingstone)
12. Feldman, E. B. (1985). Diabetes mellitus. In *Essentials of Clinical Nutrition*. (Philadelphia: F. A. Davis) (In press)
13. Feldman, E. B. (1985). Essential nutrients – vitamins, minerals. In *Essentials of Clinical Nutrition*. (Philadelphia: F. A. Davis) (In press)
14. Feldman, E. B. (1985). Special problems of the elderly. In *Essentials of Clinical Nutrition*. (Philadelphia: F. A. Davis) (In press)
15. Feldman, E. B. (1985). Nutritional assessment. In *Essentials of Clinical Nutrition*. (Philadelphia: F. A. Davis) (In press)
16. Feldham, E. B. (1985). Fads, myths and quackery. In *Essentials of Clinical Nutrition*. (Philadelphia: F. A. Davis) (In press)
17. Kuske, T. T. (1983). Quackery and fad diets. In Feldman, E. B. (ed.) *Nutrition in the Middle and Later Years*. pp. 291–304. (Boston: John Wright-PSG)
18. Korsten, M. A. and Lieber, C. S. (1983). The elderly alcoholic. In Feldman, E. B. (ed.) *Nutrition in the Middle and Later Years*. pp. 93–106. (Boston: John Wright-PSG)
19. Select Committee on Nutrition and Human Needs, U.S. Senate (1977). *Dietary Goals for the United States*, 2nd edn.
20. USDA, USDHEW (1980). Nutrition and your health: dietary guidelines for Americans. (Superintendent of Documents, US Government Printing Office)
21. Food and Nutrition Board (1980). Toward healthful diets. (Washington, DC: National Academy of Sciences)

Chapter 5

Exercise and the postmenopausal woman

B. L. Drinkwater

ABSTRACT

Chronological age and physiological age are not synonymous. In the years following menopause every woman makes daily decisions which affect her health and the quality of her life then and in the years ahead. One decision is the choice between an active or sedentary lifestyle. The woman who chooses to be sedentary has selected a course which in itself is a risk factor for chronic disease. In many respects the effects of inactivity mimic the effects of aging – and vice-versa. The physically active woman may be as much as one or two decades younger physiologically than a sedentary female of the same age. The reason is simple – physiological systems adapt to the demands placed upon them. The active woman not only reaps an immediate physiological benefit but is also helping to insure the quality of her life in the future. The best preventive medicine against some of the debilitating problems of old age may be an 'exercise prescription' for a lifetime of vigorous physical activity. Fortunately, it is never too late to benefit from an increase in physical activity. Sedentary women who embark on an exercise program will improve the functional capacity of their cardiovascular system, improve muscular strength and endurance, and increase flexibility. An individualized 'exercise prescription' from a qualified professional will insure that those benefits are obtained through a safe sound progression of activities.

When the well-informed, active woman of today reaches menopause her expectations for the future are quite different from those of women in previous generations. For one thing, she knows that she may have one-third of her life-span still ahead of her; for another, she expects those years to be good years – an enjoyable, productive period of her life. Her optimism is well-founded. Women who consistently take part in some form of vigorous physical activity may be as much as 10 to 20 years younger physiologically than sedentary women of the same chronological age. One 74-year-old Seattle woman has cycled 300 miles through China, from Fairbanks to Anchorage, and across the continental United States. A California woman in her 80s climbs Mt. Whitney (14 000 ft; 4200 m) each summer. Countless women, 50 and older, are running 10 km road races, marathons, and super-marathons. Are these exceptional women, or have we simply underestimated the capacities of this age group?

As research data accumulate it appears more and more likely that many of the debilitating problems of aging are actually problems related to inactivity. 'Hypokinesis' is the term coined to describe the sedentary life-style that so often is responsible for the diminished functional capacity of the elderly. Since active women are still a minority, there are many women entering the climacteric who have been inactive for most of their lives. Is it too late for them to benefit from an exercise program? The answer, fortunately, is 'No'.

THE ACTIVE WOMAN

What defines an active woman and how does she differ physiologically from her sedentary counterpart? In behavioral terms, a woman is 'active' if she meets the criteria recommended by the American College of Sports Medicine for developing and maintaining cardiorespiratory fitness[1]. At least three times per week she participates in an aerobic activity which maintains her heart rate at 60–90% of her maximum heart rate reserve for 15–60 min. The activities, which should involve large muscle groups, are those which can be performed continuously and rhythmically. While jogging may be the activity getting the most attention these days, any number of others meet these criteria – brisk walking, swimming, cross-country skiing, bicycling, aerobic dance, etc.

The results of this active lifestyle will be evident during an exercise stress test as a better than average aerobic power ($\dot{V}O_{2max}$) and performance time. Using a modified Balke protocol, treadmill speed at 90 m/min (3.4 miles per hour) with a grade increment of one degree per minute, active postmenopausal women, ages 50–65, will attain a $\dot{V}O_{2max}$ of ~ 30 ml kg^{-1} min^{-1} or better, while sedentary females usually fall below 25 ml kg^{-1} min^{-1}.[2] The difference in performance time on the treadmill is even more striking. Active women average 15 min while sedentary females walk ~ 9 min.[2] Active women also have a larger maximal ventilatory volume, can tolerate higher levels of lactate, and have a lower percentage body fat. The practical effect of these differences is the ability of the active woman to handle the physical demands of daily living with less fatigue. She can do more with less effort because the energy cost of any activity will represent a smaller proportion of her maximal work capacity. For example, walking at a normal pace on a hard surface would require approximately 40% $\dot{V}O_{2max}$ for an active older woman and about 50% $\dot{V}O_{2max}$ for her sedentary counterpart. The fit individual will also recover more quickly following a period of exercise. In the long term, women who maintain an active lifestyle and enjoy good health can approach their older years with confidence in their ability to remain independent and to continue the activities they enjoy.

While data on older female athletes are still scarce, two Master's swimmers in their 70s illustrate how physical conditioning programs can minimize one of the major problems of aging, the decrement in cardiovascular function. These two women have a $\dot{V}O_{2max}$ ($37.6\,\text{ml}\,\text{kg}^{-1}\,\text{min}^{-1}$) equivalent to that of the average sedentary 20-year-old female[3]!

THE SEDENTARY WOMAN

The sedentary woman is the antithesis of the active woman. She does not participate in any regular program of physical activity, has no active hobbies such as gardening, camping, backpacking, etc., and seldom, if ever, performs any physical task more demanding than the essentials of daily living.

The results are predictable. Since the body readily adapts to the demands placed upon it, the physiological systems respond to inactivity with a diminished capacity for sustained vigorous activity, a decrease in muscular strength and endurance, a loss of flexibility, and an increase in body fat. Some of these changes are a function of physiological aging, but some – perhaps as much as 50% – are due to inactivity and are reversible[4].

AGING AND INACTIVITY

One of the problems in identifying the physiological changes resulting from aging, *per se*, is the tendency of many older people, particularly women, to decrease the amount of physical activity in their lives. The decrease in physiological function associated with an aging organism is then confounded by the loss of function due to inactivity. Some physiological functions do decline with age; others do not. The question many investigators are addressing is how much of the observed decrement is due to the aging process and how much is a result of a sedentary lifestyle.

Information about age-related changes in functional capacity usually comes from cross-sectional studies rather than longitudinal studies of the same individuals as they age. The resultant averages do not necessarily represent what is normal or desirable at any given age – only what is observed. They may include data from individuals with undiagnosed pathology and certainly include many sedentary women. Unfortunately, these observations often lead to lowered expectations for the older woman who mistakes what 'is' for what 'might be'. One method of determining which changes are an irreversible result of aging is to identify a sedentary older population, measure their responses to physiological tests, enroll them in a physical conditioning program and then re-test those responses following the training period.

De Vries[5] has summarized the changes reported in six studies of physical conditioning programs which included women age 60 and older. Positive changes in the cardiovascular system included a decrease in submaximal exercise heart rate, an increase in oxygen pulse, and a marked increase in physical work capacity. Muscular strength increased by 50% in the single study reporting that variable. No improvement was reported for maximal ventilatory volume during exercise or resting systolic and diastolic blood pressure.

The responses of a younger group of women, mean age 56.4 years, included more significant changes following training[6]. In addition to a decrease in submaximal heart rate and an increase in $\dot{V}O_{2max}$, these women also increased their maximal ventilation by 14% and decreased resting heart rate and both systolic and diastolic blood pressure (139/84 to 124/77). Hematocrit (40.5%), blood volume (5 l), heart volume (656 ml) and cholesterol (279 mg/100 ml) were unchanged.

Training does not reverse the age-related decrement in vital capacity or increase in residual volume, and does not affect closing volume or pulmonary diffusing capacity[7]. It appears that the improvements in response to both submaximal and maximal exercise are related primarily to changes in cardiovascular parameters. The precise mechanisms for the improvement of oxygen transport and/or utilization in older women following training have not been identified.

A regular program of exercise may also have a beneficial effect on body composition. The gradual loss of lean body mass (LBM) with age is usually accompanied by an increase in body fat, an overall weight gain, and a decrease in the basal metabolic rate proportional to the decrease in active tissue[5]. If older women respond as younger women do, an exercise training regimen should result in an increase in LBM and a decrease in fat. Unfortunately, there are only a few studies reporting body composition changes in older women following training. While Sidney *et al.*[8] found significant losses in skinfolds and increases in LBM, most investigators report minimal and non-significant changes in these variables[7].

Part of the difficulty in identifying changes in body composition of older women may be the use of measurement sites and prediction equations validated on younger women. The site of fat depots change with age, as do the densities of bone and muscle and the amount of total water. Even hydrostatic weighing, the so-called gold standard for estimating percentage body fat, uses prediction equations which may not be valid for older age groups.

Measurable changes in body composition may require more time to become evident in an older population. In a longitudinal study[9] where average time between tests was 6.1 years, sedentary women increased percentage body fat from 27.7% to 33.3% while active women remained fairly constant at 23.9% and 25.2%. Results of cross-sectional studies also suggest that active women have less body fat[2, 10].

A decrease in muscular strength and joint range of motion can adversely affect an older woman's mobility and independence. Yet very few studies have been done to determine how much of the apparent decrement in strength and flexibility can be attributed to disuse rather than aging. It does appear, however, that older women can increase strength and improve flexibility if the exercise program includes activities designed for that purpose[11, 12]. These two aspects of physical fitness do not receive as much attention as 'aerobics' in many exercise programs but are essential for total fitness.

EXERCISE PRESCRIPTION

The cardinal rule in prescribing exercise is to fit the program to the needs, capabilities, and interests of the individual. This is particularly important for members of the 50-plus age group. Their exercise background varies from that of Sister Marion, the running nun who qualified for the women's first Olympic marathon trials, to women who are just embarking on an exercise program after years of inactivity. Many postmenopausal women have never had any experience with training programs, since sports were not encouraged for girls and women when they were coming through the education system in the 1930s and 1940s. As a result they may lack not only physical skills but the knowledge to plan a safe and effective conditioning program for themselves.

MEDICAL SCREENING

A thorough medical examination is warranted for any sedentary post-menopausal woman prior to initiating an exercise program. The inclusion of an exercise stress test is recommended as a means of identifying potential cardiac problems. Excellent sources of information about appropriate tests and contraindications to physical training are available[13-16]. Although the emphasis is on the male at risk for coronary heart disease

(CHD), there is a good deal of general information applicable to older women as well.

When a woman in encouraged to go to the point of 'volitional' fatigue, the stress test also provides a measure of her maximal heart rate (HR_{max}). Since the intensity of prescribed exercise is based on a percentage of HR_{max} or HR reserve ($HR_{max} - HR_{rest}$), it is helpful to have a more accurate estimate than can be obtained using the formula, $HR_{max} = 220 - age$, where the error of prediction can be as much as 20 beats per minute (bpm). Whether or not the woman is asked to approach her maximum depends on the judgement of the physician.

THE EXERCISE PROGRAM

The key to a successful exercise program for older women is to *gradually* adapt the body to the new demands the activity is placing upon it. The most frequent medical problems encountered by novice exercisers are not cardiovascular accidents but orthopedic problems and muscular sprains and strains. Most of these problems, which can readily discourage further participation, can be avoided by prescribing the proper type of exercise and fitting the intensity, frequency, and duration of the activity to the experience and needs of the individual woman.

While improved functional capacity of the cardiovascular system may be the ultimate goal of the conditioning program, it is important to remember that the bones and tendons – particularly of the weight-bearing extremities – also need to be 'conditioned' and that muscles long unused must become adapted to new demands. For these reasons the initial stages of an exercise program for a sedentary postmenopausal woman might well emphasize flexibility exercises and brisk walking. If conditions permit, the walking could be interspaced with other activities such as swimming or bicycling, which are non-weight-bearing and involve other muscle groups. This age group should avoid the ballistic type of flexibility exercise, where the movements are rapid and bouncy, and concentrate instead on static stretching – a slow controlled stretching movement with full extension maintained for 10–15 s.

Since the objective of these initial exercise sessions is to prepare the body for more demanding activities, the intensity of the aerobic portion (walking) can be kept low so that duration and frequency can be greater. For example, if HR is maintained at 40% HR_{res} ($HR_{rest} + (HR_{max} - HR_{rest})0.40$) during a 30 min daily walk, the gain in $\dot{V}O_{2max}$ may be minimal but the skeletal and muscular systems will be benefiting. When combined with a 10 min warm-up and a 5 min cooling down period of stretching exercises, these initial stages of an exercise program should be injury-free but effective in initiating the woman into an activity program. No specific timetable for progression can be given which would fit all

46

women, but unless a woman is obese or has orthopedic problems 2-3 weeks of this introductory program should prepare her for an exercise prescription emphasizing aerobic fitness.

The ACSM Position Statement on 'The recommended quantity and quality of exercise for developing and maintaining fitness in healthy adults' is an excellent source for detailed information and guidelines for exercise prescription. Although most of the research material was derived from studies of males, more recent reports indicate that men and women respond in a similar fashion to training regimens[10]. Some adjustments may have to be made for the older age group. The physician should feel free to adjust the three ingredients – intensity, frequency, and duration – to meet individual needs, keeping in mind that the minimal threshold for increasing $\dot{V}O_{2max}$ is about 60% HR_{res}. As a general rule, intensity and duration vary inversely for older women. The lower the intensity of the exercise, the longer it may continue, and vice-versa. Frequency is also related to intensity. At low intensity levels, exercise can be a daily occurrence; at higher intensities, rest days are indicated. One useful technique is to alternate days demanding higher levels of energy expenditure with days at reduced levels of intensity.

Since the key to determining intensity of a workout is the exercise heart rate, the women must be taught to monitor their own pulses. With practice it is possible to determine heart rate during exercise by palpating either the radial or carotid pulse for 15 s and multiplying by 4 for bpm. If an individual finds this too difficult, the rate during the first 10 s post-exercise multiplied by 6 is a close approximation of exercise rate. Knowing her target HR, the woman can then increase or decrease her pace accordingly. Using HR as a measure of intensity automatically compensates for the training effect, encouraging the woman to increase the absolute intensity of the workout as her cardiovascular fitness improves in order to maintain the same exercise heart rate.

There is no doubt that aging affects the fitness levels of active women as well as sedentary women (Fig. 5.1). Even the slope describing the decrement of $\dot{V}O_{2max}$ with time may be similar. The important point is that active women maintain a functional capacity which permits them to live active independent lives well into old age, 75 years and older. In the final analysis, the quality of life is enhanced when physical activity becomes part of the postmenopausal woman's daily life.

REFERENCES

1. American College of Sports Medicine (1978). Position statement on the recommended quantity and quality of exercise for developing and maintaining fitness in healthy adults. *Med. Sci. Sports*, **10**, vii–x
2. Drinkwater, B. L., Horvath, S. M. and Wells, C. L. (1975). Aerobic power of females, ages 10 to 68. *J. Gerontol.*, **30**, 385-94

3. Vaccaro, P., Dummer, G. M. and Clarke, D. H. (1981). Physiologic characteristics of female masters swimmers. *Phys. Sportsmed.*, **9**(12), 75–8
4. Smith, E. L. (1981). Age: the interaction of nature and nurture. In Smith, E. L. and Serfass, R. C. (eds.) *Exercise and Aging*. pp. 11–17. (Hillside, NJ: Enslow)
5. de Vries, H. A. (1984). Exercise and the physiology of aging. In *Exercise and Health*, American Academy of Physical Education Papers, No. 17, pp. 76–88. (Champaign, IL: Human Kinetics Publishers)
6. Kilbom, A. (1971). Physical training with submaximal intensity in women. I: reaction to exercise and orthostasis. *Scand. J. Clin. Lab. Invest.*, **28**, 141–61
7. Shephard, R. J. and Sidney, K. H. (1978). Exercise and aging. In Hutton, R. S. (ed.) *Exercise and Sport Sciences Reviews*, vol. 6, pp. 1–58. (Philadelphia: Franklin Institute Press)
8. Sidney, K. H., Shephard, R. J. and Harrison, J. E. (1977). Endurance training and body composition of the elderly. *Am. J. Clin. Nutr.*, **30**, 326–33
9. Plowman, S. A., Drinkwater, B. L. and Horvath, S. M. (1979). Age and aerobic power in women: A longitudinal study. *J. Gerontol.*, **34**, 512–20
10. Drinkwater, B. L. (1984). Women and exercise: physiological aspects. In Terjung, R. L. (ed.) *Exercise and Sport Sciences Reviews*, vol. 12, pp. 21–51. (Lexington, MA: Collamore Press)
11. Munns, K. (1981). Effects of exercise on the range of joint motion in elderly subjects. In Smith, E. L. and Serfass, R. C. (eds.) *Exercise and Aging*. pp. 167–78. (Hillside, NJ: Enslow)
12. Serfass, R. S. (1981). Exercise for the elderly: what are the benefits and how do we get started? In Smith, E. L. and Serfass, R. C. (eds.) *Exercise and Aging*. pp. 121–9. (Hillside, NJ: Enslow)
13. Amsterdam, E. A., Wilmore, J. H. and DeMaria, A. D. (eds.) (1977). *Exercise in Cardiovascular Health and Disease*. (New York: Yorke Medical Books)
14. Naughton, J. P. and Hellerstein, H. K. (eds.) (1973). *Exercise Testing and Exercise Training in Coronary Heart Disease*. (New York: Academic Press)
15. American Heart Association (1972). *Exercise Testing and Training of Apparently Healthy Individuals. A Handbook for Physicians*. (New York)
16. Amercian College of Sports Medicine (1976). *Guidelines for Graded Exercise Testing and Exercise Prescription, and Behavioral Objectives for Physicians, Program Directors, Exercise Leaders and Exercise Technicians*. (Philadelphia: Lea and Febiger)

Chapter 6

Health needs of climacteric women

Barry G. Wren

In addressing the problems related to the health needs of climacteric women I have used the Australian experience, particularly that of Sydney, for my data and information. The results will be very similar in all other societies in the Western world.

Australia, although approximately the same size as the United States of America, has a population of about 16 million people, most of whom live on the Eastern seaboard (Table 6.1). Of the total population, females

Table 6.1 Australian population, 1982: 15 278 409 (percentages in parentheses)

Age (years)	Males		Females	
	7 576 258	(49.6)	7 602 151	(50.4)
50–54	392 036	(51.2)	374 706	(48.8)
55–59	373 098	(50.2)	371 029	(49.8)
60–64	303 375	(47.8)	332 046	(52.2)
65–69	252 242	(46.5)	289 949	(53.5)
70–74	183 350	(43.8)	234 993	(56.2)
75–79	110 602	(40.8)	160 560	(59.2)
80 +	83 003	(31.4)	181 776	(68.6)

begin to outnumber males after the age of 60 years and of about 1 million Australians over the age of 70 years, 60% are female (Fig. 6.1). This million people over the age of 70 years make up only 6.5% of the total population, yet they are consuming over 25% of the total health care 'cake'. Not only are they requiring a disproportionate amount of money

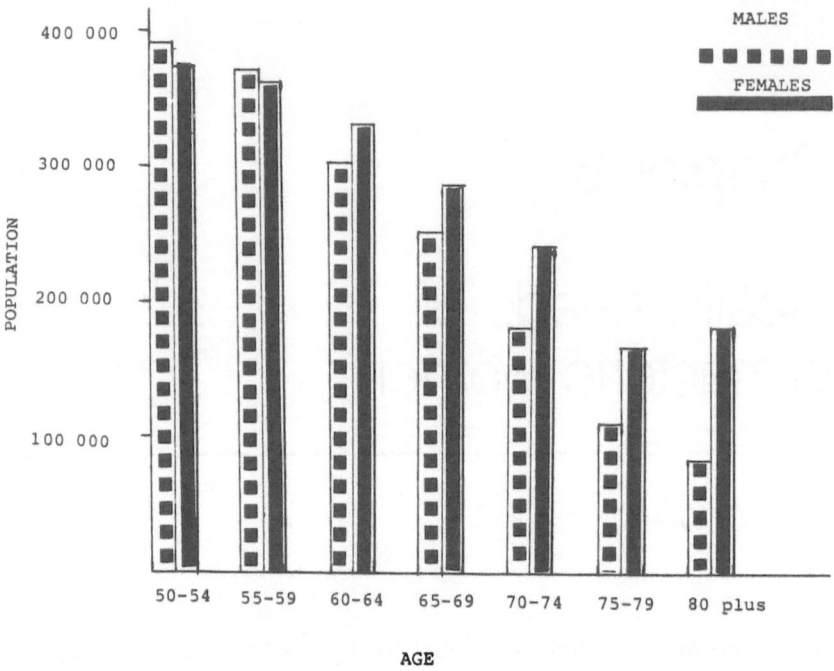

Figure 6.1   Male-female distribution, Australia, 1982

to care for them, but the females in the group are occupying over 40% of the total number of available health care beds (Table 6.2). This increased cost and bed utilization by women occurs for a number of reasons:

(a)   Women tend to live longer than men, and in Australia at present the average life expectancy for women is 78 years, compared to men who live 72 years.

(b)   Women tend to marry men who, on average, are 4 years older than themselves. When their older partner dies, the female is often left to lead a lonely and depressing life for 10–15 years.

Table 6.2   Health care details, Australia, 1982

Health care costs
  Over 70 years of age
  945 500 (6.2%) of population
  consume over 25% of health care 'cake'

Health care beds
  Females, 60 years of age and over
  1 189 500   (7.8%)
  occupy 40.2% of all available health care beds

(c) For the above reasons, women often undergo a longer senescence with a greater dependence on the community and sociological services than would be expected if they had a partner.

(d) Women are less physically active than men and quite often retire to a sedentary position within the family and society. If given the opportunity many of these women could be involved in family and societal activities.

(e) As a result of their loneliness, a greater number of women than men are placed into 'homes' and institutions as a means of senescent care. In Australia there are 3.8 women in institutional care for the elderly, for every male in such places.

WHY DO WOMEN OCCUPY INSTITUTIONAL CARE?

One might ask 'Why do women occupy so much institutional bed care?' This can be answered on three levels:

(a) There is an increase in physical and mental disability as people age. As most of the aged are females, they will occupy most of the bed space.

(b) Also, as women are often lonely, old and widowed, they tend to use their doctor and community centres as a means of making contact or attracting some interest to themselves. They often have no other sociological outlet and need to seek attention to maintain life. If they are not needed or they feel rejected, depression sets in and this, in turn, leads to more need for drug therapy and institutionalization.

(c) Estrogen insufficiency causes not only an increase in physical infirmity but an increase in certain types of diseases such as athero-sclerosis, osteoporosis and urogenital prolapse.

WHAT PROBLEMS DO POSTMENOPAUSAL WOMEN SUFFER?

The problems of postmenopausal women can be divided into those of short-term duration, such as vasovagal symptoms, urogenital atrophy and psychosexual changes; while long-term problems relate mainly to osteoporosis, atherosclerosis and psychological depression and anxiety. In a recent survey in the Menopause Clinic at the Royal Hospital for Women, Paddington, Sydney, women stated that their feelings of flushes, sweats, muscle aches and pains and formication were present in from 85% to 17% of cases (Table 6.3). Other urogenital psychological and sexual problems occurred with a degree of frequency which was much greater than expected, and which disappeared following hormonal replacement therapy (Tables 6.4-6.6). Most of these women were being treated for their symptoms with a variety of psychotrophic (35%) or other

Table 6.3 Vaso vagal symptoms (percentages)

1. Hot flushes	85
Severe	37
2. Sweats	64
3. Muscle aches and pains	34
4. Formication	17

Table 6.4 Urogenital symptoms (percentages)

1. Nocturia	34
2. Dysuria	18
3. Urinary frequency	40
4. Dry vagina	44
5. Dyspareunia	36

Table 6.5 Psychological symptoms (percentages)

1. Felt unsociable	22
2. Felt lonely	25
3. Unable to cope	21
4. Couldn't make decisions	17
5. Lacked self-confidence	21
6. Worried about self	21

Table 6.6 Symptoms of depression (percentages)

1. No energy	45
2. Irritable	45
3. Anxious	44
4. Nervous	37
5. Felt depressed	42
6. Felt like crying	30
7. Felt unloved	25
8. Insomnia	48
9. Not interested in doing things	24
10. No purpose in life	16

Table 6.7 Medications given for menopausal symptoms (percentages)

1. Sedative-hypnotics	8
2. Antidepressants	5
3. Tranquilizers	15
4. Combinations of above	7
	35
5. Hypotensives	
6. Vitamins	
7. Minerals	69
8. Other drugs	
9. No therapy	17

health-promoting drugs (69%) with only 17% of all women not taking some form of medication for postmenopausal symptoms (Table 6.7)

SEXUALITY FOLLOWING THE MENOPAUSE

A much-neglected health care problem for postmenopausal women is their changed sexuality. It is often stated by patient and doctor alike that a woman is too old to be bothered about sex following the menopause, yet in our survey we found that the major reason a diminution in sexual activity occurred was a sore, dry vagina, followed by an acceptance by both husband and wife that the ability to achieve comfortable, enjoyable sex was now lost. Most women who suffered from these atrophic changes felt a marked improvement, greater comfort, more pleasure and therefore increased desire when adequate estrogen therapy was given (Table 6.8). It is important that the sexual needs of the older woman are not neglected, and every effort should be made to encourage continued activity and enjoyment.

Table 6.8 Sexual postmenopausal women treated with estrogen (percentages)

	Before	After
1. Regular intercourse (at least weekly)	37	53
2. Desire for sex	30	56
3. Ability to achieve orgasm	37	46
4. Importance of sex	53	58
5. Enjoyment of sex	41	62

ATHEROSCLEROSIS

It has been shown consistently that women have a lower incidence of myocardial infarct than do men up to the age of 50 years. From the time

Table 6.9 Atherosclerosis: deaths from myocardial infarction, Australia, 1981 (rate per 100 000)

Age (years)	Males	Females
30–34	6.7	0.66
35–39	21.2	6.0
40–44	55.7	14.5
45–49	140.5	34.5
50–54	262	55.6
55–59	460	126.5
60–64	757	254.5
65–69	1243	491
70–74	1866	827
75–79	2713	1416
80–84	3610	2309
85 and over	5693	4316

of the menopause the incidence of infarcts increases for women but they consistently produce an incidence rate which is approximately 10 years behind those found for men (Table 6.9). Results from studies in Australia, USA and Europe, all suggest that estrogen given in adequate amounts will prevent the increased rate of atherosclerotic change, and Henderson[1] has shown that the incidence of death from myocardial infarcts is halved among these women taking estrogen from the time of the menopause.

OSTEOPOROSIS

Calcium is lost from bone at an increasing rate following the menopause, with up to 3% per year lost in the first 3 years and then settling down to about 1% loss each year thereafter. The use of estrogen has been shown to markedly inhibit the loss of calcium from bone, and when administered in conjunction with adequate amounts of calcium and with exercise, there is no increased incidence of osteoporosis.

Approximately 8000 women in Australia fracture their hips each year, about 9000 their wrists and about 15 000 suffer compression fractures of their spines. It costs almost $2000 per week to care for a person in a hospital bed, and as most women with hip fractures are hospitalized for 5 weeks and then require 7 weeks of convalescent care, it is clear that between 150 million and 200 million dollars annually is spent on this problem alone. In the USA the figure is almost certainly in the vicinity of 3 to 5 billion dollars. Not only can this crippling and financial burden be eased by administering hormonal replacement therapy, but the therapy offered leads to a more active and physically stronger woman who can participate in a normal lifestyle with no inhibitions.

THERAPY FOR POSTMENOPAUSAL PROBLEMS

It is now well established that estrogen will improve or remove the increased risks which women suffer after the menopause, so why not treat every postmenopausal woman with hormonal replacement therapy? The major problems in administering treatment have been induced by the fear of producing an increase in iatrogenic disease. Synthetic and equine estrogens have been associated with an increase in the incidence of uterine cancer, hypertension and gall bladder disease, and have been implicated as a potential cause for thrombosis and breast cancer. Now, however, the cyclical administration of estrogen with a progestogen for 10 or more days; the use of minimal dose of hormones; the use of better, more physiological hormones and the close monitoring of the effect of hormones, has dramatically changed the situation.

We are now employing types of estrogens which are almost identical to natural estrogen, which can be easily metabolized, and have no greater effect than when produced in young menstruating women. Non-androgenic progestogens are being used and the sex hormones are being developed in forms which can be easily absorbed from sites other than the gut to avoid liver protein synthesis.

Risks must be continually avoided, and for women who are overweight, hypertensive, suffer from hypercholesterolemia, have varicose veins, or who smoke cigarettes, the estrogen employed should be an easily metabolized 'natural estrogen', as these have little or no effect on liver synthesis and therefore do not increase clotting factors or renin-substrate.

Of the risks, cancer of the uterus is normally found in about 1 : 1500 postmenopausal women and may increase to 1 : 250 when unopposed estrogen is used. The use of progestogen has reduced the risk to negligible proportions. Cancer of the breast normally occurs in 90 per 100 000 premenopausal women in Australia but increases to 475 per 100 000 when the climacteric arrives. The influence of hormonal replacement therapy on induction of cancer is controversial but recent papers suggest that there is no change in the incidence, or that estrogens may even be protective against carcinoma[2,3].

NEEDS OF POSTMENOPAUSAL WOMEN

The needs of postmenopausal women can be summarized as follows:

(a) Sympathy to their plight and their problems.
(b) Understanding of the cause of their problems.
(c) Education both of the patient and of the doctor.
(d) Hormonal replacement therapy. It must be realized that the postmenopause is a sex-linked female-dominant endocrine deficiency disease and must be treated as such.
(e) Care must be exercised in the regime and dosage of treatment and there must be careful and continual monitoring of all patients on therapy.
(f) Full use must be made of social support systems other than inpatient institutions.
(g) Improved facilities must be made available for occupational and leisure activities for these old but significant members of our community.

REFERENCES

1. Henderson, B. (1984). Estrogen replacement therapy and the risk of arteriosclerotic cardiovascular disease. Proceedings from a symposium on Estrogen Replacement Therapy, San Francisco. Abbott Laboratories–Ogen Round Table Conference.

THE CLIMACTERIC IN PERSPECTIVE

2. Kaufman, D. W., Miller, D. R., Rosenberg, L., Helmrich, S. P., Stolley, P., Schottenfeld, D. and Shapiro, S. (1984). Noncontraceptive estrogen use, and the risk of breast cancer. *J. Am. Med. Assoc.*, **252**, 63–82
3. Vakil, D. V., Morgan, R. W. and Halliday, M. (1983). Exogenous estrogens and development of breast and endometrial cancer. *Cancer Detect. Prevent.*, **6**, 415–24

Chapter 7

Health status and health care utilization by menopausal women

Sonja M. McKinlay and John B. McKinlay

ABSTRACT

This chapter challenges the prevailing perception that the 'typical' meno-pausal woman suffers from a 'syndrome' or 'deficiency disease' – is beset with complaints, experiencing major physical changes, evidences regret-fulness and even depression and is generally a burden on medical care resources. As a move towards correcting this imbalance in knowledge, this chapter focuses on three interrelated themes:

(1) A vast majority of mid-aged women do *not* express regret at reaching menopause, do *not* report more symptoms or poorer health status and do *not* evidence increased use of medical services. The 'typical' menopausal woman is neither sick nor a high user of medical care.

(2) Women who experience an artifical menopause (cessation of menses through surgery) constitute an atypical subgroup, which differs from the vast majority of women in important ways unrelated to the menopause. These are the women who have been extensively studied and discussed in the professional and popular literature.

(3) It is this atypical subgroup which physicians tend to see (as patients) and from whom they understandably derive their statistically biased image of the 'typical' menopausal woman.

INTRODUCTION

According to the popular view and many experts, the menopause, or so-called 'change of life', is thought to represent a major cultural, psychological and physiological milestone for women during the middle years. It signifies the end of reproduction in societies such as the United States, where sexuality and reproduction are considered evidence of personal success and fulfillment. It is a prominent biological marker for an aging process in cultures which extoll youthfulness. The menopause is even perceived as a major negative life event of the same magnitude as, for example, job loss or loss of a spouse. Consequently, it is thought to be accompanied by increases in morbidity and health care utilization, commensurate with the increases observed for such other negative life events.

Associated with these perceptions surrounding the menopause, this normal physiological event has been viewed as a 'syndrome'[1-3], and more recently, as a newly discovered 'deficiency disease'[4]. Women experiencing this normal end of reproduction are thought to experience regretfulness, to evidence signs of clinical depression (involutional melancholia), to present with a broad range of accompanying symptoms, to be high utilizers of physicians' services and generally to consume a disproportionate share of medical resources. The 'typical' menopausal woman, then, is perceived as growing old, beset with psychosocial complaints, experiencing major physical changes, losing cultural significance, evidencing regretfulness and depression and generally being a burden on medical care resources[5, 6]. Such a characterization would appear to receive reinforcement both from pharmaceutical advertisements in professional medical journals[7, 8] and from patient images used and developed during the course of medical education[9, 10].

While remaining the predominant view, it has evolved from biased clinical encounters and is actually without epidemiological foundation. Studies of health status and health service utilization in adult populations show no evidence of increased morbidity or health service use in this mid-aged population beyond expected increases with age[11, 12]. Most of the work to date which focuses on the menopause tends to be based on hospital/clinic populations or general-practice settings which, by definition, represent patients presenting complaints[13, 14]. This view is equally attributable to the practice of reporting only positive findings or association between the menopause and, for example, CHD, osteoporosis or depression[15].

As a move towards correcting the present imbalance in scientific knowledge concerning the menopause, this chapter focuses on three interrelated themes, which may be summarized as follows:

(1) A vast majority of mid-aged women do *not* express regret at reaching menopause, do *not* report more symptoms or poorer health status

and do *not* evidence increased use of medical services. The 'typical' menopausal woman is neither sick nor a high user of medical care.

(2) Women who experience an artificial menopause (cessation of menses through surgery) constitute an atypical subgroup, which differs from the vast majority of women in important ways unrelated to the menopause. These are the women who have been extensively studied and discussed in the professional and popular literature.

(3) It is this atypical subgroup which physicians tend to see (as patients) and from whom they understandably derive their statistically biased image of the 'typical' menopausal woman.

METHODS

The data reported in this chapter were obtained through mailed questionnaires and telephone interviews completed by 8050 women aged 45–55 years (as of 31 December 1981) and residing in Massachusetts at the time of the survey (September 1981 to May 1982). Simple random samples of eligible women were selected in each of 38 towns and cities in a two-stage cluster sampling design, with a response rate of 77%.

Self-report data were obtained on a range of sociodemographic, health and employment variables using, in all cases, the most reliable methodologies available. The *sociodemographic* variables considered include age, education (in three categories), number of regular contacts per week with friends or relatives not living with the respondents, and household composition. Occupation and per capita income were considered as socioeconomic indicators but regarded as inappropriate for this analysis. Occupation was relatively invariant in this population of mid-aged women, even though 67% were currently working for pay (54% of these were in clerical or service jobs). Per capita income could not be assessed for a substantive proportion (14%) of women due to missing information on total household income. Many women simply do not know what their husbands earn. Educational status, which is strongly associated with per capita income in this sample, was therefore chosen as the most reliable socioeconomic indicator for this population. The number of contacts with relatives or friends was used as a crude measure of social network size, which has been shown to correlate strongly with health behavior in other populations[16, 17]. Household composition rather than marital status was thought to provide more sensitive information on the respondent's nurturing role (including children as well as other, usually elderly, adult relatives) as a potential source of stress for mid-aged women. At the same time, this variable includes most information on marital status which has been well-documented as related to health and health behavior[18–21]. Elsewhere it has been reported that employment status is unrelated to health and health behaviors in this same population[22] and was, therefore, not included here. A small subgroup of 721 women, not in the labor force primarily for health reasons, was identified in the earlier analysis as contributing all of the apparent difference in health status between employed and unemployed women. This subgroup, however, although more likely to have an early surgical menopause, was too small to affect results by menopausal status, in the sample.

Five measures of *health status* were included in this investigation. Self-assessed health in relation to one's peers is the primary measure, which is highly correlated with all others and has been shown to be a reliable indicator of actual health status[23]. Women were also asked if they currently had, or were receiving treatment for, any of the following common chronic conditions which usually require clinical diagnosis: diabetes (4%), high blood pressure (19%), asthma (4%), allergies or eczema (14%), heart disease (4%), ulcer (4%), arthritis or rheumatism (23%) and cancer (1%). The third health status variable is the number of restricted activity days in the prior 2 weeks due to some aspect of the respondent's health. This measure is comparable to that used in the National Center for Health Statistics' ongoing Health Interview Survey. Finally, respondents were asked to indicate whether or not each on a list of common symptoms had been experienced in the past 2 weeks. Eliminating those listed which related to either menstruation or the menopause (hot flushes/flashes, cold sweats, menstrual problems, fluid retention), the remaining symptoms were divided into two groups. Common physical symptoms included: diarrhea and/or constipation, persistent cough, upset stomach, backaches, headaches, sore throat and aches/stiffness in the joints. A group of symptoms of a less obviously physical origin, especially in the absence of other physical signs or diagnosed disease, included: dizzy spells, lack of energy, irritability, feeling blue or depressed, shortness of breath, trouble sleeping and loss of appetite. This latter group was labeled as primarily psychological in origin, given the low prevalence of heart disease and cancer in this sample.

Five measures of *utilization* of formal and informal health care resources were included. Prescribed and over-the-counter (OTC) medications reportedly taken in the prior 2 weeks were classified separately. Respondents were also asked if they had consulted either a health professional (nurse, nurse practitioner, physician assistant, physician, pharmacist, etc.) and/or relative or friend concerning a problem with their health in the prior 2 weeks. Consultation with one or more health professional indicated formal health service use, while consultation with a friend or relative indicated use of their informal or lay helping resources. Finally, reported breast surgery for cysts or benign tumors was used as an additional indicator of formal health service use. The use of a 2-week time frame for the first four of these variables has been shown by NCHS to ensure reliable recall.

Menopausal status was reliably determined from a combination of questions on current menstrual status and changes in the past 12 months. *Natural menopause* was considered to have occurred if no menses were reported for 12 months, in the absence of surgery which would terminate menstruation. Twelve months of amenorrhea is the widely accepted definition used in European studies since the 1950s (see, for example, ref. 24) and is recommended by Treloar[25] on the basis of his prospective study of normal menstrual patterns. Women are classified as *perimenopausal* if menses have been reported in the past 12 months, but with periods of amenorrhea and/or changes in regularity or flow. Again, this is consistent with prior research[24-26]. Women are *still menstruating* if they report regular menses in the past 3 months. *Artificial menopause* is considered to have occurred if menses were surgically stopped by either a hysterectomy (with or without removal of the ovaries) (26%) or a bilateral oophorectomy (2%).

A final variable included in this analysis was the response to an *attitudinal question* on how respondents felt about the time when menstrual periods stopped altogether. Four pre-coded options were provided: 'relief', 'regret', 'mixed feelings' and 'no particular feelings at all'.

The analytical approach followed a logical sequence of steps involving primarily contingency table methods and stepwise discriminant modeling. Initial cross-tabulations of menopausal status by each of the health status and health behavior variables indicated that women with an artificial menopause reported health status and health-related behavior which was markedly different from the other three menopausal groups. Perimenopausal women showed selected differences compared to women still menstruating or who had experienced a natural menopause. Given the very different age distributions in each menopausal group (see Fig. 7.1), Fisherian discriminant functions[27] were estimated, using a stepwise procedure[28], between: (a) artifically and naturally menopausal women; and (b) perimenopausal and still menstruating women. These estimated functions indicated which sociodemographic variables required control in final comparisons, and which health status and health behavior variables contributed significant differences in the two comparisons. Differences in combined proportions, adjusted for sociodemographic factors, were tested for significance in the final comparisons[29].

RESULTS

Figure 7.1 presents the distribution of the four menopausal status groups by age for the sample cases with complete data. As expected, the proportions of still menstruating and perimenopausal women decrease with age, the latter group more slowly. The proportion reporting a natural menopause increases rapidly in this cohort, while the proportion reporting a

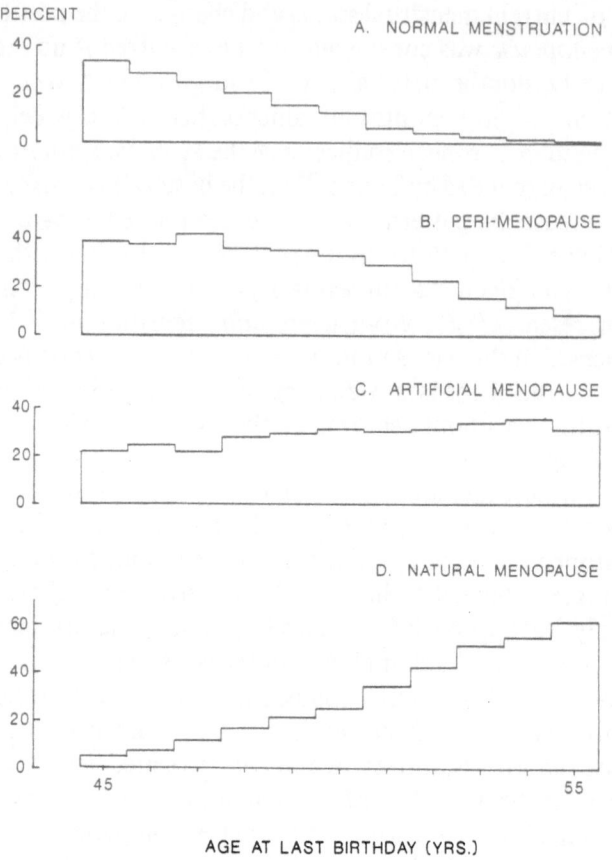

Figure 7.1 The distribution of menopausal status by age

surgical menopause increases somewhat before age 50, then remains constant at about 30%, indicating that the majority of women undergo this surgery before the age of 50 and, therefore, before the occurrence of a natural menopause (median age 51.4 ± 0.19 years in this sample).

A summary of the distributions of selected sociodemographic characteristics is presented in Table 7.1. As anticipated from Fig. 7.1, the mean ages in each of the four menopausal status groups are significantly different with increments of 1.5 years, going from still menstruating to perimenopausal to artificially and finally to naturally menopausal women, in that order.

The proportion reporting more than 12 years of education, however, does not decrease with age as expected from survey and census data in adult populations[30]. The decline in education with increasing age is evident when the artificial menopause group is excluded. This latter group, however, is not only *younger* than naturally menopausal women

Table 7.1 The distribution of selected sociodemographic characteristics by menopausal status

	Menopausal status			
Characteristic	Still menstruating	Peri- menopausal	Artificially menopausal	Naturally menopausal
(1) Mean age (years) (SE)	48.0 (0.07)	49.5 (0.06)	51.1 (0.06)	52.6 (0.05)
(2) Percentage >12 years education	44.3	39.6	29.6	31.7
(3) Percentage 10+ weekly contacts	57.8	57.8	63.4	58.5
(4) Household Composition				
Living with spouse and children	59.3	55.3	45.3	44.7
Living with spouse only	11.2	14.7	21.1	20.5
Living alone	4.1	6.4	8.6	9.0
Total (100%)	994	2113	2223	2421

All differences are significant at $\alpha = 0.001$; all tests included adjustments for age or age and education differences as appropriate

by 1.5 years, but is less well-educated than the otherwise oldest, least-educated group of menopausal women. Such a reversal of the expected trend indicates that women with an artificial menopause have received markedly less education than women the same age who are at risk to or experiencing a natural menopause.

The distribution of the number of weekly contacts with friends and relatives is independent of both age and education, with non-significant chi-square values. When compared to all other women in the sample, however, those with an artifical menopause are significantly more likely to report ten or more weekly contacts. This difference indicates that frequent contact with relatives or friends is, in some way, associated directly with a surgical menopause but is otherwise unrelated to menopausal status in this sample of women.

The atypical sociodemographic profile in the artificially menopausal subgroup, when compared to the rest of the sample, is repeated with respect to household composition. When this subgroup is excluded, the expected trend with age is toward a two-fold increase in the proportion living alone (reflecting an increase in widowed, divorced or separated women), an increase in the proportion living with a spouse only (11% to 20%) and a corresponding decrease in the proportion with both a spouse and children still living at home (59% to 45%). It should be noted that the artificial menopause subgroup reports the same distribution for household composition as the older, more educated, naturally menopausal women. This equivalence is partly due to the higher rate of divorce in artificially menopausal women (12% compared to 9% in the rest of the sample), offsetting a lower proportion of never-married women in this group (4% compared to 7% in naturally menopausal women). The comparably low proportion of artificially menopausal women with both children and a spouse at home appears to contradict the higher parity in this group (92% with at least one child compared to 88% among naturally menopausal women). A possible explanation (not verifiable in this data set) is that the artificially menopausal women began childbearing considerably earlier than did women with a natural menopause.

When these sociodemographic characteristics (age, education, number of contacts with relatives/friends and household composition) were entered stepwise into the two discriminant functions described above, age and number of contacts with friends and relatives were the two significant discriminators between artificially and naturally menopausal women (Table 7.2). The variables significantly discriminating between the two younger groups were, as expected, age and educational status, although almost all the R^2 value (0.69) was contributed by age alone, with education adding little information to the discriminant. The lack of comparability in these two discriminants underscores the atypical sociodemographic profile of the artificial menopause group.

Table 7.2 Summary of stepwise Fisherian discriminant analyses

	Comparison			
	Perimenopausal v still-menstruating		*Artificially v. naturally menopausal*	
Variable group	*Variables entered (in order)*	R^2	*Variables entered (in order)*	R^2
A. Sociodemographic	1. Age 2. Educational status	0.69	1. Age 2. Number of relatives/ friends	0.47
B. Health status	3. Number of physical symptoms 4. General health status 5. Number of psychological symptoms	0.70	3. Number of physical symptoms 4. Number of chronic conditions 5. Number of restricted activity days	0.48
C. Health care behavior	No variables entered (none met minimum criterion)		6. Number of prescribed medications 7. Breast surgery 8. Consulting with relative or friend	0.49

These sociodemographic variables were then held constant in the discriminants while all five health status measures were added, stepwise. From Table 7.2 it is evident that health status variables add little to the discrimination of the two pairs of menopausal groups. Moreover, two of the three discriminatory variables added are different in the two comparisons. While both comparisons include physical symptoms as the primary discriminator, the younger premenopausal groups differ primarily on

Table 7.3 The distribution of selected measures of health status, by menopausal status

Health status measure	Menopausal status			
	Still menstruating	Peri- menopausal	Artificially menopausal	Naturally menopausal
Percentage health worse than peers	3.8	6.3	10.6	7.9
Percentage reporting two or more chronic conditions	9.7	14.9	21.3	16.6
Percentage reporting one or more restricted activity days	11.7	15.8	18.2	12.6
Percentage reporting two or more physical symptoms	34.8	46.7	52.8	41.8
Percentage reporting two or more psychological symptoms	35.9	46.9	48.9	43.5
Total (100%)	989	2113	2218	2430

All differences are significant at $\alpha = 0.001$; all comparisons are adjusted for age and education differences.

measures of acute health status, while the older groups differ on more chronic health measures.

The differences between all four menopausal groups are summarized in Table 7.3, which shows that, irrespective of the sociodemographic differences already discussed, the artificial menopause subgroup reports consistently worse health on all five measures. The differences are particularly marked when this subgroup is compared to the rest of the sample with respect to measures of long-term health status (perceived general health and reported chronic conditions). The reporting of recent symptoms and restricted activity days also shows increases in this atypical subgroup, but they are not as marked and, as expected, are accompanied by increased reporting among the perimenopausal women. The increases in the latter group are associated with increases in menstrual flow problems and the hot flashes and sweats which are typical of this transitional phase preceding cessation of menses (see Table 7.4). The measure showing the least differences among the four groups is the number of psychological symptoms, although all three measures based on reporting in the prior 2 weeks show elevation in the perimenopausal and menopausal women compared to those still menstruating naturally. This pattern indicates that the experience of menopause has some immediate but short-term effect on reported health, but is certainly not of the magnitude reported by the artificial menopause subgroup and is primarily associated with expected increases in menstrual flow problems, hot flashes and the accompanying sweats. These findings provide some cross-cultural corroboration for the studies by Flint[31] (of 483 Indian women of the Rajput caste) and Maoz and his colleagues[32] (of five ethnic groups of women in

Table 7.4 The percentage reporting flushes/sweats and menstrual problems/fluid retention, by the number of other physical symptoms and menopausal status

	Menopausal status							
	Still menstruating		Peri- menopausal		Artificially menopausal		Naturally menopausal	
	Number of physical symptoms*							
	<2	⩾2	<2	⩾2	<2	⩾2	<2	⩾2
Percentage reporting flushes/sweats	7.2	26.2	30.4	45.2	33.5	54.1	33.4	55.1
Percentage reporting menstrual problems/ fluid retention	17.5	43.0	28.4	50.8	–	–	–	–
Total (100%)	645	343	1121	981	1037	1157	1404	1001

*Other than flushes, sweats, menstrual problems or fluid retention

Israel). Although women from different cultures may exhibit differences in attitudes towards the menopause, they are similar in their reporting of symptomatology – especially hot flashes/sweats and menstrual cycle changes.

The transient nature of the increases in symptomatology among peri-menopausal women is reflected in the lack of a corresponding increase in the use of formal health care by this group, as summarized in Tables 7.2 and 7.5. In marked contrast, the relatively poorer health of the surgical menopause subgroup is accompanied by a two-fold increase in prescribed medication (primarily estrogen replacement therapy), a 75%

Table 7.5 The distribution of selected measures of health care utilization behavior, by menopausal status

| | Menopausal status | | | |
Health care utilization measure	Still menstruating	Peri- menopausal	Artificially menopausal	Naturally menopausal
Percentage reporting one or more prescribed medications	11.6	15.5	34.8	16.1
Percentage reporting one or more OTC medications	77.0	83.0	84.7	78.7
Percentage reporting breast surgery	9.2	11.6	17.8	11.0
Percentage consulting one or more health professionals	19.1	22.3	28.8	21.0
Percentage consulting a relative/friend	20.4	26.6	29.0	22.2
Total (100%)	981	2098	2197	2400

All differences are significant at $\alpha = 0.001$; all comparisons are adjusted for age and education or age and number of relatives/friends higher rate of reported breast surgery, a 30–50% increase in consultations with a health professional, and a 10–40% increase in lay consultation.

Both the perimenopausal women and those who are artificially menopausal show slight but insignificant increases in the use of OTC medications, as well as correspondingly higher rates of informal consultation with relatives or friends concerning a health problem.

The health behavior variables which significantly added to the discriminant (artificial versus natural menopause) were, in order of entry, the number of prescribed medications, breast surgery and consultation with a relative or friend (Table 7.2). Almost all the increase (2%) in R^2 (0.49) was contributed by the first variable, as anticipated. In comparing perimenopausal and menstruating women, none of the health behavior variables considered added significantly to the discriminant, confirming the lack of impact of the menopause on health behavior, evident in Table 7.5. Only the use of OTC medications even approached significance in the discriminant.

Given the two-fold higher rate of prescribed medication use by women with an artificial menopause, a more detailed analysis of this relationship was undertaken and the results are summarized in Fig. 7.2. The two primary types of prescribed medication were estrogens (for hormone replacement therapy) and tranquilizers such as valium and librium. Because the primary motivation for estrogen therapy is castration (bilateral oophorectomy), the artificial menopause group was further classified according to whether or not both ovaries had been removed.

As expected, those most likely to be currently using estrogens (alone or combined with a tranquilizer) were castrated women (one-third of this group). However, even among hysterectomized women with at least one ovary intact, nearly 16% were also using estrogens. These rates are in marked contrast to the remaining groups in which the rate of estrogen use varies from just over 6% (natural menopause group) to less than 2% (among menstruating women).

It is notable that there is no elevation of tranquilizer use in either surgical menopause group if it is not combined with estrogen prescription, the rates remaining remarkably constant at about 10% across all menopausal groups. However, when combined with estrogen prescription, tranquilizers are more likely to be used by women with an artificial menopause. This pattern could indicate that physicians who are likely to prescribe estrogen are more likely to prescribe other drugs. Alternatively, it could reflect demands from a subset of women who are high drug users.

The remaining differences of interest are the rates of formal and informal consultation of relatives and friends concerning a health problem. From Table 7.5 it appears that the perimenopausal women show some increase in informal consultation only, while the artificial menopause group shows higher rates of both formal and informal consultation.

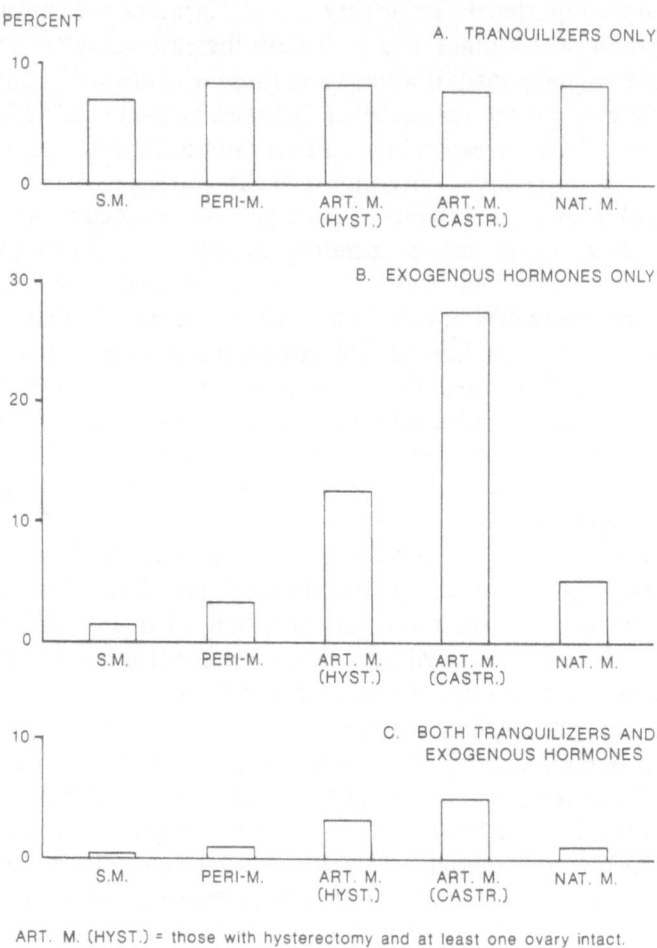

Figure 7.2 Prescribed exogenous hormone and tranquilizer use, by menopausal status

The relationship of these two outcomes was further explored by considering their joint distribution by menopausal status (Fig. 7.3). From this figure it is evident that the perimenopausal and artificially menopausal women exhibit quite different consulting behavior patterns, as suggested in Table 7.5. The younger, perimenopausal group shows a modest increase in lay consultation only, with no increase in either the use of health professionals only, or of both sources. In contrast, the artificially menopausal women show a clear increase in the use of both formal and informal consultation, rather than independent increases in the use of each source separately.

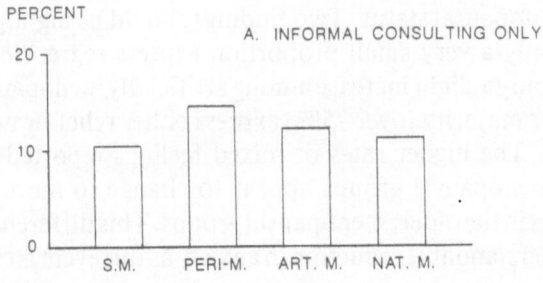

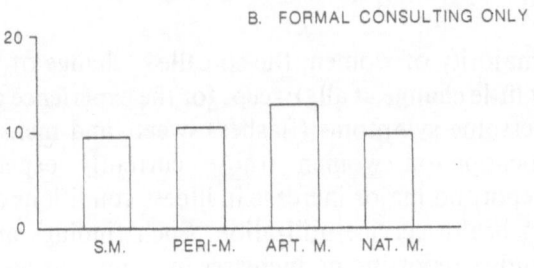

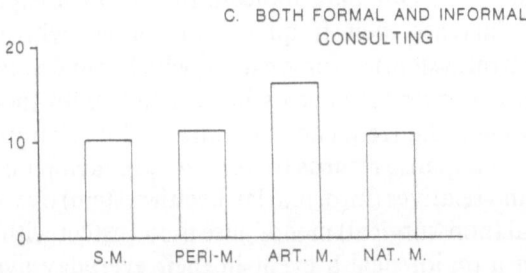

Figure 7.3 Consultation concerning health, with professionals (formal) and/or with relatives/friends (informal), by menopausal status

Table 7.6 Percentage distribution of attitude to cessation of menses, by menopausal status

	Menopausal status			
Attitude	Still menstruating	Peri- menopausal	Artificially menopausal	Naturally menopausal
Relief or no feelings at all (combined)	73.5	74.0	79.5	80.8
Mixed feelings	23.5	23.6	17.0	17.0
Regret	3.0	2.4	3.4	2.2
Total (100%)	935	2037	2130	2409

$\chi^2(9) = 137.2$; $p < 0.0001$ (including all four attitude categories)

Finally, Table 7.6 summarizes women's feelings about cessation of menses, by menopausal status. Two findings should be highlighted in this table. *First*, only a very small proportion express regret (less than 3% overall), with only a slight increase among artificially menopausal women. *Second*, a clear majority (over 75%) express either relief or no particular feelings at all. The higher rates of mixed feelings reported by the two younger, premenopausal groups appear to change to more positive or neutral feelings in the older, menopausal groups. This difference probably reflects an understandable reduction in anxiety as this event is experienced.

DISCUSSION

For the vast majority of women, the so-called 'change of life' actually produces very little change at all. Except for the experience of some temporarily bothersome symptoms (flashes, sweats and menstrual irregularity), perimenopausal women (those currently experiencing the menopause) report no major increase in illness conditions and evidence no increase in health service utilization. Such findings are consistent with earlier studies reporting no increases in symptoms associated with the menopause[1, 34–36]. Our data indicate that women experiencing the menopause do increase their frequency of contact with relatives and friends (lay referral system) to some extent, which is understandable since most people discuss everyday events in their lives with their significant others. As expected, the frequency of contact with relatives and friends after a natural menopause returns to its lower premenopausal level. This use of friends and relatives (informal lay health system) by women experiencing a natural (non-surgical) menopause is consistent with our findings that this is not a major health event in their everyday lives. It can be understood and coped with through lay resources, rather than formal health care services.

Just over a quarter of women in Massachusetts experience an artificial menopause (i.e. surgical cessation of menses). These are a distinctly atypical subgroup who differ from the majority of women sociodemographically, and perceive their health as worse than their peers, report a higher incidence of chronic conditions, experience more restricted activity days and report more physical symptoms. They tend to be younger, of lower socioeconomic status (as measured by educational level) and more likely to be divorced than are their naturally menopausal counterparts. Understandably, they are significantly more likely to consult health professionals for these problems, undergo breast surgery, consume prescription drugs and consult relatives and friends concerning their health problems.

For these atypical, artificially menopausal women, reported morbidity appears to be quite independent of the menopause itself. That is, they report higher rates of diagnosed chronic conditions (e.g. diabetes, asthma, allergies and cancer) which are independent of the menopause. For whatever reason (whether a direct result of their poorer health status or whether due to their consequent increased exposure to medical care) the artificially menopausal subgroup appears to be at increased risk to medical intervention. This is strongly suggested by their higher rate of breast surgery and increased use of estrogen replacement therapy and tranquilizers, in the absence of bilateral oophorectomy. It should be noted that the artificially menopausal women are higher users of *both* the formal health care system and their informal lay system of friends and relatives – perhaps signifying the more serious morbid episodes they encounter. Some studies of utilization behavior suggest that the use of one system tends to substitute for the other. For example, high use of relatives and friends is associated with low use of formal health services[16, 37, 38]. For the artificially menopausal women, however, the lay resources of friends and relatives are used in addition to, rather than instead of, formal medical care.

Health care workers are often criticized for their patient stereotypes – for example, the image of the 'typical' menopausal woman[39]. It is possible that this clearly erroneous image derives from frequent contact with the selected subgroup of atypical women whose major differences from the majority of women experiencing the menopause have been described in this chapter. This subgroup clearly forms the core of the clinical caseload and remains the population most often studied and referenced[40].

The substantive findings presented here highlight two fairly obvious, but important, methodological requirements for further work in this area. *First*, epidemiological studies of representative samples of apparently healthy women experiencing normal aging are required to offset and complement the statistically biased portrait which understandably derives from highly selective clinical encounters with predominantly sick individuals (in, for example, general practice or clinic settings). It is axiomatic in epidemiological research that more can be learned about the sick by studying the well, than by studying the sick themselves.

Secondly, only static associations can be presented here (an unavoidable limitation of cross-sectional designs) which raise rather than resolve questions concerning causality, that can only be definitively addressed by longitudinal or prospective data. For example, the analysis presented here associates a surgical menopause with poorer health and higher health care utilization. However, the most likely causal sequence of these three factors remains to be determined. The results shown in this chapter indicate that poorer health *may* be independent of (and therefore possibly precede), a surgical menopause. However, it is not clear whether or not increased exposure to the health care system resulting from poorer health intervenes to increase the risk of a surgical menopause.

Which of these possible causal explanations is the most likely can only be decided by appropriate analyses of longitudinal data. Such data are being obtained from the Massachusetts Women's Health Study which is following a large sample of 2600 women every 9 months. These subsequent data will permit definitive answers to the derivative questions raised by the cross-sectional results presented in this chapter.

Acknowledgements

The research for this paper is supported by Grant No. AG-03111 from the National Institute on Aging, National Institutes of Health. All inquiries should be directed to Dr Sonja M. McKinlay (Principal Investigator) at the Cambridge Research Center/AIR, 22 Hilliard Street, Cambridge, MA 02138, USA. The authors would like to acknowledge the contribution of Christine A. Crandall to the preparation of this chapter.

REFERENCES

1. McKinlay, S. M. and Jefferys, M. (1974). The menopausal syndrome. *Br. J. Prev. Soc. Med.*, **28**, 108-15
2. Townsend, J. M. and Carbone, C. L. (1980). Menopausal syndrome: illness or social role – a transcultural analysis. *Culture, Med. Psychiatry*, **4**, 229-48
3. Greenblatt, R. (1974). *The Menopausal Syndrome.* (New York: Medcom Press)
4. McCrea, F. (1983). The politics of menopause: the discovery of a deficiency disease. *Soc. Problems*, **31**, 111-23
5. Wilson, R. (1966). *Feminine Forever.* (New York: Evans)
6. Reuben, D. (1969). *Everything You Always Wanted to Know About Sex, But Were Afraid to Ask.* (New York: David McKay)
7. Chapman, S. (1979). Advertising and psychotropic drugs: the place of myth in ideological production. *Soc. Sci. Med.*, **13A**, 751-64
8. Prather, J. and Fidell, L. (1975). Sex differences in the content and style of medical advertisements. *Soc. Sci. Med.*, **9**, 23-6
9. Scully, D. and Bart, P. (1973). A funny thing happened on the way to the orifice: women in gynecology textbooks. *Am. J. Sociol.*, **78**, 1045-51
10. Howell, M. C. (1974). What medical schools teach about women. *N. Engl. J. Med.*, **291**, 304-7
11. Anderson, R. and Anderson, O. W. (1979). Trends in the use of health services. In Freeman, H. E. *et al.* (eds.) *Handbook of Medical Sociology.* pp. 371-91. (Englewood Cliffs, NJ: Prentice Hall)
12. Maurana, C. A., Eichhorn, R. L. and Lonnquist, L. F. (1981). *The use of health services: indices and correlates.* (Washington, DC: Government Printing Office)
13. Shephard, M. *et al.* (1966). *Psychiatric Illness in General Practice.* (London: Oxford University Press)
14. Skegg, D. C. *et al.* (1977). Use of medicine in general practice. *Br. Med. J.*, **1**, 1561-3
15. Kuller, L. H., Meilahn, E. N. and Costello, E. J. (1984). Relationship of menopause to cardiovascular disease. *Behav. Med. Update*, **5**, 35-47
16. McKinlay, J. B. (1981). Social network influence on morbid episodes and help-seeking behavior. In Eisenberg, L. and Kleinman, A. (eds.) *The Relevance of Social Science for Medicine.* pp. 77-107. (The Hague: D. Reidel)
17. Broadhead, W. E. and Kaplan, B. H. (1983). The epidemiologic evidence for a relationship between social support and health. *Am. J. Epidemiol.*, **117**, 521-37

18. Verbrugge, L. M. (1983). Multiple roles and physical health of women and men. *J. Health Soc. Behav.*, **24**, 16–30
19. Haynes, S. G. and Feinleib, M. (1980). Women, work and coronary heart disease: prospective findings from the Framingham Heart Study. *Am. J. Publ. Health*, **70**, 133–41
20. Haynes, S. G., Eaker, E. D. and Feinleib, M. (1984). The effect of employment, family and job stress on coronary heart disease in women. In Gold, E. B. (ed.) *The Changing Risk of Disease in Women: an Epidemiological Approach.* pp. 37–48. (Lexington, MA: Collamore Press)
21. Berkman, L. F. and Syme, S. L. (1979). Social networks, host resistance and mortality: a nine-year follow-up study of Alameda County residents. *Am. J. Epidemiol.*, **109**, 186–204
22. Jennings, S., Mazaik, C. and McKinlay, S. (1984). Women and work: an investigation of the association between health and employment status in middle-aged women. *Soc. Sci. Med.* **19**, 423–31
23. Maddox, G. L. and Douglass, E. (1973). Self-assessment of health: a longitudinal study of elderly subjects. *J. Health Soc. Behav.*, **14**, 87–93
24. Magursky, V., Mesko, M. and Sokolik, L. (1975). Age at menopause and onset of the climacteric in women of Martin District. *Int. J. Fertil.*, **20**, 17–23
25. Treloar, A. E. (1974). Menarche, menopause and intervening fecundability. *Human Biol.*, **46**, 89–107
26. Jaszmann, L., VanLith, N. D. and Zaat, J. C. A. (1969). The age at menopause in the Netherlands. *Int. J. Fertil.*, **14**, 106–17
27. Mosteller, F. and Tukey, J. W. (1977). *Data Analysis and Regression.* (Reading, MA: Addison-Wesley)
28. SAS Institute (1982). *The User's Guide*, 1982 edition. (Raleigh, NC: SAS Institute)
29. Cochran, W. G. (1954). Some methods for strengthening the common χ^2 tests. *Biometrics*, **10**, 417–51
30. US Department of Commerce, Bureau of the Census (1980). *Statistical Abstract of the US: 1980*, 101st edition. (Washington, DC: Government Printing Office)
31. Flint, M. P. (1975). The menopause: reward or punishment. *Psychosomatics*, **16**, 161–3
32. Maoz, B., Antonovsky, A., Apter, A. Wijsenbeek, H. and Datan, N. (1977). The perception of menopause in five ethnic groups in Israel. *Acta Obstet. Gynecol. Scand. Suppl.*, **65**, 69–76
33. Neugarten, B. L. and Kraines, R. J. (1965). Menopausal symptoms in women of various ages. *Psychosom. Med.*, **27**, 266–73
34. Greene, J. G. (1976). A factor analytic study of climacteric symptoms. *J. Psychosom. Res.*, **20**, 425–30
35. Hallstrom, J. (1973). *Mental Disorders and Sexuality in the Climacteric.* (Goteberg, Sweden: Orstadius Boktrgstreu A.B.)
36. Winokur, G. (1973). Depression in the menopause. *Am J. Psychiatry*, **130**, 92–3
37. McKinlay, J. B. (1973). Social networks, lay consultation and help-seeking behavior. *Social Forces*, **51**(3), 275
38. Tennstedt, S. (1984). Informal care of frail elders in the community. Unpublished doctoral dissertation, Boston University, Boston, MA
39. Ruzek, S. B. (1978). *The Woman's Health Movement.* (New York: Praeger)
40. McKinlay, S. M. and McKinlay, J. B. (1973). Selected studies of the menopause: a methodological critique. *J. Biosoc. Sci.*, **5**, 533–55

Section 2
Osteoporosis

Chapter 8

Pathogenesis of postmenopausal osteoporosis

R. Lindsay, D. M. Hart, H. Abdalla and D. Dempster

The presentation of osteoporosis to the clinician relies on the chance occurrence of fracture. Such events are sufficiently commonplace to allow identification of osteoporosis as a major public health problem. In 1986 in the USA, we expect more than 300 000 fractures of the femoral neck, and one woman in four over the age of 60 years will have a vertebral crush fracture. In 1983 it has been estimated that the USA spent $5.8 billion for health care of patients with osteoporosis. Recent evidence from both the USA and the United Kingdom suggests that the frequency of fractures occurring secondary to osteoporosis may be increasing[1-3]. In the USA femoral neck fracture frequency has increased from 176 000 per year in 1970 to 267 000 per year by 1980 (Fig. 8.1). If the present trend continues, by the end of the century there will be approximately 500 000 hip fractures annually.

Fracture occurrence is preceded by a prolonged asymptomatic period of loss of bone tissue. This bone loss is universal in all cultures studied thus far and is greater among women than men. Since bone mass at maturity is greater in men than in women, it is perhaps not surprising that women reach an assumed, but theoretical, fracture threshold at a considerably younger age than their male counterparts.

Among the fracture population, the amount of bone lost probably exceeds 30% of the maximum skeletal mass at maturity (estimated from average bone mass at 30 years). The majority of this loss occurs as a biphasic, exponential process following the cessation of ovarian function. Liability to fracture therefore depends both on initial bone mass and

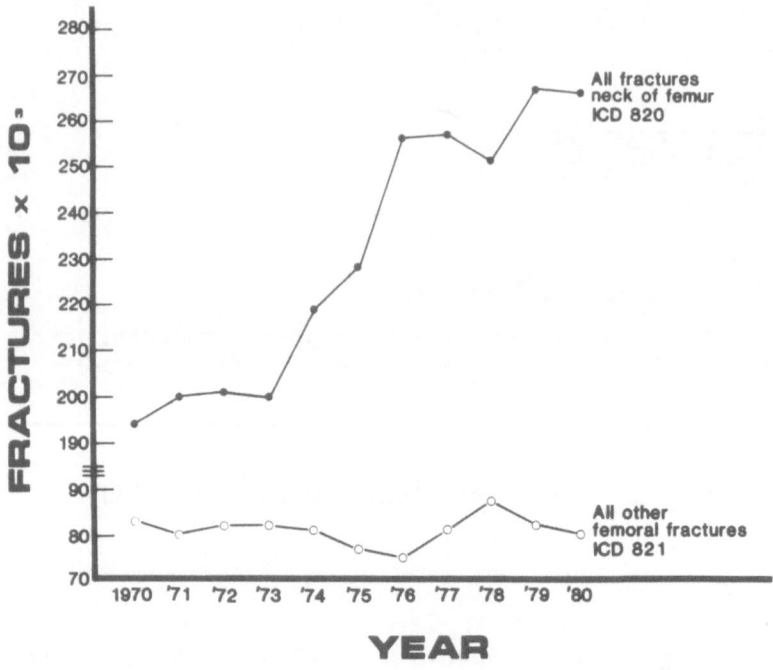

Figure 8.1 Estimated total fractures of the femoral neck (ICD 820) in the USA from 1970 through 1980. For comparison, all other femoral fractures (ICD 821) assumed to be traumatic are shown.

subsequent rates of loss. To date, no pathological changes have been described in osteoporotic bone, apart from a reduced mass of bone tissue per unit volume. The data available, however, suggest that a threshold exists below which the likelihood of a fracture occurrence rises rapidly. Scanning electron micrographs of normal and osteoporotic bone demonstrate how this might occur. Normal trabecular bone consists of a honeycomb of plates and bars surrounding the marrow cavities (Fig. 8.2a). As bone loss occurs, the plates of bone become increasingly replaced by rods, and eventually these rods may become completely eroded through (Figs 8.2b and 8.2c), effectively providing no structural support. At some critical point, as the frequency of these eroded trabeculae increases, the fracture threshold is surpassed. The corollary to this observation relates to the question of treatment of established disease. Even if satisfactory methods of increasing trabecular bone mass can be achieved, it seems unlikely that normal trabecular architecture will be restored. Therefore, an increase in mass may not be accompanied by a corresponding increment in strength.

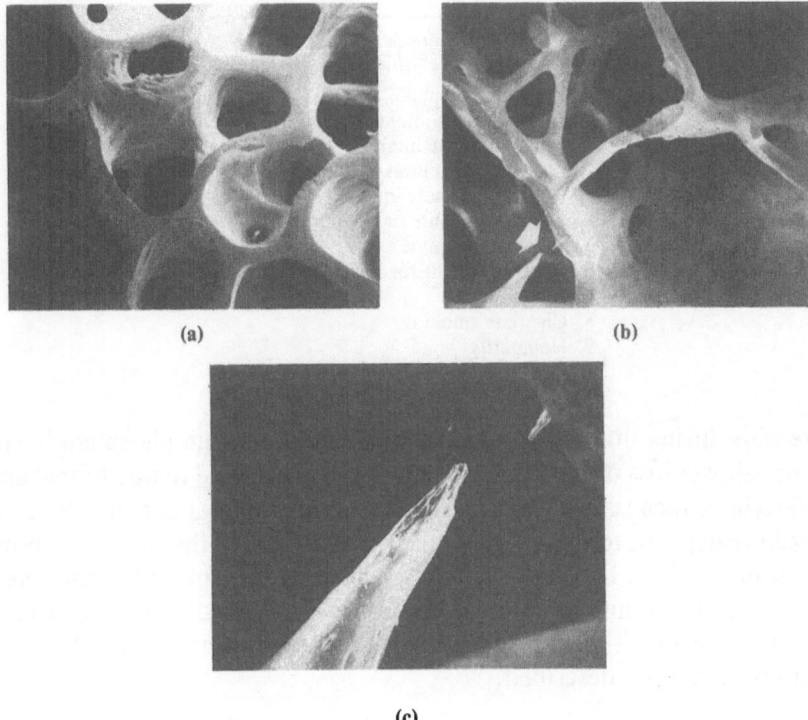

Figure 8.2 Scanning electron micrographs of iliac crest trabecular bone from a normal, 44-year-old male (a) and a 47-year-old osteoporotic female with multiple vertebral crush fractures (b and c). Note that the bone from the patient with osteoporosis consists primarily of rods. A higher-power view (c) of the tip of a disconnected rod (b, arrow) reveals the characteristic hallmarks of osteoclastic erosion as seen in the scanning electron microscope. Field width: a and b = 3.1 mm, c = 0.54 mm. The specimens were prepared by a method that allows iliac crest bone biopsies to be viewed in the scanning electron microscope after the traditional histomorphometric analysis has been performed. (Published with permission from Mary Ann Liebert Publishers Inc., New York, from *J. Bone Min. Res.* **1**, 1)

RISK FACTORS

Many so-called 'risk factors' have been described in publications reviewing not only fracture patients but also younger women actively losing bone. The commonly quoted risk factors are listed in Table 8.1. Several of these may be causally related to the disorder; however, many seem likely to be associated only by chance. Presently, however, distinction is often difficult. Undoubtedly, genetic influences, diet, and lifestyle during childhood and early adult life impact on bone mass at maturity (maximum skeletal mass and density achieved between ages 25 and 40). Menstrual status, pregnancy, and oral contraceptive use as well as, possibly, diet and lifestyle influence bone mass at menopause. The early loss of bone after menopause or oophorectomy is dependent on circulating levels of sex

Table 8.1 Risk factors for osteoporosis

1. Females of white or oriental origin
2. Positive family history for osteoporosis
3. Poor diet, including:
   low calcium intake
   high caffeine intake
   high protein intake
   high phosphate intake
4. Early menopause or oophorectomy
5. Sedentary lifestyle
6. Reduced weight for height
7. Alcohol abuse
8. Cigarette smoking
9. Nulliparity

steroids during that period, and perhaps also on serum phosphate[4]. The later, slower loss of bone appears more closely related to nutritional and lifestyle influences, as well as the initial bone mineral content. Finally, fracture depends to some extent on chance, as well as the amount of bone present. With at least two periods of skeletal loss and different determinants of rate and amount of loss for each, it is not surprising that a plethora of nutrition, lifestyle, environmental and pathological associations have been described.

Nutrition

The concept that osteoporosis may be a nutritional deficiency disease has been a long-standing discussion. In many animal species, calcium deficiency clearly causes osteoporosis. However, the human data to support this concept are less certain. Lifelong calcium deficiency, in one study, appears to result in lower bone mass at maturity and reduced fracture frequency at the other end of the age spectrum[5]. Nonetheless, a preponderance of studies, often compounded by other variables, have failed to show a demonstrable effect of dietary calcium. The most convincing data come from Heaney, who demonstrated a positive relationship between calcium intake and balance, which suggested that premenopausal women would require approximately 1 g of dietary calcium to obtain balance, while postmenopausal women would require nearly 1.8 g (at the 95% confidence limit) to obtain zero balance. Even so, intervention with calcium has not been universally successful in preventing bone loss, especially in the trabecular bone of the spine[6]. This is of particular importance since the Matkovic study referred to above failed to detect any difference in fractures of wrist or spine at differing calcium intakes. The role of phosphorus is even less clear. Heaney's data[7] and that from Spencer et al.[8] suggest that there is no effect of phosphorus on calcium homeostasis. Yet phosphate lowers urinary calcium and impairs the hydroxylation of 25-hydroxyvitamin D^9.

Recent epidemiological evidence suggests that high intakes of caffeine and alcohol have deleterious effects on the skeleton. Indeed, when osteoporosis is seen in young males, a high alcohol intake is often evident. Calcium intake is often low among alcoholics, and heavy alcohol intake is associated with hypercalciuria. The relative importance of caffeine as a pathogenetic risk factor is difficult to define. High protein intakes, by increasing calcium losses, undoubtedly raise calcium requirements. However, again the relative importance of protein within the normal range of protein intakes is not clearly established. In all nutritional surveys, dietary protein, phosphate, and calcium correlate well together, a factor which must be taken into account in the analyses of the data.

Lifestyle

A sedentary or inactive lifestyle appears to play a permissive role in the phenomenon of bone loss. The majority of evidence to support this comes from the opposite ends of the activity spectrum. Bed rest or space flight is associated with loss of trabecular bone, while athletes have greater bone mass, most evident in the exercised limbs. Animal experiments confirm that bone mass responds to mechanical stress both directly and perhaps also indirectly by induction of growth hormone secretion. In our experience, the effects of exercise are most evident at high calcium intakes (above the RDA)[10].

Endocrine status

Examination of the factors affecting axial bone mass in young individuals and at the time of the menopause has emphasized the role of sex steroids in both the younger as well as the peri- and postmenopausal populations. Pregnancy and oral contraceptive use are positive indicators of bone mass, as is postmenopausal estrogen use. Oophorectomy or an early menopause are risk factors both for bone loss and fracture. Periods of amenorrhea in younger women are also associated with reduced bone mass, apparently not offset by exercise. The mechanisms by which lack or loss of sex hormones might act as pathogenetic risk factors are discussed in detail in Chapter 9, by John Stevenson.

Other risk factors

Other potential pathogenetic risk factors include genetics, coexisting disease, chronic use of aluminum antacids, corticosteroid and other drug therapies. Low bone mass by itself is a risk factor, and the acceleration of bone turnover in a situation of negative bone balance must, therefore, also be a risk factor (i.e. postmenopause or in thyrotoxicosis, hyperpara-thyroidism, etc.).

Other risk factors for osteoporosis have been described, including race; tooth loss in adult life and alveolar ridge resorption; cigarette smoking; and in the elderly, stability in the erect position. The presence of osteoarthrosis of significant degree may be a protective feature in the aging population.

RISK ASSESSMENT

For those women who are approaching or at the menopause, some assessment of risk can be made simply and easily by nutritional and life-style history and simple examination of body habits. The presence of a preponderance of factors increasing the risk of fracture suggests that there would be value in obtaining a bone mass measurement. This should be an estimate of bone in the axial skeleton, since peripheral measurements are relatively poor indicators of the status of the axial skeleton. For this younger population, dual photon absorptiometry is to be preferred since the radiation dose is significantly less than that from CT measurements. Even if normal bone mass is found in the presence of a high-risk assessment, such individuals should be followed closely with repeat measurements at 6-monthly or annual intervals. Prophylactic measures should include the removal of those risk factors which can be corrected and consideration for prescription of small but effective doses of estrogen.

REFERENCES

1. Lindsay, R., Dempster, D. W., Clemens, T., Herrington, B. S. and Wilt, S. (1984). Incidence, cost, and risk factors of fracture of the proximal femur in the U.S.A. In Christiansen, C. *et al.* (eds.) *Osteoporosis: Copenhagen International Symposium on Osteoporosis.* pp. 311-15
2. Fenton-Lewis, A. (1981). Fracture of neck of the femur: changing incidence. *Br. Med. J.*, **283**, 1217-20
3. Wallace, W. A. (1983). The increasing incidence of fractures of the proximal femur: an orthopaedic epidemic. *Lancet*, **1**, 1413-14
4. Abdalla, H., Hart, D. M. and Lindsay, R. (1984). Determinants of bone mass at menopause and subsequent rate of bone loss. Fourth International Symposium on the Menopause, Florida
5. Matkovic, V., Kostial, K., Simanovic, I., Buzine, R., Brodarec, A. and Nordin, B. E. C. (1979). Bone status and fracture rates in two regions of Yugoslavia. *Am. J. Clin. Nutr.*, **32**, 443-52
6. Genant, H. K., Cann, C. E., Ettinger, B., Gordan, G. S., Kold, F. O., Reizer, U. and Arhaud, C. D. (1984). Quantitative computed tomography for spinal mineral assessment. In Christiansen, C. *et al.* (eds.) *Osteoporosis: Copenhagen International Symposium on Osteoporosis.* pp. 65-71
7. Heaney, R. P., Recker, R. R. and Saville, P. D. (1977). Calcium balance and calcium requirement in middle aged women. *Am. J. Clin. Nutr.*, **30**, 1603-11

8. Spencer, H., Kramer, L., Osis, D. and Narvis, C. (1978). Effect of phosphorus on the absorption of calcium and on the calcium balance in man. *J. Nutr.*, **108**, 447-57

9. Clemens, T. C., Silverberg, S., Dempster, D. W., Shane, E., Williams, G. V., Segre, G. V., Lindsay, R. and Bilezikian, J. P. (1985). Oral phosphate depresses serum 1,25-dihydroxy-vitamin D concentrations in osteoporotic patients. In Norman, A. W., Schaefer, K., Grigioleit, H. G. and Herratt, D. V. (eds.) *Vitamin D: Chemical, Biochemical and Clinical Update.* pp. 1010-11

10. Kanders, B., Lindsay, R., Dempster, D. W. and Markhard, L. (1984). Determinants of bone mass in young healthy women. In Christiansen, C., Arnaud, C. D., Nordin, B. E. C., Partitt, A. M., Peck, W. A. and Riggs, B. L. (eds.) *Proc. Copenhagen International Symposium on Osteoporosis.* pp. 337-40

11. Dempster, D. W., Shane, E. S., Horbert, W. and Lindsay, R. (1986). A simple method for correlative light and scanning electron microscopy of human iliac chest bone biopsies: qualitative observations in normal and osteoporotic subjects. *J. Bone Min. Res.* (In press)

Chapter 9

Etiology of postmenopausal osteoporosis

J. C. Stevenson

Osteoporosis is a diminution of skeletal mass in which bone is normally mineralized but the amount of bone tissue in a given volume of bone is reduced compared with normal. The major consequence is an increase in certain fractures which occur spontaneously or with minimal trauma. Osteoporosis is by far the most common metabolic bone disease in the Western world. In terms of morbidity, mortality and cost, its consequences are devastating[1]. Whilst some bone is lost as a consequence of the aging process in both sexes, it is the superimposition of rapid bone loss in the early postmenopause which leads to the marked increase in the incidence of osteoporosis in women. In general, two factors will determine whether and when a woman will develop osteoporosis: the initial amount of skeletal mass, and the amount and rate of bone loss following the onset of the menopause.

CELLULAR MECHANISMS

As with any living tissue, there is a continuous turnover of bone through removal and replacement. In adult life this turnover is usually very slow. Under normal circumstances the processes of formation and resorption of bone, which are linked or 'coupled', are in equilibrium and hence there is no net gain or loss of bone. The process of bone remodeling occurs sequentially with the involvement of a group of different cell types, known as a basic multicellular unit or BMU[2]. Firstly, an amount of bone is removed by an osteoclast. A reversal phase then occurs, when a cement substance is deposited on the resorption surface. After a fixed interval, bone formation is initiated by osteoblasts which have been recruited by the prior initiation of osteoclastic resorption. The resorption cavity is thus filled in. Bone loss will occur if there is an increase in resorption or decrease in formation, either absolute, or relative if the sequential process is disrupted or impaired – 'uncoupled'. It is likely that the following mechanisms may be involved.

Firstly, there is a decrease in bone formation with aging which occurs in both sexes. This means that osteoblasts are unable to completely replace bone lost by osteoclastic resorption, and may be a result of a shortened effective lifespan of osteoblasts[3]. Secondly, there is an increase in bone resorption in women following the menopause[4]. This is probably due to an increase in the activation of the basic multicellular units[5]. Whilst both these processes are undoubtedly involved in the development of osteoporosis, it appears that increased resorption is more important in postmenopausal osteoporosis[6].

FACTORS DETERMINING INITIAL SKELETAL MASS

There are probably a number of factors which can influence the maximum skeletal mass achieved, including racial, genetic and environmental factors. Black people have a greater bone density than whites[7], which is one reason why postmenopausal osteoporosis is hardly ever seen in blacks[8]. There is probably a familial tendency to osteoporosis and some individuals may have a genetically determined smaller bone mass throughout life, rendering them particularly prone to the development of postmenopausal osteoporosis. Thus, for example, women of small stature may be more at risk of developing osteoporosis.

Environmental factors are more difficult to assess, but physical exercise and dietary calcium deserve special consideration. There is a correlation between bone mass and muscle mass[9], and long-term physical exercise can result in regional increases in bone mass. Exercise may also be of some benefit in aiding maintenance of skeletal mass. However, there is no evidence that exercise alone can prevent osteoporosis and its attendant fractures, and the major factor contributing to osteoporosis in women, postmenopausal bone loss, occurs independently of exercise levels. Whilst exercise should be encouraged, particularly to build up skeletal mass earlier in life, it is not a substitute for appropriate hormonal therapy to prevent bone loss. It should also be remembered that athleticism in women can sometimes lead to secondary amenorrhea and a decrease in bone mass.

There has been much speculation on possible links between dietary calcium intake and skeletal mass. Any correlations between bone mass and calcium intake are extremely weak. Certainly the geographical variations in osteoporosis do not support the importance of dietary calcium since the disease is less common in areas where dietary calcium is low[10]. A higher bone mass was found in people with a high calcium intake compared with another group of people on a lower calcium intake in Yugoslavia[11], but other factors may have been involved. Probably the most extensive studies have been conducted by Garn and co-workers, who have concluded that peak bone mass and adult bone loss are not products of low or inadequate calcium intake[12, 13]. At present there are insufficient data to warrant widespread dietary manipulation in young adults as an attempt to increase peak bone mass.

FACTORS DETERMINING BONE LOSS

Trabecular bone mass in women starts to decline in the 5th decade[14], and cortical bone mass in the 6th decade[15]. For trabecular bone at least, despite a report to the contrary[16], there is increasing evidence that the most rapid loss occurs exponentially following the menopause[17] and that initial losses may be quite substantial. Thus following the menopause the so-called 'fracture threshold' of bone density may be approached quite rapidly but actually passed more slowly. Hence fractures may not occur until 10–15 years or more after the onset of the menopause. The greater importance of the menopause rather than aging process in determining bone loss in women is illustrated by its severity following oophorectomy[14] or an early menopause[18, 19]. The exact mechanism by which the loss of ovarian function leads to mobilization of bone is still not established. Indeed, it is not known if estrogen can exert a direct effect on bone since repeated studies have failed to demonstrate receptors for estradiol in bone[20, 21]. The pathogenesis of postmenopausal bone loss is discussed in detail by Rober Lindsay in Chapter 8 of this book, but part of the action of estrogen on bone might be explained by changes in calcitonin secretion[22]. Changes in other calcium regulating hormones probably occur as a result of, rather than prior to, bone mobilization. Some of the hormonal changes may be exaggerated in the established osteoporotic. For example, some osteoporotic women are less well estrogenized than their peers[23, 24], and they may develop osteoporosis because they lose bone at a faster rate postmenopausally[25]. Similarly, calcitonin levels may be lower in osteoporotics than in age-matched non-osteoporotic controls[26]. Evidence that calcitonin may be involved in the pathogenesis of osteoporosis is suggestive although not conclusive. Throughout adult life men have higher calcitonin levels than women[27], and this may explain why the female skeleton is more severely affected in bone resorbing disorders[28]. Calcitonin secretion appears to be regulated by estrogen[29] and there is a fall in its secretion following the loss of ovarian function[30]. This may explain the postmenopausal 'sensitization' of the skeleton to the actions of the bone-resorbing hormones. Evidence that changes in calcitonin secretion influence skeletal mass comes from the fact that totally thyroidectomized, and hence calcitonin-deficient, patients have a reduced bone mineral content[31]. Furthermore, an association between complete calcitonin deficiency and osteoporosis has been reported[32]. It is well known that estrogens can prevent bone loss in osteoporosis[33] and a similar effect has been shown for calcitonin[34]. Finally, in addition to having a greater skeletal mass, black women may also lose bone more slowly than white women after the menopause[35]. This in turn may be due to the higher calcitonin levels found in black people[36].

The possible involvement of calcium malabsorption in the pathogenesis of postmenopausal osteoporosis is still controversial. The hypothesis, based on animal studies[37], is that increased intestinal calcium malabsorption, perhaps together with an increase in obligatory urinary calcium losses, causes skeletal mobilization to maintain the plasma calcium level. Certainly intestinal calcium absorption is reduced and urinary calcium excretion increased in osteoporotics although there is considerable overlap with non-osteoporotics. Plasma calcium levels, however, are not reduced in osteoporotics. They actually increase following the menopause[38], but are not different from controls in osteoporotic women[39]. The reduction in intestinal calcium absorption can be entirely explained by a reduction in 1,25-dihydroxyvitamin D levels which is also found in osteoporotics, both parameters being reduced by approximately 20%[39]. The reduced 1,25-dihydroxyvitamin D levels can in turn be explained by suppression of production secondary to increased bone mobilization. The capacity of the kidney to produce 1,25-dihydroxyvitamin D is not impaired[40] when osteoporotics are compared with age-matched controls.

Although PTH levels tend to increase with age[41], this increase is not substantial. There may be a small fall in PTH levels at the time of the menopause[42], and the levels are lower in osteoporotic women compared with controls[39]. Together with increased bone mobilization, this latter finding may explain the increased urinary calcium excretion seen in some osteoporotics. Increased PTH levels have been reported in a very small subset of osteoporotics[43], but for the great majority of patients elevated PTH levels are not found and cannot account for the increased bone resorption.

Finally, there are a number of less specific factors that have been associated with the development of osteoporosis. Some, such as body fat, are due to their influence on estrogen metabolism whilst others, such as cigarette smoking, have a less clear role. Undoubtedly, a combination of many factors is ultimately responsible for determining which women will eventually develop osteoporosis. Of those, the peak skeletal mass and the onset of the menopause are the most important. It is not clear as to whether the former can be influenced; it is quite clear that the latter can be influenced, and hormone replacement therapy still remains the single most effective therapy in the prevention and treatment of osteoporosis.

ACKNOWLEDGEMENTS

It is a pleasure to acknowledge the help of many colleagues in some of the studies referred to above. In particular I thank my colleagues in the Endocrine Unit, Royal Postgraduate Medical School, London, UK, and Mr Malcolm Whitehead and colleagues in the Academic Department of Gynaecology, King's College Hospital, London, UK.

REFERENCES

1. Stevenson, J. C. and Whitehead, M. I. (1982). Postmenopausal osteoporosis. *Br. Med. J.*, **285**, 585–8
2. Frost, H. M. (1970). Tetracycline-based histological analysis of bone remodelling. *Calcif. Tissue Res.*, **3**, 211–37
3. Arlott, M., Edouard, C., Meunier, P. J., Neer, R. M. and Reeve, J. (1984). Impaired osteoblast function in osteoporosis: comparison between calcium balance and dynamic histomorphometry. *Br. Med. J.*, **289**, 517–20
4. Heaney, R. P., Recker, R. R. and Saville, P. D. (1978). Menopausal changes in bone remodelling. *J. Lab. Clin. Med.*, **92**, 964–70
5. Parfitt, A. M., Mathews, C. H. E., Villanueva, A. R. *et al.* (1983). Microstructural and cellular basis of age-related bone loss and osteoporosis. In Frame, B. and Potts, J. T. (eds.) *Clinical Disorders of Bone and Mineral Metabolism*. pp. 328–32. (Amsterdam: Excerpta Medica)
6. Nordin, B. E. C., Aaron, J., Speed, R. and Crilly, R. G. (1981). Bone formation and resorption as the determinants of trabecular bone volume in postmenopausal osteoporosis. *Lancet*, **2**, 277–9
7. Cohn, S. H., Abesamis, C., Yasumura, S., Aloia, J. F., Zanzi, I. and Ellis, K. J. (1977). Comparative skeletal mass and radial bone mineral content in black and white women. *Metabolism*, **26**, 171–8
8. Gyepes, M., Mellins, H. Z. and Katz, I. (1981). The low incidence of fracture of the hip in the Negro. *J. Am. Med. Assoc.*, **181**, 1073–4
9. Doyle, F., Brown, J. and Lachance, C. (1970). Relation between bone mass and muscle weight. *Lancet*, **1**, 391–3
10. Chalmers, J. and Ho, K. C. (1970). Geographical variations in senile osteoporosis. *J. Bone Jt Surg.*, **52B**, 667–75
11. Matkovic, V., Kostial, K., Simonovic, I., Buzina, R. Brodarec, A. and Nordin, B. E. C. (1979). Bone status and fracture rates in two regions of Yugoslavia. *Am. J. Clin. Nutr.*, **32**, 540–9
12. Garn, S. M. (1970). *The Earlier Gain and Later Loss of Cortical Bone.* (Springfield: CC Thomas)
13. Garn, S. M., Solomon, M. A. and Friedl, J. (1981). Calcium intake and bone quality in the elderly. *Ecol. Food Nutr.*, **10**, 131–3
14. Genant, H. K., Gordan, G. S. and Hoffman, P. G. (1983). Osteoporosis: Part I. Advanced radiologic assessment using quantitative computed tomography. Medical Staff Conference, University of California, San Francisco. *West J. Med.*, **139**, 75–84
15. Doyle, F. H. (1972). Involutional osteoporosis. In MacIntyre, I. (ed.) *Clinics in Endocrinology and Metabolism*. pp. 143–67. (London: Saunders)
16. Riggs, B. L., Wahner, H. W., Seeman, E. *et al.* (1982). Changes in bone mineral density of the proximal femur and spine with aging. *J. Clin. Invest.*, **70**, 716–23
17. Krolner, B. and Nielsen, S. P. (1982). Bone mineral content of the lumbar spine in normal and osteoporotic women: cross-sectional and longitudinal studies. *Clin. Sci.*, **62**, 329–36
18. Aitken, J. M. (1976). Osteoporosis and its relation to oestrogen deficiency. In Campbell, S. (ed.) *The Management of the Menopause and Postmenopausal Years*. pp. 225–36. (Lancaster: MTP Press)

19. Stevenson, J. C. (1985). Inter-relation of oestrogen and the major calcium-regulating hormones. In van Herendael, H., van Herendael, B., Riphagen, F. E., Goessens, L. and van der Pas, H. (eds.) *The Climacteric: an update.* pp. 199-206. (Lancaster: MTP Press)

20. Nutik, G. and Cruess, R. L. (1974). Estrogen receptors in bone. An evaluation of the uptake of estrogen into bone cells. *Proc. Soc. Exp. Biol. Med.*, **146**, 265-8

21. Chen, T. L. and Feldman, D. (1978). Distinction between alpha-fetoprotein and intracellular estrogen receptors: evidence against the presence of estradiol receptors in rat bone. *Endocrinology*, **102**, 236-42

22. Stevenson, J. C., Abeyasekera, G., Hillyard, C. J. *et al.* (1981). Calcitonin and the calcium-regulating hormones in postmenopausal women: effect of oestrogens. *Lancet*, **1**, 693-5

23. Marshall, D. H., Crilly, R. G. and Nordin, B. E. C. (1977). Plasma androstenedione and oestrone levels in normal and osteoporotic postmenopausal women. *Br. Med. J.*, **2**, 1177-9

24. Davidson, B. J., Ross, R. K., Paganini-Hill, A., Hammond, G. D., Siiteri, P. K. and Judd, H. L. (1982). Total and free estrogens and androgens in postmenopausal women with hip fractures. *J. Clin. Endocrinol. Metab.*, **54**, 115-20

25. Christiansen, C. (1982). Osteoporosis and vitamin D metabolites. A status report. In Norman, A. W., Schaefer, K., Herrath, D. V. and Grigoleit, H. G. (eds.) *Vitamin D: Chemical, biochemical and clinical endocrinology of calcium metabolism.* pp. 915-20. (Berlin: Walter de Gruyter)

26. Taggart, H. Mc. A., Chesnut, C. H., Ivey, J. L. *et al.* (1982). Deficient calcitonin response to calcium stimulation in post-menopausal osteoporosis. *Lancet*, **1**, 475-8

27. Hillyard, C. J., Stevenson, J. C. and MacIntyre, I. (1978). Relative deficiency of plasma calcitonin in normal women. *Lancet*, **1**, 961-2

28. Pak, C. Y. C., Stewart, A., Kaplan, R., Bone, H., Notz, C. and Browne, R. (1976). Photon absorptiometric analysis of bone density in primary hyperparathyroidism. *Lancet*, **2**, 7-8

29. Stevenson, J. C. (1982). Regulation of calcitonin and parathyroid hormone secretion by oestrogens. *Maturitas*, **4**, 1-7

30. Stevenson, J. C., Abeyasekera, G., Myers, C. H. *et al.* (1984). Comparison of the influence of ovarian function and age on calcium metabolism in women. In *Abstracts. 7th International Congress of Endocrinology.* p. 1969. (Amsterdam: Excerpta Medica)

31. McDermott, M. T., Kidd, G. S., Blue, P., Ghaed, V. and Hofeldt, F. D. (1983). Reduced bone mineral content in totally thyroidectomized patients: possible effect of calcitonin deficiency. *J. Clin. Endocrinol. Metab.*, **56**, 936-9

32. Stevenson, J. C., White, M. C., Joplin, G. F. and MacIntyre, I. (1982). Osteoporosis and calcitonin deficiency. *Br. Med. J.*, **285**, 1010-11

33. Nordin, B. E. C., Horsman, A., Crilly, R. G., Marshall, D. H. and Simpson, M. (1980). Treatment of spinal osteoporosis in postmenopausal women. *Br. Med. J.*, **1**, 451-4

34. Chesnut, C. H., Baylink, D. J., Roos, B. A. *et al.* (1981). Calcitonin and postmenopausal osteoporosis. In Pecile, A. (ed.) *Calcitonin 1980: chemistry, physiology, pharmacology and clinical aspects.* pp. 247-55. (Amsterdam: Excerpta Medica)

35. Garn, S. M. (1975). Bone loss and aging. In Goldman, R. and Rockstein, M. (eds.) *The Physiology and Pathology of Human Aging.* pp. 39-54. (New York Academic Press)

36. Stevenson, J. C., Myers, C. H. and Ajdukiewicz, A. B. (1984). Racial differences in calcitonin and katacalcin. *Calcif. Tissue Int.*, **36**, 725-8

37. Nordin, B. E. C. (1960). Osteomalacia, osteoporosis and calcium deficiency. *Clin. Orthop.*, **17**, 235-57

38. Young, M. M. and Nordin, B. E. C. (1967). Effect of natural and artificial menopause on plasma and urinary calcium and phosphorus. *Lancet*, **2**, 118-20

39. Gallagher, J. C., Riggs, B. C., Eisman, J., Hamstra, A., Arnaud, S. B. and DeLuca, H. F. (1979). Intestinal calcium absorption and serum vitamin D metabolites in normal subjects and osteoporotic patients. *J. Clin. Invest.*, **64**, 729-36

40. Riggs, B. L., Hamstra, A. and DeLuca, H. F. (1981). Assessment of 25-hydroxyvitamin D 1 α-hydroxylase reserve in postmenopausal osteoporosis by administration of parathyroid extract. *J. Clin. Endocrinol. Metab.*, **53**, 833-5

41. Marcus, R., Madvig, P. and Young, G. (1984). Age-related changes in parathyroid hormone and parathyroid hormone action in normal humans. *J. Clin. Endocrinol. Metab.*, **58**, 223-30

42. Stevenson, J. C. (1983). Vitamin D in postmenopausal women. In Duursma, S. A. and Sluys, Veer J. v. d. (eds.) *Vitamine D.* pp. 43–55. (Utrecht: Wetenschappelijke uitgeverij Bunge)
43. Riggs, B. L., Gallagher, J. C., DeLuca, H. F., Edis, A. J., Lambert, P. W. and Arnaud, C. D. (1978). A syndrome of osteoporosis, increased parathyroid hormone, and inappropriately low 1,25 dihydroxyvitamin D. *Mayo Clin. Proc.*, **53**, 701–6

Chapter 10

Bone mineral assessment: a practical guide for primary care physicians

B. Ettinger, H. K. Genant and C. E. Cann

INTRODUCTION

In the past 10 years there has been an extraordinary expansion in the field of non-invasive bone mineral determination. As the number of articles appearing in the medical literature is increasing, there has been a parallel increase in newspaper and magazine articles emphasizing the dire consequences of osteoporosis. In an era of expanding women's rights, osteoporosis prevention has become a prominent social and political issue. Our patients are responding to the media's messages and are expressing greater demands for information and guidance about ways to protect themselves from osteoporosis.

How shall we respond to our patients' concerns about 'the bone drain' and the 'crippling effects of osteoporosis'? A reasonable approach consists of three steps: (1) a balanced presentation of the real risks involved; (2) general advice regarding prevention; and (3) assessment of bone mineral, when indicated.

Proper counseling is the first step. We find that accurate information regarding the natural history and epidemiology of osteoporosis helps to allay the unrealistic fears created by the distorted lay literature. We describe the dynamic nature of bone turnover, emphasizing the balance between bone resorption and formation; we explain that 20% of the skeleton is composed of highly active spongy bone which is eight times more actively turning over than the dense cortical bone which makes up 80% of the skeletal mass.

We help our patients recognize the difference between the two types of osteoporosis – one which is called 'postmenopausal', the other 'senile'. The former results from the rapid loss of spongy bone in the 10–15 years following menopause, and causes wrist and vertebral fractures in a small fraction of women, while the latter results from loss of cortical and spongy bone in the femur and causes a geometrically increasing rate of hip fractures, reaching 1% per year by the age of 80. Women who are upset about the prospects of death and disability from 'osteoporosis' are grateful to know that vertebral compression fractures are usually asymptomatic and self-limited, while hip fracture morbidity and mortality are largely the problem of infirm octagenarians (75% of hip fracture deaths occur in women beyond the age of 80). We encourage women to reduce those factors associated with a higher risk of osteoporosis (smoking, alcohol, sedentary lifestyle, glucocorticoids, etc.) and explain the possible benefits of factors which may prevent bone loss (exercise, calcium and estrogen). The relative contribution of these factors is also discussed elsewhere is this book.

The purpose of this review is to suggest guidelines for the use of quantitative measurements of bone mineral in the clinical management of patients. First, we shall review those methods which are currently available, offering brief descriptions of the technical aspects and practical considerations (time, cost, availability, and sensitivity). Finally, we will use two common clinical situations to illustrate a practical approach to decision-making regarding bone mineral assessments.

METHODS OF BONE MINERAL ANALYSIS

Standard radiography

Many patients are referred for bone mineral assessment after routine radiographs of the chest or lower spine show either a 'washed-out' appearance, deformity of the endplates (biconcavity) or wedging (loss of anterior vertebral height only). We find that these all are unreliable indicators of reduced bone mass. The results of standard X-ray exams are based on subjective criteria, greatly affected by body habitus and technical factors relating to radiographic exposure. On the other hand, we see normal-appearing spinal X-rays in women with significant loss of spinal mineral, and it is generally accepted that about 30% of bone mineral must be lost before standard X-rays indicate osteopenia. There is considerable radiation dose from spinal X-rays, including gonadal dosage. The thoracic spine is a more sensitive region for detection of osteoporosis than the lumbar. Crush fractures in the mid-thoracic spine are seen earlier and more frequently than in the lumbar spine, and there is an excellent correlation between fracture severity and spinal mineral content. The average cost for a lateral X-ray of the thoracic spine is US$40.

Radiogrammetry

A standard radiograph of the hand provides a cheap, safe and reasonable assessment of cortical bone mass. Using calipers or a magnifying loupe with a reticule, it is easy to measure the combined cortical thickness at the midshaft of the second metacarpal. There are convenient tables of normative data and the film is always available for re-reading if it needs to be compared to past or future films. The method is precise (3–5%), but it is not as sensitive as methods which assess spongy bone. It corre lates poorly with spinal mineral content. The cost is low (about US$30) and its universal availability makes it a reasonable screening test in certain cases.

Photodensitometry

This method also requires a simple hand X-ray but quantitates the density of bone by comparing the amount of photographic density produced by the bone to the density produced by an aluminum reference wedge exposed on the same film. A photodensitometer is used to scan over the image of the fingers and the wedge. Despite the ease of performing this measurement, it is losing popularity among the experts who study bone diseases. Photon absorptiometry (see below) appears to be replacing this method by providing the same type of quantitative density measurement with better accuracy and less radiation.

Single energy photon absorptiometry

This method measures the mass of a bone by the degree to which it blocks (attenuates) a beam of radiation. A gamma ray source (usually iodine 125) is placed on one side of the bone and a scintillation detector on the other. The Norland-Cameron absorptiometer has been in wide clinical use for over 10 years but recently developed rectilinear scanners are gaining in popularity. The forearm must be carefully positioned and surrounded by a water bag or water bath. The source and the detector are moved across the arm and the changes in the strength of the radiation beam are measured. The test takes about twenty minutes to perform and costs about US$50– 75. Two sites are commonly measured; the mid-radius which is nearly all cortical bone and the distal radius which has a spongy component of approximately 25%. The usual precision is 2–4% and the rate of loss detected in menopausal women is 1.5–3.0% per year.

The distal radius appears more sensitive to bone loss and may correlate better with changes in spinal mineral but positioning errors are often quite a problem at this site. The rectilinear scanner provides a number of measurement 'tracks' across the arm proceeding from mid-shaft to the distal end resulting in much improved precision and sensitivity.

Dual energy photon absorptiometry (DPA)

This technique is similar to single energy absorptiometry but uses 153 gadolinium as the gamma ray source. The gamma emissions are at two energies, so one energy can be used to correct for the beam length, eliminating the need for a water bath. A rectilinear scanner usually scans across and down the lumbar spine but this technique can also be used to scan the entire body. The attenuation of the beam measures the sum total of all mineral within its path and hence is a measure of spongy and cortical bone in the spine. The highly active spongy bone makes up about 50–60% of the vertebral mass in younger women and less than 50% in older women. The scan is also affected by osteoarthritic changes and calcifications in the discs and aorta. In younger healthy menopausal women the precision is 2–3% and the accuracy is good. The radiation dose is low (less than 20 millirems), the cost about US$150, and time in the scanner is usually 25 min although improved precision can be obtained by doubling the number of 'tracks' and scanning for 45 min. The annual rate of loss seen in cross-sectional studies of menopausal women has usually been reported as 1.5% but recent longitudinal studies show rates of 3–5%. Younger women with low bone mass can be discriminated by this test, while in osteoporotic women DPA correlates, to a modest degree, with the severity and number of vertebral compression fractures.

Neutron activation analysis

Neutron activation depends on the ability to change stable 48 calcium in the body to an unstable isotope, 49 calcium. This reaction can be brought about by neutron bombardment coming from any of three sources: a cyclotron, a reactor or a portable source such as plutonium–beryllium. 49 calcium undergoes rapid decay (half-life 8.8 min), giving off a characteristic gamma ray, which can be counted outside the body. The patient is irradiated (dose varies from 300 to 3000 mrem depending on the source of neutrons) and then quickly moved to a counting device. The precision and accuracy of this method is 2–5%. It is largely a measure of cortical bone, since 80% of the skeleton is composed of cortical bone. The annual rate of loss for women in the menopause is 1.5%, similar to that obtained using other cortical measurements. Although there is a poor correlation with spinal mineral content, this method appears to discriminate younger women with osteopenia from normals. In the near future this method may become available as portable isotope sources are developed and lower doses are employed for measurement of local regions of the skeleton rather than the entire body.

Quantitative computed tomography

A relatively simple adaptation of most commercially available CT scanners can provide a quantitation of spinal trabecular mineral (QCT). A lateral scout view is made and serves to localize the subsequent scans through the midplanes of the lumbar vertebrae. A region of interest is identified within each vertebral body and the density of spongy bone found in a 3–4 cm^3 volume is compared to the density of potassium phosphate solutions in a phantom which is scanned with the patient. The examination takes 10–15 min (1 min for the scout view and 3 min for the measurement scan). Radiation exposure is 200 mrem (about one-tenth of the dose usually required for abdominal CT scans) and the cost is US$150.

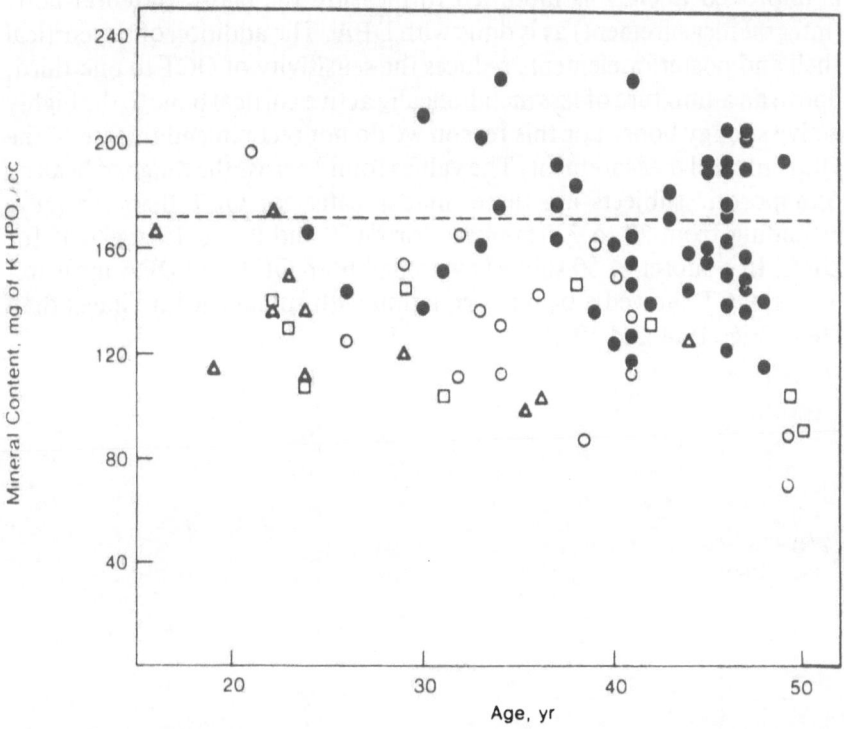

Figure 10.1 Spinal mineral content (QCT) of young normal women and those with amenorrhea of various etiologies. ● = Normal; ○ = premature ovarian failure; □ = prolactinomas; △ = hypothalamic amenorrhea

QCT has a precision of 1–3% and is quite sensitive to changes in spinal mineral. Menopausal women show 7–9% annual loss and young women with low bone mass can easily be distinguished from normals (Fig. 10.1). The accuracy varies from 5–10% in young women to 20–25% in elderly osteoporotic women, largely because of an underestimation of bone mineral due to fat in the marrow. However, the sensitivity of QCT is so great that the inaccuracy caused by fat does not limit its usefulness. The degree of bone loss seen with QCT correlates well with bone loss measured by iliac crest biopsy, and in clinical applications it is not necessary to use dual energy QCT to correct for the fat-induced error. In a large number of patients with various metabolic bone disorders we found that a QCT level of $105\,mg/cm^3$ was the fracture threshold, while levels below $60\,mg/cm^3$ were frequently associated with fracture (Fig. 10.2). QCT examinations in 90 women, 6–36 months after menopause, showed that approximately 1 in 5 had spinal mineral mass at or below the fracture threshold, $105\,mg/cm^3$ (Fig. 10.3).

QCT and DPA correlate moderately well with each other, as might be expected, since both methods examine the lumbar spine. The correlation is improved if QCT is modified to measure the entire vertebral body (integral measurement) as is done with DPA. The addition of the cortical shell and posterior elements reduces the sensitivity of QCT to one-third, due to an admixture of less metabolically active cortical bone to the highly active spongy bone. For this reason we do not recommend the use of the QCT integral measurement. The values found across the range of healthy osteoporotic subjects are three times greater for QCT than for DPA extending from 20 to $220\,mg/cm^3$ for QCT and 0.4 to $1.2\,mg/cm^2$ for DPA. In a subset of 50 subjects who had both QCT and DPA measurements, QCT showed a better correlation with spinal fracture index than DPA (Figs 10.4 and 10.5).

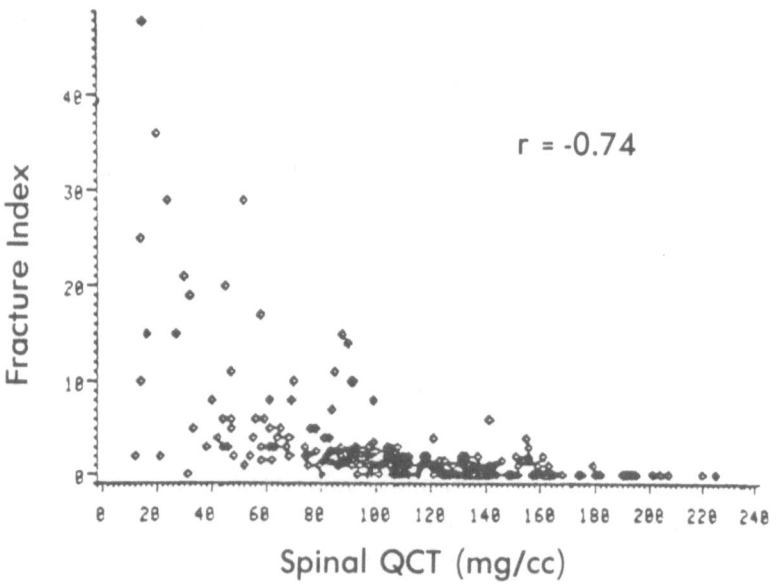

Figure 10.2 Relationship between spinal fracture index and spinal mineral content (QCT) in 269 male and female subjects with various metabolic bone disorders

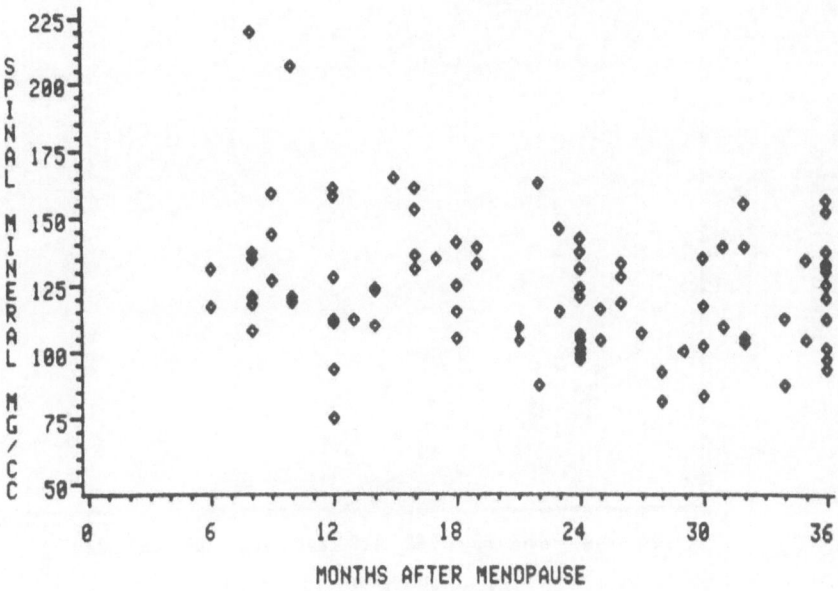

Figure 10.3 Spinal mineral content (QCT) in the early postmenopausal period

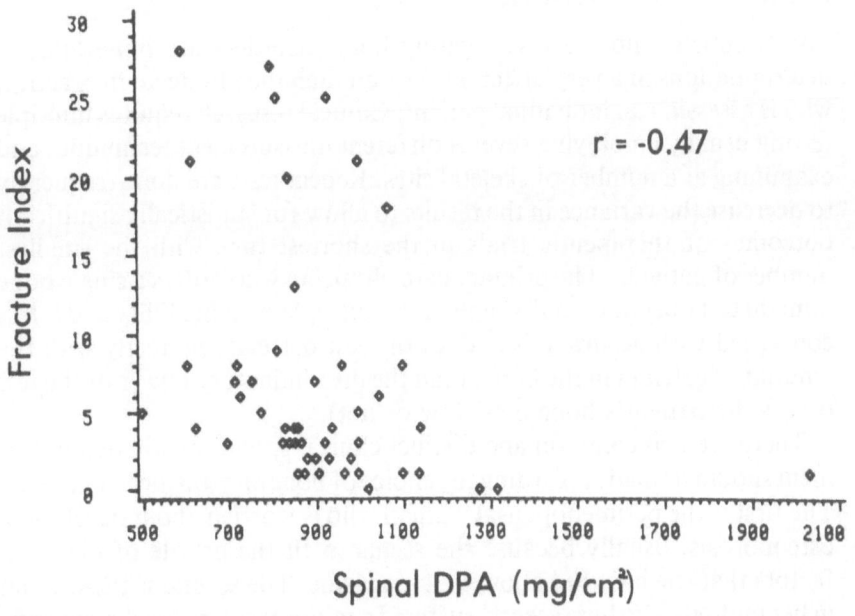

Figure 10.4 Relationship between spinal fracture index and spinal mineral content (DPA) in 50 subjects

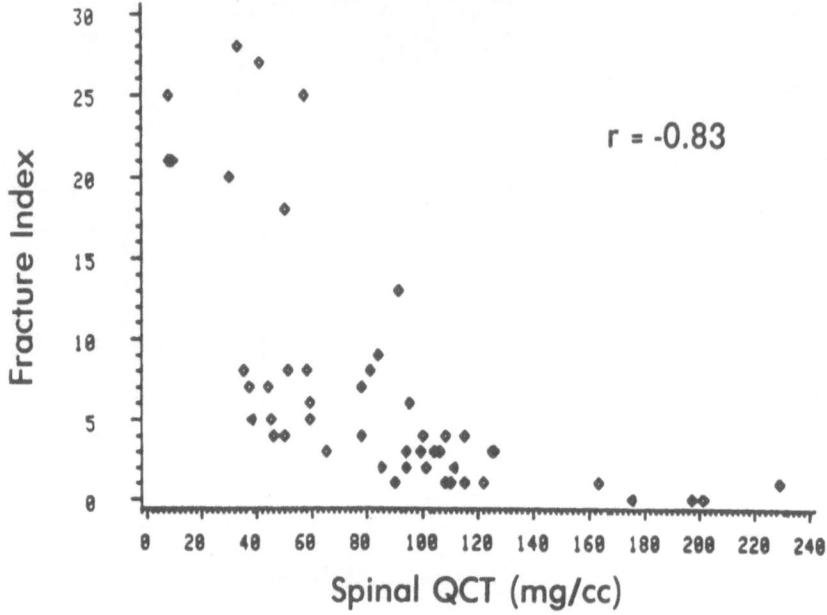

Figure 10.5 Relationship between spinal fracture index and spinal mineral content (QCT) in same subjects as in Fig. 10.4

CLINICAL APPLICATIONS

The scientists who are investigating bone disorders use bone mineral determinations in a very different fashion than the physician in practice, who is assessing an individual patient. Clinical research requires multiple testing usually employing several different measurement techniques and examining at a number of skeletal sites. Repeat tests are done frequently to decrease the variance in the results to allow for statistically significant outcomes of therapeutic trials in the shortest time with the smallest number of patients. The primary care physician who orders a single bone mineral test does not require high precision and reproducibility and is less concerned with accuracy (i.e. does the test correlate perfectly with the amount of calcium in the bone) than the discriminatory power of the test (i.e. is the patient's bone mass low or not).

There are two common and distinct clinical situations where a judgement should be made regarding the choice of bone mineral measurements. The first is the perimenopausal woman who is worried about developing osteoporosis, usually because she seems to fit the profile of high-risk factors that she has read about in a magazine. The second is the woman in her mid-60s who has recently suffered a minor fracture or who has been found to have an asymptomatic 'washed-out' spine on a chest X-ray.

In the first case the area of interest should be the spine, since it is this site which will suffer a major loss of mineral in the 10–15 years following menopause. Although some women appear to lose bone faster than others, there does not seem to be a distinct 'rapid-losing' group of women. If the patient's initial bone mass determination is borderline, it would be of value to have a repeat test done in 2 years. Although availability, cost and radiation exposure all may enter into the choice of test, the ultimate decision whether to do any test rests on its practical usefulness. We do not recommend that bone mineral tests be done in women who are already committed to using estrogen replacement therapy – since we know that they are being protected against bone loss. Similarly perimenopausal women who are totally opposed to using estrogen need not have their bone mineral measured. They can simply be provided with an assessment of risk and be advised of the general measures which may retard the loss of bone. They can be told that the risk of having a vertebral crush fracture is about 1 in 200 patients, every year, beginning 5-10 years after menopause. Multiple vertebral fractures occur at about half this rate. It is important to emphasize that only a small percentage of these crush fractures will cause any back symptoms and long-term disability from spinal osteoporosis is rare. The perimenopausal woman who is 'on the fence' about long-term estrogen therapy, who is also concerned about the possible risks of estrogen, may have her quandary resolved by a spinal mineral measurement.

The second example, the woman in her mid-60s, who has already lost a major part of her spinal mineral in the 10-15 years since menopause, is an altogether different problem. She does not need a spinal mineral assessment. Our knowledge of the natural history of osteoporosis predicts that the spongy bone in her skeleton is, on the average, 50% lower than her youthful level and that it will probably decrease only a little more in the years to come. Treatment to maintain spinal bone mass in a woman of this age offers very little benefit against significant risk of side-effects. We presently have no clinically acceptable means of increasing spinal mineral (although research is actively proceeding in this area). Our attention, in this patient, should be focused on the prevention of hip fracture. The incidence rate of this fracture doubles every 5 years after age 60 so that by age 80, 1% of women will suffer a hip fracture each year.

None of our presently used bone mineral tests can discriminate between women who have suffered a hip fracture and age-matched controls (although QCT of the spine has not been evaluated in this regard). Even quantitative histologic bone methods show that the amount of bone in the femur is not less in hip fracture patients than elderly women without a hip fracture. Some experts believe that bone mass is not the crucial factor in hip fracture causation. They suspect that chronic illness, infirmity and an increased tendency to fall cause the increasing rate of hip fracture in the elderly who are already osteopenic.

Of greater importance is the ability to identify, at the earliest time, the woman who is at increased risk for hip fracture – so that prophylactic measures can be instituted. Up to this time, no prospective studies have been done to answer this question and it is not known whether any bone mineral test applied to menopausal women would yield useful predictive information.

Bone mineral tests are of unproved value in the 65-year-old woman, but measurement of urinary calcium may be useful. We suspect that maintenance of the remaining bone mineral in women who have already suffered 10–15 years of postmenopausal bone loss is much less dependent on estrogen than on calcium. We find that a large percentage of older women being evaluated for osteoporosis have malabsorption of calcium. If adequate amounts of calcium are ingested and absorbed, at least 75 mg will be excreted in a 24 h urine sample. Treatment with additional calcium (up to 1500 mg daily) and modest doses (400–2000 units) of vitamin D are indicated if calcium malabsorption is found. This therapy is certainly safe and perhaps is effective in reducing bone loss and fractures in the elderly.

CONCLUSIONS

Our knowledge regarding prevention and treatment of osteoporosis is largely due to the expansion of non-invasive bone mineral assessment technology. Now these same tests will be evolving from limited investigational tools into widespread general clinical use. Their proper applications in clinical practice require an understanding of the techniques as well as the natural history of osteoporosis.

There is growing evidence that the most important risk factor for the development of osteoporosis is a low bone mass at the time of menopause, with a second factor being the rate of loss after menopause. We know that estrogen therapy, begun within a few years of menopause, is effective in preventing bone loss. By directing our efforts towards the early detection of that fraction of women with reduced bone mass, we can provide appropriate therapy to the patients most likely to benefit from it.

Quantitative bone mineral tests are unlikely to be of clinical benefit in the elderly patient and are presently too costly and time-consuming to be used in mass screening of all women going through the menopause. Considerable effort is being directed towards adaptation of present methods to mass screening (e.g. a limited QCT or DPA scan might be done in 5–10 min at a cost of US$50–75). At the present time it is reasonable for primary care physicians to limit the use of these tests to women who are near the time of their menopause and who are undecided about taking estrogen prophylaxis.

Acknowledgement

This work was sponsored in part by the Community Services Program of the Kaiser Foundation Hospitals.

Chapter 11

Prophylactic treatment for age-related bone loss in women

C. Christiansen

INTRODUCTION

Women lose a considerable amount of calcium from the bones after the menopause. The clinical manifestations of this negative calcium balance are fractures, collapse of one or more vertebrae, and reduced body height. Treatment is largely ineffective once the symptoms have set in and preventive treatment, if it exists, should therefore be instituted at the start of the menopause.

Calcium metabolism

A healthy subject in the steady state has a daily intake of about 1000 mg calcium. Out of this amount, there is a net absorption of 250 mg, which is the difference between absorption and resorption. The amount excreted with feces is thus 750 mg calcium. In the steady state, the 250 mg has to be excreted again: about 200 mg via the kidneys and about 50 mg with the sweat. In addition, calcium is transported from the extracellular fluid to the bones (*bone formation*) and in the opposite direction (*bone resorption*). The amount of calcium involved in this exchange transport is the same in healthy adults. In women after the menopause the calcium balance becomes negative, with a mean daily loss from the bones of about 50 mg. The calcium content in extracellular fluid is extremely well regulated, and two of the regulatory influences on the calcium exchange are the parathyroid hormone and vitamin D.

Normal bony tissue is formed from an organic matrix in which inorganic constituents are deposited, principally calcium phosphate and in particular hydroxyapatite. When the absolute amount of bone mineral content is reduced, this is called *osteopenia*. This may be due to a reduction in both the organic and inorganic constituents, although the ratio between the two remains unchanged (*osteoporosis*). With *osteomalacia*, the organic constituents of the bone are unaffected, but there is a loss of inorganic material. To date osteoporosis is virtually untreatable, whereas osteomalacia responds well to treatment with vitamin D, calcium, or phosphate, depending on the pathogenesis.

Vitamin D metabolism

Intensive research on vitamin D metabolism over the last decade has succeeded in clarifying the metabolic pathways of these biologically important compounds. At the same time several metabolites of vitamin D have been synthesized, so we now have potential agents for the treatment of disturbances in the calcium metabolism. Man normally obtains vitamin D_2 (*ergocalciferol*) and D_3 (*cholecalciferol*) from food. Vitamin D is also synthesized in the human body through ultraviolet irradiation of the skin. The D vitamins are hydroxylated in the liver to *25-hydroxy-ergocalciferol* or *25-hydroxycholecalciferol*, depending on which of the two is the parent compound. Further hydroxylation takes place in the kidneys, thereby forming *1,25-dihydroxy-D* or *24,25-dihydroxy-D*. Today most scientists believe that 1,25-dihydroxy-D is the active metabolite of vitamin D. The pharmaceutical industry now synthesizes and markets all these substances; but since 1,25-dihydroxy-D_3 is difficult to synthesize, a substance called 1-α-OHD$_3$ has become available. Treatment with this preparation enables subjects with normal liver function to synthesize 1,25-dihydroxy-D_3 *in vivo*.

Recent years have seen the successful development of specific analytical methods for determining the blood concentrations of these vitamin D metabolites. It appears that the concentration of 1,25-dihydroxy-D falls with age after the menopause. Correspondingly, the intestinal absorption of calcium also falls. On this background research groups throughout the world have suggested treatment with 1-α-OHD$_3$ or 1,25(OH)$_2$D$_3$ for postmenopausal osteoporosis. A few preliminary reports indicate that the calcium balance becomes positive in women treated with these agents.

Fracture prevalence

We studied the incidence of different fractures occurring in 285 70-year-old women who were selected as being representative of the corresponding Danish population[1] (Fig. 11.1): 125 out of the 285 (44%) women had fractures after the start of the menopause without known trauma. Figure 11.2 shows the cumulated number of fractures as a function of age in the

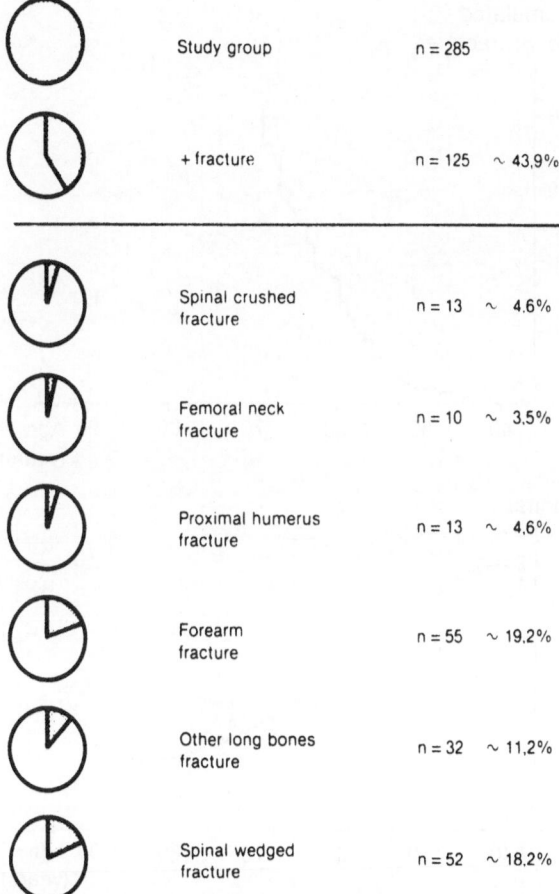

Figure 11.1   Prevalence of fractures in 70-year-old females

70-year-old women, and bone mineral content as a function of age in a group of normal subjects. There is an exponential rise in the number of cumulated fractures as a function of age after the menopause and a corresponding loss of bone mineral content[2].

The Department of Clinical Chemistry at Glostrup Hospital has attempted to probe deeper into the pathophysiological mechanisms behind postmenopausal osteoporosis. We have also tried to find the optimal prophylaxis of this disease.

PARTICIPANTS AND METHODS

Participants

With these aims we carried out two large, controlled clinical studies:

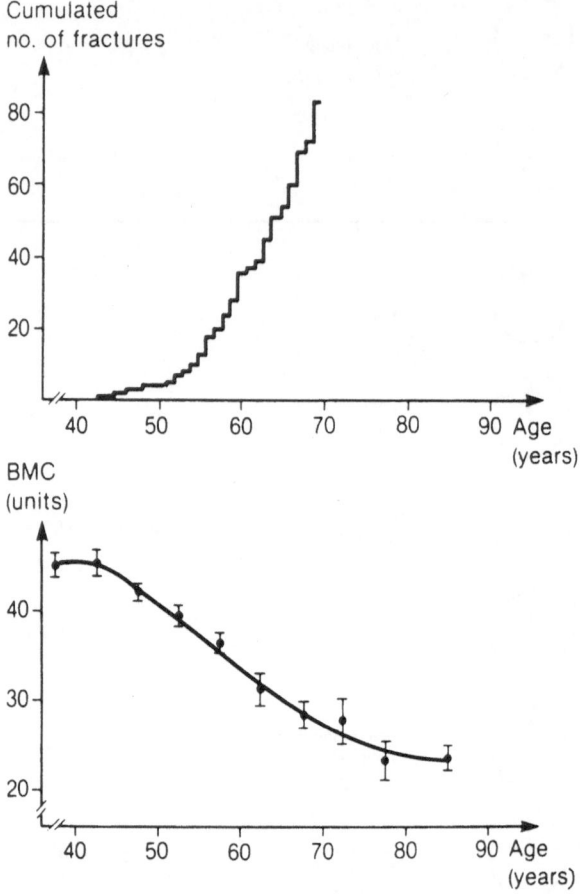

Figure 11.2 Cumulated number of fractures and bone mineral content in women after the menopause

Study I comprised 315 women aged 45–54 years, who had just passed the menopause. This study ran for 2 years and all the women were examined every 3 months – altogether nine times. 264, or 85%, completed the study. The aim of study I was primarily to establish the *optimal preventive treatment of osteoporosis.*

Study II comprised 213 healthy women, aged 47–56 years, who had passed the menopause 3 years before. This study ran for 1 year and 94% .completed it. The principal aim of study II was to establish the *optimal dose of the optimal prophylaxis.*

Methods

The women in both studies were examined every 3 months and after the first examination they were randomized to different treatment regimens. At each examination the procedure was as follows: bone mineral content, height, weight, and blood pressure were measured; all the women filled in a questionnaire which included the Kupperman index, a measurement of postmenopausal subjective symptoms; blood samples were taken for the determination of serum calcium, phosphate, creatinine, alkaline phosphatases, parathyroid hormone, lipids, vitamin D metabolites, pro- lactin, androstenedione, estrone, estradiol, FSH, and LH; the 24 h urine was collected for the determination of calcium, phosphate, and creatinine.

Figure 11.3 shows schematically how the bone mineral content (BMC) is measured. The apparatus consists of a Plexiglass container with water, in which the patient places her forearm. The U-shaped frame round the container is the scanner, with the radioactive source which emits photons on one side and on the other side the detector which registers the number of photons passing through the forearm. The higher the calcium content in the bones, the greater the number of photons absorbed. The right side of the picture shows the scanning movement on the distal part of the forearm. The *long-term precision* of this method is about 1% in healthy subjects; its *accuracy* is about 3%. The site measured is reasonably representative of the total body calcium, since estimation of the amount of calcium measured in the distal part of the forearm from the total body content has an unreliability in the order of 10%. This means that when the technique is applied to a group of subjects, we can obtain an exact measure- ment of the changes in the calcium balance during a given treatment.

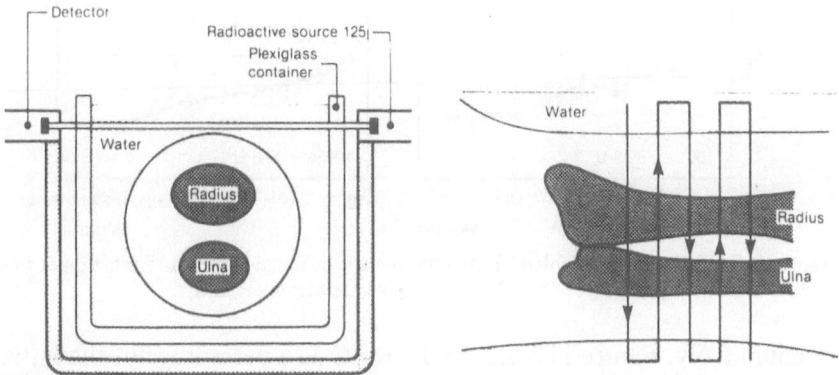

Figure 11.3 Schematic diagram illustrating the principles used in measuring bone mineral content with photon absorptiometry

RESULTS

Study I[3-9]

Four of the groups in study I were given: an estrogen/gestagen combi- nation (Table 11.1); fluoride and vitamin D_3; the active metabolite of vitamin D, 1-α-OHD_3; and placebo. The women also received 500 mg

Table 11.1 Combination of hormones (mg)

		12 days	10 days	6 days
High dose	17-β-estradiol	4.0	4.0	1.0
(Horm. forte)	estriol	2.0	2.0	0.5
	norethisterone acetate	–	1.0	–
Medium dose	17-β-estradiol	2.0	2.0	1.0
(Horm.)	estriol	1.0	1.0	0.5
	norethisterone acetate	–	1.0	–
Low dose	17-β-estradiol	1.0	1.0	–
(Horm. mite)	estriol	0.5	0.5	–
	norethisterone acetate	–	1.0	–

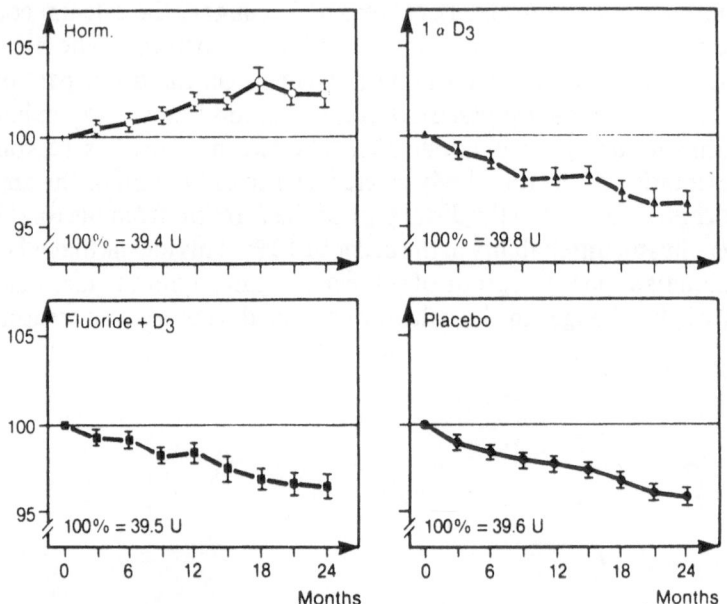

Figure 11.4 Bone mineral content (BMC) (percentage of initial values) as a function of time in four treatment groups (see text). Values are given as mean ± 1 SEM

calcium daily. Figure 11.4 shows the BMC as a percentage of the initial value as a function of time on these four groups during the treatment. The mineral content in the hormone group rose about 2% during the course of the 2 years. This corresponds to a positive calcium balance of about 25 mg daily during the study period. The BMC in the groups receiving fluoride + vitamin D_3 and 1-α-D_3 fell linearly, which was identical with the fall in BMC in the placebo group. The mean loss in all three groups was about 4% over 2 years, corresponding to a mean negative calcium balance in the individual women of about 50 mg daily.

Figure 11.5 shows the relationship between urinary calcium as a percentage of the initial value and corrected for creatinine excretion, and

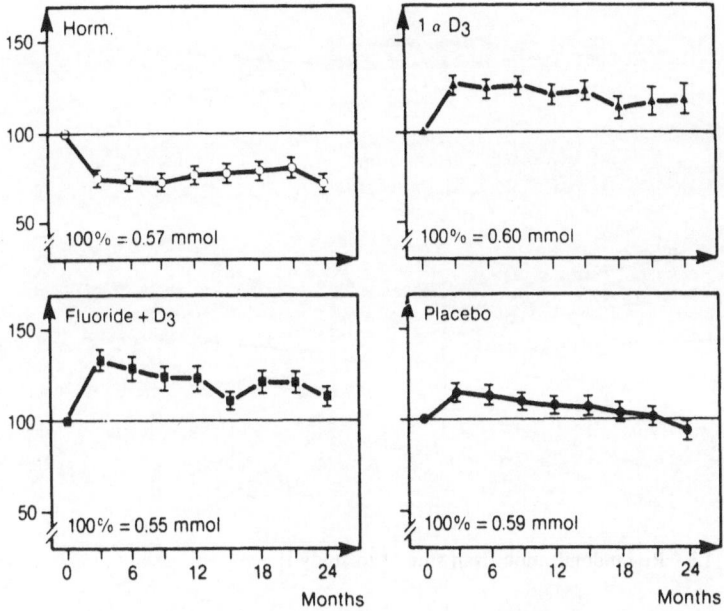

Figure 11.5 Urinary calcium mmol/mmol creatinine (percentage of initial values) as a function of time in four treatment groups (see text). Values are given as mean ± 1 SEM

time in the same four groups. The urinary calcium excretion fell by about 25% in the hormone group. If hormones do not induce increased calcium absorption in the gut, this reduction in urinary calcium corresponds to a positive calcium balance of about 25 mg daily, or exactly the same amount that we found when we calculated the calcium balance from the BMC values measured. The two groups receiving fluoride + vitamin D_3 or 1-α-D_3 exhibited increased urinary excretion of calcium. Thus, both vitamin D_3 and its metabolites seem to increase intestinal absorption of calcium, but this increased amount is excreted with urine, and has no effect on the metabolic condition of the bone.

Study II[10–14]

At the completion of study I, 213 women were randomized to new treatment groups (Fig. 11.6). The women who had received hormones in study I were collected in one group and then randomized to two new treatment groups. One continued the hormone treatment and the other received placebo. All the women who had been given inactive substances in study I, i.e. placebo, fluoride, vitamin D_3, and 1-α-D_3, were collected in one group and then randomized to seven new treatment groups. Three groups were treated with three different doses of estrogen/gestagen (see Table 11.1); one group received the estrogen/gestagen combination without estriol; two groups were given 1,25(OH)$_2$D$_3$ either alone or in combination with hormones; and the last group was given placebo.

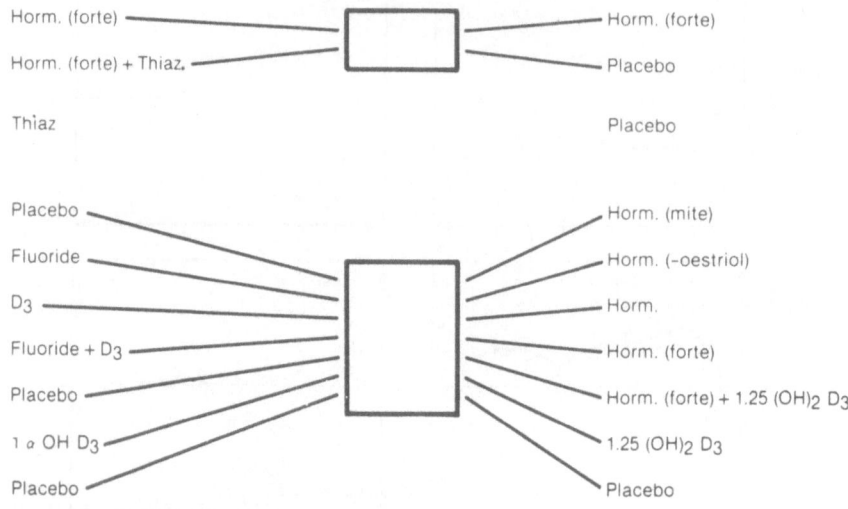

Figure 11.6 Re-randomization from study I to study II

Two reports in the literature have postulated that the benefits con-
ferred by estrogen treatment on the bones are rapidly lost when the
estrogen treatment is withdrawn. Figure 11.7 gives the combined results
of studies I and II. The fall in BMC after estrogen withdrawal is entirely
parallel to that observed with placebo. After 3 years of estrogen treatment

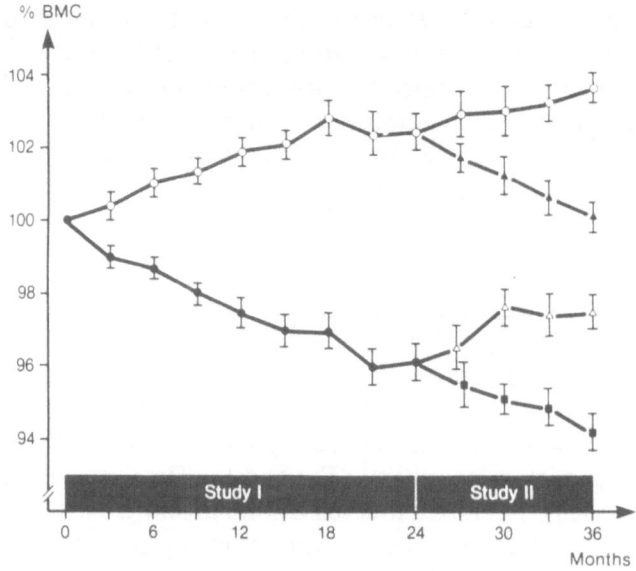

Figure 11.7 Bone mineral content (BMC) (percentage of initial values) during treatment (O, △)
and after withdrawal (▲) of hormones. Values are given as mean ± 1 SEM

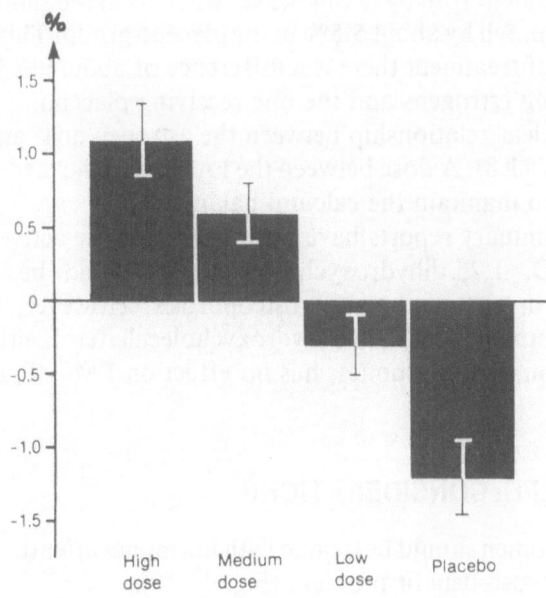

Figure 11.8 Dose response on BMC during treatment with different doses of hormones. Values are given as mean ± 1 SEM

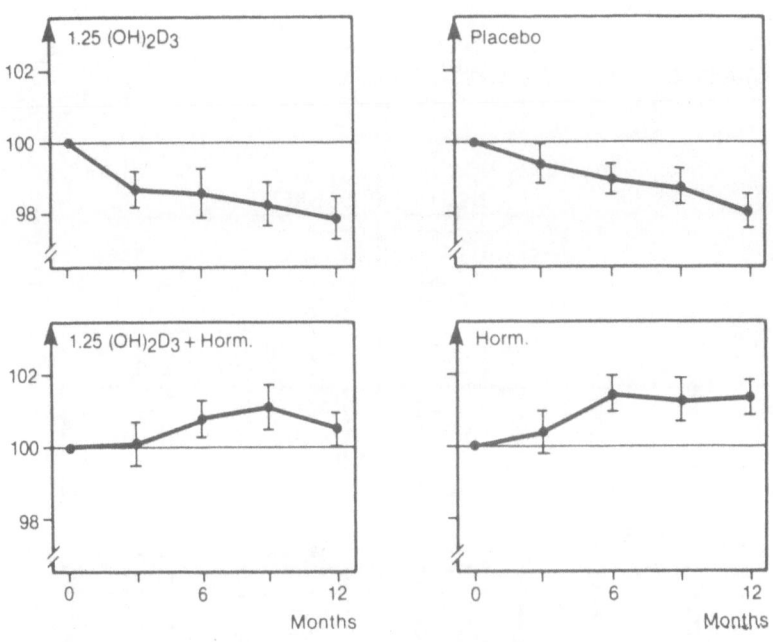

Figure 11.9 Bone mineral content (BMC) (percentage of initial values) as a function of time in four treatment groups (see text). Values are given as mean ± 1 SEM

the mineral content rose by about 3.5%, whereas in the same period the mineral content fell by about 5.5% in the placebo group. This means that after 3 years of treatment there is a difference of about 9% between the group receiving estrogens and the one receiving placebo.

There is a clear relationship between the estrogen dose and the BMC response (Fig. 11.8). A dose between the lowest and the medium one will thus be able to maintain the calcium balance.

A few preliminary reports have postulated that the active metabolite of vitamin D, 1,25-dihydroxycholecalciferol, could be a potential *prophylactic* in postmenopausal osteoporosis. However, our studies show that treatment with 1,25-dihydroxycholecalciferol, either alone or in combination with hormones, has no effect on BMC (Fig. 11.9).

COST-BENEFIT CONSIDERATIONS

Whether all women should be treated with hormones after the menopause is naturally a cost–benefit problem (Fig. 11.10).

(1) There can now be little doubt that estrogen treatment prevents osteoporosis and reduces the number of osteoporotic fractures.

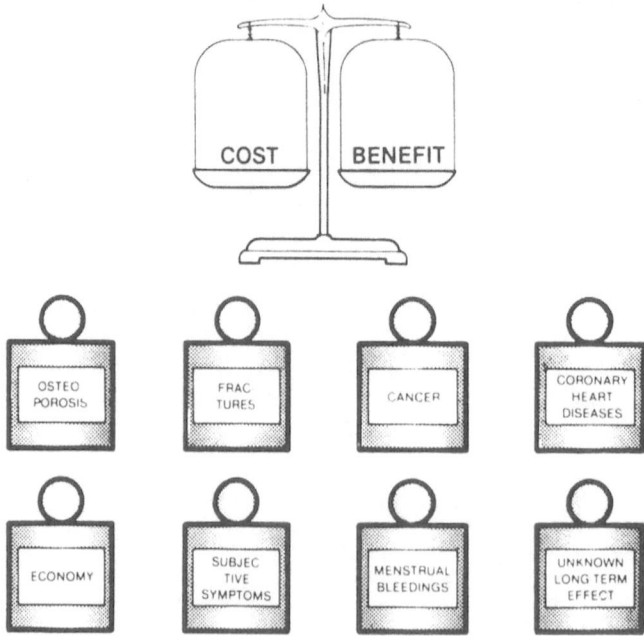

Figure 11.10 Cost–benefit considerations

(2) Nor can there be much doubt that, although the studies are retrospective, pure estrogen treatment increases the risk of uterine cancer. On the other hand, some studies indicate that combined estrogen/gestagen treatment does not increase this risk. A few reports have postulated a greater risk of breast cancer.

(3) Hormonal activity on serum lipids has been the object of considerable interest in recent years. The mean change in serum cholesterol during the 2 years of hormonal treatment in study I was highly significant with a fall of about 12% ($p < 0.001$); in the other treatment groups serum cholesterol remained unchanged compared with the placebo group. Moreover, the relationship between serum cholesterol and dose response in study II was found to be significant. The serum concentration of cholesterol as a function of time during the 3 years of treatment is illustrated in Fig. 11.11 where the results of studies I and II are combined. Figure 11.12 shows the mean change in the diastolic blood pressure (upper) and body weight (lower) during the 2 years of treatment. The group treated with hormones exhibited a significant fall in both parameters, whereas they were unchanged in the two treatment groups compared with the placebo group.

(4) Preventive treatment of a large population over a period of years will naturally have enormous economic consequences.

(5) Hormonal treatment indisputably reduces subjective postmenopausal symptoms. We found a highly significant dose response to

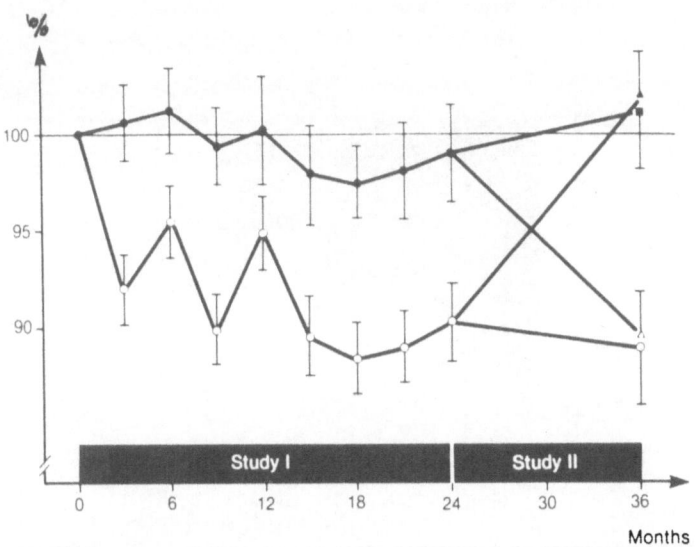

Figure 11.11   Serum cholesterol during treatment (O, △) and after withdrawal (▲) of hormones

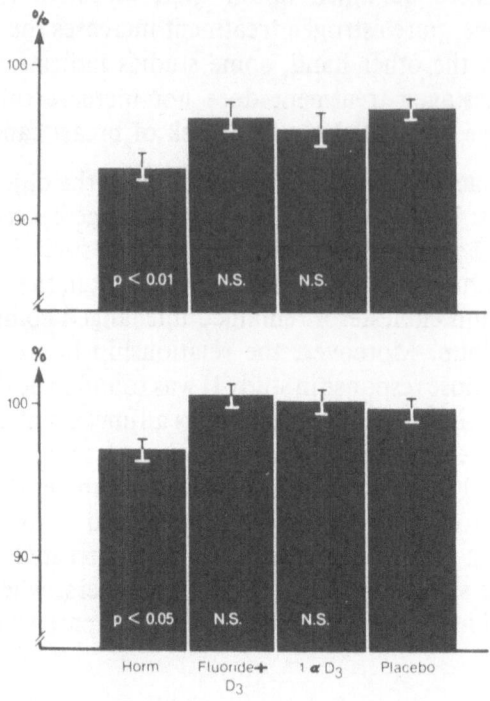

Figure 11.12 Response on diastolic blood pressure (above) and body weight (below) during different treatments. Values are given as mean ± 1 SEM

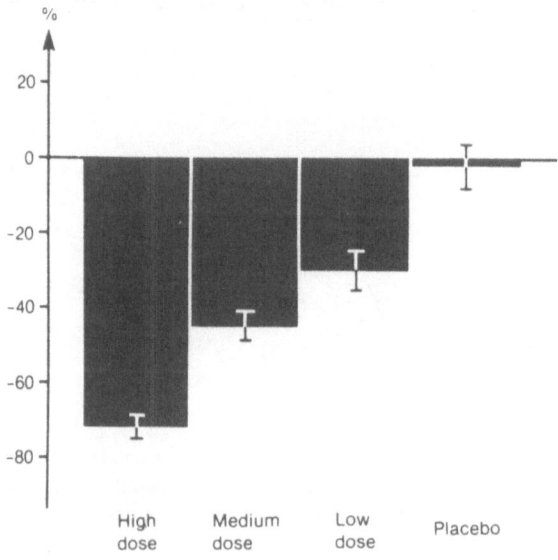

Figure 11.13 Response on Kupperman index during treatment with difference doses of hormones. Values are given as mean ± 1 SEM

116

the Kupperman index during the given treatment (Fig. 11.13). All three doses of estrogen reduce the Kupperman index in varying degrees: about 70% by the highest dose and about 35% by the lowest dose.

(6) The estrogen/gestagen treatment we gave induces regular menstruation.

(7) From a clinical-pharmacological point of view, preventive long-term treatment of large populations should always be approached very cautiously, owing to the possibility of unknown side-effects occurring later on.

REFERENCES

1. Jensen, G. F., Christiansen, C. and Transbøl, I. (1982). Fracture frequency and bone preservation in postmenopausal women treated with estrogen. *Obstet. Gynecol.*, 60, 493–6
2. Jensen, G. F., Christiansen, C., Boesen, J., Hegedüs, V. and Transbøl, I. (1982). Epidemiology of postmenopausal spinal and long bone fractures. A unifying approach to postmenopausal osteoporosis. *Clin. Orthop. Rel. Res.*, 166, 75–81
3. Christiansen, C., Christensen, M. S., McNair, P., Hagen, C., Stocklund, K.-E. and Transbøl, I. (1980). Prevention of early postmenopausal bone loss. Controlled 2-year study in 315 normal females. *Eur. J. Clin. Invest.*, 10, 273–9
4. Christiansen, C., Christensen, M. S., Hagen, C., Stocklund, K.-E. and Transbøl, I. (1981). Effects of natural oestrogen/gestagen and thiazide on coronary risk factors in normal postmenopausal women: A 2-year double-blind placebo study. *Acta Obstet. Gynecol. Scand.*, 60, 407–12
5. Hagen, C., Christensen, M. S., Christiansen, C., Stocklund, K.-E. and Transbøl, I. (1982). Effects of two years oestrogen–gestagen replacement on climacteric symptoms, gonadotrophins and prolactin in the early postmenopausal period. *Acta Obstet. Gynecol. Scand.*, 61, 237–41
6. Christiansen, C., Mazess, R. B., Transbøl, I. and Jensen, G. F. (1981). Factors in response to treatment of early postmenopausal bone loss. *Calcif. Tissue Int.*, 33, 575–81
7. Hagen, C., Christiansen, C., Christensen, M. S. and Transbøl, I. (1982). Long-term effect of oestrogens in combination with gestagen on plasma prolactin and FSH levels in postmenopausal women. *Acta Endocrinol.*, 100, 486–91
8. Christiansen, C., Christensen, M. S., Rødbro, P., Hagen, C. and Transbøl, I. (1981). Effect of 1,25-dihydroxyvitamin D_3 in itself or combined with hormone treatment in preventing postmenopausal osteoporosis. *Eur. J. Clin. Invest.*, 11, 305–9
9. Transbøl, I., Christensen, M. S., Jensen, G. F., Christiansen, C. and McNair, P. (1981). Thiazide and oral calcium for the postponement of postmenopausal osteoporosis. *Metabolism*, 31, 383–6
10. Christiansen, C., Christensen, M. S. and Transbøl, I. (1981). Bone mass in postmenopausal women after withdrawal of oestrogen/gestagen replacement therapy. *Lancet*, 1, 459–61
11. Christiansen, C., Christensen, M. S., Larsen, N.-E. and Transbøl, I. (1982). Pathophysiological mechanisms of estrogen effect on bone metabolism. Dose-response relationships in early postmenopausal women. *J. Clin. Endocrinol. Metab.*, 55, 1124–30
12. Christensen, M. S., Hagen, C., Christiansen, C. and Transbøl, I. (1982). Dose-response evaluation of cyclic estrogen/gestagen in postmenopausal women: placebo-controlled trial of its gynecologic and metabolic actions. *Am. J. Obstet. Gynecol.*, 144, 873–9
13. Christiansen, C. and Rødbro, P. (1983). Does postmenopausal bone loss respond to estrogen replacement therapy independent of bone loss rate? *Calcif. Tissue Int.*, 35, 720–2
14. Christiansen, C., Christensen, M. S., Grande, P. and Transbøl, I. (1984). Low-risk lipoprotein pattern in post-menopausal women on sequential oestrogen/progestogen treatment. *Maturitas*, 5, 193–9

Section 3

Climacteric in the cultural context

Chapter 12

The climacteric syndrome: historical perspectives

J. Wilbush

The history of medicine traditionally concentrates on the achievements of its distinguished practitioners. Often it traces the progress of medical concepts in the changing contexts of prevailing ideas. Alternatively it recounts the development of diagnostic or therapeutic methods and operative procedures. There are, however, only few histories of behavioral disorders. There is no clear model to follow.

Our predecessors were faced with many problems similar to the ones which face us today. They solved them in their way, in accordance with their resources and circumstances. History can best be regarded as an account of those solutions. It is an attractive way, at least for the scientifically inclined: for history then becomes a series of reports of scientific experiments. We do not choose the variables but that does not make these experiments less valid.

The story of the climacteric syndrome can be told through the historical records: of references, publications and books. Attention can be focused on its place in the development of medical thought on practical therapeutics. The emphasis can be shifted to the social and economic forces which have attended its recurrent appearances. On the other hand it is possible to concentrate more on its changing semeiology.

In a general outline like this it may be best to mention something of each. The main points are also summarized in Table 12.1.

Table 12.1 The changing faces of the climacteric syndrome (a generalized outline)

Epoch	Chief complaints	Social class or background	Specialized sources of help	Cultural/scientific explanations	Curative treatment	Palliative treatment
Climacteric disorders prior to the 18th century	Loss of beauty, *personal* degradation resulting in loss of status	Upper class. Roman patrician. European nobility	Female healers (also barber–surgeons)	Retention of poisons normally excreted by the menses	Emmenagogues, purgatives, issues, cauteries, phlebotomies	Rich clothing, jewelry, wigs, dentures, and cosmetics
Climacteric ills, 18th century	Personal degradation, loss of beauty and status. Illness. Menorrhagia	Nobility. Upper class	Female healers but increasingly male doctors	Theory of retention of poisons questioned towards end of century. Solidist explanations. Awareness of social stresses	Various methods promoting excretion of poisons (see above). Purgatives, cauteries, etc.	Rich clothing and jewelry, cosmetics, wigs
La ménopause. Early 19th-century France	Loss of beauty, status and influence. Illness. General symptoms. Menorrhagia	Deposed royalist, later Napoleonic aristocracy	Medical men also female healers	Upheaval of body balance. Crisis of change. Solidist explanations. Social stress mentioned	Rest. Restrictive regimens. Persistance of (mild) elimination of toxins	Dresses, cosmetics
The Change of Life. Tilt[1] and others	'Female disorders'. Depression. Bleeding. Cancer. Loss of role in *family*	Upper-middle and middle class	Medical men. Physicians specializing in diseases of women.	Change of uterine and ovarian function. Influence on nervous system. Social factors recognized	Rest. Restrictive regimens. Exclusion of organic diseases[2]. Sedatives[1]. Laxatives, bathing, sweating	General measures. Intellectual pursuits.
The menopausal syndrome. Last quarter 19th and 1st this century	Loss of role; 'empty nest'. Hot flushes, other symptoms, depression	All classes. Symptoms vary with background	Physicians, gynecologists (hysterectomy for menorrhagia)	Change of ovarian and uterine functions. Hormones suspected. Male prejudice blames female 'hypersensitivity'	Awareness of concurrent disease. Sedatives (new synthetic compounds lead to addiction). Operative procedures	Dresses, cosmetics. General measures. Travel
The climacteric syndrome; modern era	Anxiety, depression. Hot flushes. Physical degradation. Loss of coital capacity (dry vagina). Loss of role. Discrimination in the work place	All classes. Symptoms vary with subculture	Physicians, gynecologists, health gurus	Ovarian involution. Estrogen deprivation and change in hormone balance. Confusion over behavioral aspects.	HRT modified by inclusion of other hormones (testosterone, progesterone). Psychotrophic drugs	Attention to image. Arts of the beautician, couturier and plastic surgeon

CLIMACTERIC DISORDERS PRIOR TO THE 18TH CENTURY

I have not, as yet, come across any medical description of disturbances in the female climacteric dating prior to the 18th century. Whatever I have been able to assemble derives either from non-medical sources or from material found in later writings.

The first successful 'women's lib. revolution' was won by the patrician ladies of Rome. Though they never gained political rights, they achieved economic independence by retaining control over their share of the family property. This gave them social, including sexual, freedom. Body image, as a consequence, became very important. They dressed in rich clothes, wore extravagant jewelry and extensively used cosmetics and other beauty aids. Ovid, Martial and others tell us that older women continued to use these aids in an effort to look young and attractive. They probably employed emmenagogues, ostensibly because of suppression of the menses, secondary amenorrhea, for the same purpose. It is tempting to hypothesize they also used other means at the same time.

A parallel situation developed among upper-class women during the late and post-renaissance. Once an aristocratic lady produced an heir or heirs, she was, at least informally, allowed to follow the inclinations of her heart. Considered as created for love and not for the exclusive pleasure of one man, she had, whatever her position in law, the same or even greater rights than the male. She could, therefore, choose and change lovers at will (see chap. 46 of ref. 3). Yet to be successful she had to be young and preferably pretty. Climacteric degradation could mean an end to her status, and adventures.

THE POISONOUS MENSTRUAL BLOOD

Science, medicine and women believed that the sexual aging which accompanied the climacteric was due to the toxic effects of the 'retained' menstrual blood. Latin traditions regarded the menstrual discharge as poisonous. This attitude was transferred to European medicine. These are well-known views. They even persist today.

After the cessation of the menses, toxins previously excreted through them were 'retained'. They then destroyed the body from within. Female healers first tried to prolong natural 'excretion' by emmenagogues, leeches applied to the genitalia and, with the help of surgeons, directional phlebotomies. The latter, performed on a vein below the genitalia, 'drew' the blood, which, according to classical ideas, ebbed and flowed, towards the uterus. (Incidentally, their strong condemnation, as late as the mid-19th century, shows medical men did not understand Harvey's work until very recently.) When these measures failed, alternative routes for excretion were tried; purgation, issues, cauteries, setons and others. The latter

Table 12.2 Methods of promoting excretion of 'toxins' retained after the menopause (18th century)

(a) *Encouragement of the menstrual flow*
    (1) Emmenagogues (frequent renal iatrogenic effects)
    (2) ˅ Directional phlebotomies
    (3) Induced vicarious menstruation, e.g. via hemorrhoids, also leeches to cervix or external genitalia

(b) *Promotion of excretion through other venues*
    (4) purgation, *evacuations remplaçantes*
    (5) phlebotomy
    (6) excretion through skin:
        (i) vesicatories, cupping;
        (ii) issues, cauteries, setons;
        (iii) sweating, bathing

---

promoted pus, considered proof-positive of excreted toxins. The novelist LeSage describes in his book *Gil Blas* (1715) a lively woman of indeterminate age who kept her youth through two issues, one on each buttock (Table 12.2).

CLIMACTERIC ILLS DURING THE 18TH CENTURY

Economic conditions in Europe improved greatly by the end of the 17th and beginning of the 18th century. Better agricultural practices, such as the Norfolk system, and the introduction or improvement of cultigens, especially the turnip and potato, eliminated the recurrent winter scarcity of food. The plagues which regularly devastated the continent subsided. The expectation of life, both at birth and of adults, rose. That of aristocratic ladies at marriage, or the age of 20, jumped[4] (Table 12.3). By the next century this applied to all women[5]. Most women were reaching the menopause and many more living for a number of years past the climacteric. Concurrently women, at first among the upper classes and later more generally, began to visit doctors instead of, or in addition to, their female healers.

Table 12.3 Expectation of life at 20 years of age, English ducal families[4]

Historical period	1330–1479	1480–1679	1680–1729	1730–1779	1780–1829	1830–1879	1880–1949
Average age attained by a lady of 20 years	51.1	49.1	55.4	64.2	66.2	66.2	74.3

The first thesis dealing with disturbances of the climacteric was defended at the University of Magdeburg at Halle in February 1710. Its author was Simon Daniel Titius, a Silesian from the city of Wroclaw now in Poland[6]. This was followed by two theses presented at the University of Leiden, by Germans, in 1722 and 1737[7,8].

The first reference to climacteric discomforts in English is on a much more practical level[9]. It occurs in a 'physical directory' soliciting women to buy purging pills or uterine drops at three shillings and six pence an item, a very considerable sum in those days. The anonymous physician-entrepreneur refers to various, apparently well-known, molimena of the climacteric but obviously not to an established or named syndrome.

More theses were defended in other universities, especially in France. By the second half of the century *le temps critique* was being discussed in most French books dealing with women (e.g. ref. 10). In 1776 John Fothergill wrote on the management at the cessation of the menses in the *Medical Observations and Inquiries* (**5**, 160-186) of London[11]. The unknown *maux secrets*, secret ills, of women were being medically exposed.

This open discussion finally separated the older syndrome of suppression of the menses, i.e. secondary amenorrhea, from that of the climacteric. The latter eventually crystallized in the beginning of the next, the 19th, century. Its main characteristics were, however, being defined already in the 18th; so were the controversies surrounding it.

The French physicians generally empathized with their women patients. They realized the social factors in their illnesses. They saw them, in the climacteric, as '*des reines dethronées*', dethroned queens abandoned by their subjects – their lovers[12]. They called the climacteric *l'enfer des femmes*, women's hell[10]. Not so Fothergill who, on the other side of the Channel, was surrounded by the wives of the new industrial 'aristocracy'. Godfearing nonconformists, often Quakers like himself, they accepted their fate. The climacteric was a God-ordained, natural event to them. They did not complain. They needed minimal treatment; and Fothergill said so.

These arguments were rejected by Jeannet des Longrois[12], who urged physicians to help every woman in the climacteric. This author asserted that 'The maxim that nature is the best healer of women in the climacteric, as, indeed, ailing women at any time, is as false as it is heartless. Nature can heal only simple ills, due to fortuitous physical causes. Women's maladies are, however, always complex – affected by their sensitivity and their mental state' (pp. 9-10).

THE FRENCH REVOLUTION AND EARLY 19TH CENTURY IN FRANCE

Much has been written about the French Revolution, but little about its effects on the ladies of '*l'ancien regime*'. Most younger women somehow managed. Others, not so young, did not. These climacteric women were subjected to a historical experiment on a grand scale.

It did not stop there. French women were repeatedly adversely affected as they reached the climacteric. The free society which rose from the ashes of the Revolution and Terror encouraged sexual licence. Women who were young and attractive did very well – those in the climacteric did not. Finally, on the fall of Bonaparte, the Napoleonic elite suffered the same fate as the royalist nobility – its climacteric women joining the ranks of others subject to the '*ménopause*'.

During the waning years of the 18th century, and even the beginning of the 19th, these women were exposed to aggressive medication by emmenagogues, purgatives and phlebotomies (e.g. as typified by Broussais). Climacteric ills were thus often exchanged for gross iatrogenic diseases. The greater frequency of climacteric disorders was therefore followed by an increase in complications. French physicians realized their treatment was wrong.

It was then that a small pamphlet[21], printed in 1788, caught their attention. It was a translation of Fothergill's article of 1776. It caused a revolution in the therapy of the climacteric in France. Indeed, in this, Fothergill probably became much more influential in France than in his own country.

The visibility of climacteric disturbances and the controversy surrounding their treatment soon became hot medical items in France. More than 30 theses on the subject were presented in French universities during the first quarter of the 19th century. One was by de Gardanne (1812)[13] who later wrote the first book entirely dedicated to it (1816)[14]. It was, in fact, he who originally coined the term ménèspausie, which he subsequently shortened to ménopause (1821)[15].

The activity of this period lasted for the first half of the century. Another major work was published in 1839[16] and translated into German as were other French books. Yet hardly any papers on the subject were published in the Continental medical press. British and US doctors who, up to the 1860s, used to visit Paris for postgraduate study, learned of the condition there. It was 'promoted' by some, almost invariably looked upon as quacks[17]. Only few in the main stream of medicine wrote about it when they returned home. The climacteric was a French 'disease'.

TILT'S 'CHANGE OF LIFE' (1857) AND ATTITUDES IN BRITAIN AND THE USA

In 1857 Edward Tilt wrote the first, and for over a century the only, English book dealing with climacteric disorders. Subsequent editions appeared in both Britain and the USA up to the mid-1880s[18]. It was still being quoted in the second quarter of this century.

Tilt was the first to suggest climacteric symptoms were due to ovarian involution. He was the first to offer a statistical analysis of symptoms. He was the first to mention the influence of the empty nest. He was the first to insist on proper sedation as help for the nervous tension of this stage of life. He was the first to accept alcoholism in climacteric women as due to medical factors. He was one of the first to describe climacteric symptoms among the urban poor. On the other hand he was still, subconsciously, tied to the past, to the necessity to encourage excretion of toxins, by baths, sweating, even phlebotomy.

His work, however, had relatively little impact. British doctors continued to follow Fothergill, whose article was republished only a few years prior to Tilt's book[20]. Tilt had greater influence in North America where he was extensively quoted by Skene (1889)[22] and others. The groundwork here was prepared by Meigs (1848)[2], who was one of the first to teach his students about the change of life.

As long as British and North American women accepted their fate, be it biological or social, without protest, their climacteric years remained relatively symptom-free. They ceased to be so when women became more assertive.

THE LAST QUARTER OF THE 19TH AND THE FIRST OF THE PRESENT CENTURY

The assertiveness of women at the end of the last century did not express itself solely in political protest, clamouring for votes. It had other aspects. In one of these they were actively supported by their husbands. Times were tough, a long economic depression settled over Europe. No-one could any longer afford the large families of the early Victorian era.

The techniques of contraception, for nearly two centuries largely the preserve of upper-class ladies and their lovers, finally percolated to the middle classes. Their dissemination in Britain was helped by various pamphlets which gained wide publicity through the Bradlaugh-Bessant obscenity trial (1876). Families became smaller. Sons and daughters, following economic opportunities, increasingly moved away from their home towns. Towards the end of the century women in the climacteric often found themselves alone, their role in the family gone. Unable to stand the stresses of their position they became ill.

Tilt published a few articles[23, 24] and a revised edition of his book[18] was also serialized in the French medical press[19]. Other works appeared in Germany and elsewhere. By the beginning of this century almost every gynecological book included a chapter dealing with the climacteric.

THE MODERN ERA

The various ovarian hormones were identified, synthesized and refined in the 1920s. The first injections of estrogens were attempted in Germany and the USA in the 1930s. Stilbestrol was synthesized in Britain in 1939. The 1940s and 1950s saw an increase in experimental and therapeutic hormone therapy. This exploded into a flood by the demand created through Wilson's book 'Feminine Forever' (1966)[25]. Climacteric research, previously a sideline, became a promising field[26]. The first international congress on the menopause was held at La Grande Motte, France, in 1976. Climacteric studies are now an accepted part of both the medical and behavioural sciences.

CONCLUSIONS

There is little space left for the many conclusions which can be drawn from the 'historical experiments' I have so rapidly sketched. The climacteric syndrome had, apparently, been evident mostly in times when women gained relatively high status, but had to forgo their privileges on aging. Western women, who willingly acquiesced with their fate, submitted to an inferior social status and accepted a premature biological change which made them less attractive, were not subject to climacteric disorders. Those who enjoyed their influence over the opposite sex and wished to continue to do so, had always, on the contrary, been very much at risk. This is not just a matter of social status. The often narcissistic factor of body image is apparently much more important than the role allotted it by modern research. There are, of course, many other matters to be learned. Their elucidation will, however, take far too long. I shall leave the reader to ponder about them. I hope he does and develops an interest in the history of the subject.

REFERENCES

1. Tilt, E. J. (1857). *The Change of Life in Health and Disease. A practical treatise on the nervous and other affections incidental to women at the decline of life.* (London: Churchill)
2. Meigs, C. D. (1848). *Females and their Diseases: a series of letters to his class.* (Philadelphia: Lea & Blanchard)
3. Lewinsohn, R. (1956). *Eine Weltgeschichte der Sexualität.* (Hamburg: Rowahlt) 1958 trans. Mayce, A. *A History of Sexual Customs.* (New York: Longmans Green)
4. Hollingsworth, T. H. (1957). A demographic study of British ducal families; revised 1965 and reprinted in Glass, D. V. and Eversley, D. E. C. (eds.) (1965) *Population in History.* pp. 354–78. (London: Arnold)
5. Pressat, R. (1971). *Population.* (Penguin Books: Harmondsworth) (trans. from the French by R. and D. Atkinson)
6. Titius, S. D. (1710). *De fine mensium initiis morborum variorum opportuno* (Magdeburg: Chris. Henckel, Halae)
7. Buhl, J. C. (1722). *De praeservatione morborum post-plenarium mensium cessationem.* (Leiden: Lugdunum Batavorum)
8. Regemann, J. L. (1737). *De morbis ex menstruis per aetatem cessatibus.* (Leiden: Lugdunum Batavorum)
9. A Physician (1727). *The Ladies' physical directory or a treatise of all the weaknesses, indispositions and diseases peculiar to the female sex from eleven years of age to fifty or upwards.* (London)
10. Roussel, P. (1775). *Système physique et moral de la femme, ou tableau philosophique de la constitution, de l'état organique, du temperament, des moers et des fonctions propre au sexe.* (Paris: Vincent)

11. Fothergill, J. (1776). On the management proper at the cessation of the menses. *Medical Observations and Inquiries*, **5**, 160–86
12. Longrois, Jeannet des (1787). *Conseils aux femmes de quarante ans* (1st edn 1781). (Paris: Méquignon-Marvis)
13. Gardanne, C. P. L. de (1812). *Dissertation sur les avis à donner aux femmes qui entrent dans l'âge critique*. (Paris: Didot Jeune)
14. Gardanne, C. P. L. de (1816). *Avis aux femmes qui entrent dans l'âge critique*. (Paris: Gabon)
15. Gardanne, C. P. L. de (1821). *De la Ménopause, ou de l'âge critique des femmes (ed. 2)*. (Paris: Méquignon-Marvis)
16. Menville, C. F. de Ponsan (1839). *Conseils aux femmes à l'époque de l'âge de retour, ou de l'âge critique et des moyens de combattre et prévenir les maladies qui peuvent survenir à cette époque de la vie*. (Paris: Baillière)
17. Parrish, J. (1854). 'The Change of Life', in women; with remarks on the periods usually called 'critical'. *The New Jersey Medical Reporter* and *Transactions of the New Jersey Medical Society*, vol. 7. (This series of articles was cut short by the author's illness; little is said about climacteric disorders)
18. Tilt, E. J. (1882). *The Change of Life in Health and Disease. A clinical treatise on the diseases of the ganglionic nervous system incidental to women at the decline of life* (4th edn). (London: Churchill)
19. Tilt, E. J. (1883-85). *De l'âge critique, état de santé - état de maladie*, trans. R. Fauquez. *Rev. Méd. Chirurg. Malad. Femmes*, **5**, 301–13, 426–38, 486–500, 548–65, 606–24, 665–81; **6**, 5–25, 64–79, 133–53, 185–97, 265–79, 312–27, 431–53; **7**, 141–54, 246–63, 369–87, 493–506, 665–77
20. Fothergill, J. (1849). As ref. 11, reprinted in Churchill, F. (ed.) *Essays on the Puerperal Fever and other Diseases Peculiar to Women*. Selected from the writings of British authors prior to the close of the 18th century, pp. 503–16. (London: Sydenham Society Publications)
21. Fothergill, J. (1788). Conseils pour les femmes de 45 à 50 ans, ou conduite à tenir lors de la cessation des règles: par le célèbre practicien de Londres le D. Fothergill. Extrait des observations et recherches de la Société Medicale de Londres. (London and Paris: Briand). The name of the translator, Petit-Radel, P., appears only as initials on this edition. It appears in full on the 2nd (1800) edition, published by Gabon, Paris, and on the 3rd (1812) edition, published by Méquignon-Marvis, Paris
22. Skene, A. J. C. (1889). *Treatise on the Diseases of Women, for the Use of Students and Practitioners*. (New York: D. Appleton & Co.)
23. Tilt, E. J. (1870). On uterine pathology at the change of life and after the menopause. *Br. Med. J.*, **2**, 435–6
24. Tilt, E. J. (1879). Three articles, all in the *Medical Press and Circular*: The right understanding of the change of life, **27**, 419–20; Uterine inflammation at the change of life, **27**, 481; On uterine inflammation after the menopause, **28**, 103–4 and **28**, 201–2
25. Wilson, R. A. (1966). *Feminine Forever*. (New York: Evans)
26. Cyran, W. (1973). Estrogen replacement and publicity. In Keep, P. A. Van and Lauritzen, C. (eds.) *Ageing and Estrogens*. pp. 152–9. (Basel: Karger)

Chapter 13

The climacteric in different cultural contexts

P. A. van Keep and T. Abe

INTRODUCTION

Epidemiological studies have traditionally held little interest for clinicians, except in those cases where the findings confirm the clinicians' own preconceived and sometimes ill-founded ideas. This may be disappointing for the epidemiologist, but it is understandable and to some extent even justifiable, particularly in the case of climacteric complaints. The clinician is confronted with the individual patient who presents with complaints for which she seeks relief. It is of little consolation to her to be told that she is only one of many sufferers and there is little therapeutic value in telling her that some women do not suffer at all. We nevertheless feel that studies on the incidence of female climacteric complaints in the 40–60 age group serve a useful purpose.

WHAT IS THE VALUE OF EPIDEMIOLOGY IN THE STUDY OF THE CLIMACTERIC?

(1) There is a *public health* aspect. When it is known what percentage of women around 50 years of age will suffer from climacteric symptoms and what percentage will ask – at some stage during the climacteric experience – for medical help, it is possible to plan accordingly. Such knowledge may be important when decisions have to be taken on whether or not to open special menopausal clinics.

(2) There is an *economic* aspect. Women who seek medical advice and treatment for climacteric complaints contribute to the total health bill, and it could be useful to know by how much.

(3) There is a *health policy* aspect. Prevention of some of the consequences of the climacteric, particularly osteoporosis, is, to some
extent at least, an issue that calls for decisions at the political level.

(4) There is a *scientific* aspect. Insight into the incidence of climacteric
symptoms in different subgroups, cultures and subcultures will
enable us to understand the mechanisms of symptom formation,
and may make it possible to predict which individuals will suffer
most.

(5) Finally there is an *educational* aspect. When it is known which
women suffer most and why, it might be possible, through health
education and information, to reduce or even eliminate such
suffering.

METHODOLOGICAL PITFALLS

The literature on the climacteric syndrome reflects the many pitfalls and
difficulties involved in research in this area. Many of the older reports are
just statements, impressions or, at best, reflections of clinical experience.
Moreover, global studies of all patients attending gynecology outpatient
departments provide little insight into the incidence and severity of
climacteric complaints in the total female population concerned. It is
obvious that the only way to obtain reliable data is to investigate a representative sample from the age group concerned in the population under
study. Another approach is to study *all* the women in this age group in a
community – preferably a community that is representative of the
population as a whole.

Jaszmann's study is an example of this approach[1]. By means of a postal
questionnaire he interviewed all women aged between 40 and 60 living in
Ede (Netherlands), a city which may, from the sociodemographic point
of view, be regarded as representative of the whole country. Interviews
may be carried out by postal questionnaire or in person by a trained interviewer. The latter approach is more time-consuming and more expensive
than the former, but yields more details.

In developing countries, illiteracy can be a problem, and the self-
administered questionnaire is of limited value. It must be borne in mind
that women do not always know their age, and that data on the age at which
the first and last menstrual periods occurred are at best approximations.

Whatever the technique used, care must be taken that the terms employed are understood by respondents of different social and cultural
backgrounds. For example, vernacular words for dyspareunia may vary
considerably!

Non-response may distort the findings, but the impression exists that in most published studies the motives for failing to respond were such that the results and conclusions were unlikely to have been influenced.

CULTURAL DIFFERENCES

We have on several previous occasions stressed the differences between the ways women go through the climacteric phase in different cultures[2]. Marcha Flint[3], and more recently Maoz[4], have both provided evidence that points towards the underlying mechanisms. In societies where women gain in status with advancing age – and the cessation of the menses is a milestone in this regard – the menopause is experienced in a different way from that in societies where a woman's status decreases when she ceases to be fertile. Although this hypothesis is questioned by Wilbush[5], we feel that it is still valid. Van Keep and Kellerhals[2] have advanced the hypothesis that it is primarily the significance that a culture attaches to the phenomenon of menstruation which determines that culture's attitude to the menopause, a hypothesis which partly coincided with that of Flint[3].

From studies carried out in Western Europe and in North America, as well as in related cultures such as Australia, New Zealand and South Africa, a rather uniform picture emerges. Whereas 20% of women sail serenely through the climacteric without noticeable symptoms, the other 80% suffer symptoms for varying periods of time. Half of these, i.e. 40% of the total group, will at some stage ask for medical help and 40% will not. There are, of course, national deviations from this general pattern, particularly as regards the percentage that seek medical help. Factors such as a general tendency to seek aid, stoicism and levels of awareness concerning the availability of therapy are obviously of importance.

THE CLIMACTERIC IN THE WEST

Several large-scale studies have been carried out in various countries, and although the results are not always the same, the differences are of minor importance only. The most comprehensive study performed so far is that of Jaszmann[1], referred to earlier. It is on this study that we base the general picture. Jaszmann interviewed, by means of a postal questionnaire, the total female population aged between 40 and 60 in the community of Ede (Netherlands). He grouped his respondents according to their menstrual pattern and, if they were postmenopausal, to the number of years that had elapsed since the menopause. The most prominent symptom was the hot flush, this being reported by two-thirds of the women interviewed, who were in the early postmenopausal phase.

The second most frequently reported symptom was pain in the bones and joints, the third being bouts of perspiration.

Jaszmann grouped the reported symptoms according to the menstrual age at which their incidence was highest. The vasomotor symptoms, viz. hot flushes, perspiration, tingling sensations and pains in muscles, bones and joints were most prominent in the early postmenopausal phase. Other symptoms, such as fatigue, headaches, irritability, mental imbalance and feelings of being depressed, were more frequent in the years before the menopause occurred. Even though this study was a synchronous one – that is to say that many women were interviewed at the same time, but at different stages in the aging process – it nevertheless provides us with some idea of how long symptoms persist in the group as a whole. However this does not necessarily tell us how long such symptoms last in individual cases. The paper by McKinlay and Jefferys[6] provides some clues in this regard. Of a group of British women who were at least 5 years postmenopausal, 82% had had hot flushes over a period of more than 1 year and 6% for more than 5 years. Thompson *et al.*[7] found that of their patients who were still having hot flushes, 17% had been having them for more than 1 year, 50% for 3–7 years and 19% for more than 5 years. Of those respondents who had previously, but no longer, suffered from hot flushes, 15% reported having had them for more than 1 year, 25% for 2–5 years and 19% for more than 5 years.

SOCIOECONOMIC FACTORS

The influence of socioeconomic factors on the climacteric syndrome was first studied by Van Keep and Kellerhals[2], their findings later being confirmed by others[3, 4]. Briefly, the picture is as follows: women in the lower socioeconomic groups have more climacteric complaints than those in the higher groups. Women who are well integrated into their environment, and women who still have a maternal role – either as a mother or as a grandmother – suffer fewer complaints than lonely women and women whose children have just left home. Childless women, or those whose children leave home well before the menopause, have fewer problems than those whose children leave the parental home in the perimenopausal years. When the last child to leave home is a daughter, the climacteric complaints are more pronounced than when it is a son[8].

In general, women who have a job have fewer problems than women who are housewives, although Liesbeth Severne[9] is of the view that this is true only in the higher socioeconomic groups, the opposite being the case in the lower groups, where working women experience a more difficult climacteric. She also pointed out that the variations observed were due mainly to differences in the secondary, psychic complaints of the climacteric syndrome and not to differences in somatic complaints such as hot flushes and bouts of perspiration. We may conclude from this that what holds for the climacteric in different cultures also holds for different subcultures within the Western culture, although here the difference between a premenopausal and a postmenopausal woman does *not* depend on whether she is still menstruating and therefore still perceives herself as being fertile and relatively young. The difference lies in the role from which she derives her identity and self-esteem. This may be the traditional female role as mother and homemaker, which is generally more valued in the lower socioeconomic groups, or her role in her profession. It stands to reason that the *types* of job performed by women in the higher socioeconomic groups differ in general from those of women in the lower groups.

Jobs in the higher groups may be more intellectually rewarding and constitute a more valued alternative to the maternal role.

THE CLIMACTERIC IN OTHER CULTURES

Practically all epidemiological studies on the incidence of climacteric complaints have been carried out in women living in North American and west European societies, and little work has been reported from comparable studies in developing countries. Recently, however, some other interesting studies have been published.

Sharma and Saxena studied 405 married women aged between 40 and 55 living with their husbands in Varanasi City in India[10]. Interestingly enough, the incidence of climacteric complaints was more or less the same as that seen in western European samples of similar size. This is at variance with the findings of Flint[11]. Sharma and Saxena's sample was made up of urban, middle-class women of at least college education level. Could it be that these women are so westernized that their climacteric also resembles that of western women

Moore interviewed women in the rural areas of Zimbabwe (Africa)[12]. All the subjects were illiterate. A total of 43% were experiencing symptoms attributed to imbalance of the autonomic nervous system, such as hot flushes, sweating, palpitations and dyspepsia. Fifty-eight percent were experiencing 'psychogenic' symptoms such as insomnia, depression, anxiety, irritability, fear of aging, poor memory and reduced libido, and 42% were experiencing physical symptoms such as dyspepsia, vaginal dryness, hair or skin changes, headaches, backache, joint pains and urinary problems.

Van Keep, working in cooperation with Agoestina, carried out a study in Bandung in Indonesia in 1982[13]. A questionnaire was completed by 1025 women. This was the first time that such a study had been done in Indonesia. The age at menopause was found to be 48–49 years. There was not much difference between the incidence of climacteric complaints in this study group and their prevalence in the West. However, there were a few striking features. In contrast with the findings from European studies, it emerged that the hot flush was not the most typical single symptom mentioned by 13% of premenopausal women, compared to 28% of postmenopausal women.

It was also observed that the period of transition from a regular menstrual pattern via an irregular pattern to complete amenorrhea was shorter than that seen in western Europe. A relatively large percentage of Indonesian women continue to menstruate regularly until the menopause suddenly occurs and the postmenopausal phase commences.

According to Ikeda (personal communication) about 45% of Japanese women have no symptoms, 43% have symptoms but do not seek medical help and about 10% have complaints that lead them to see a doctor.

Abe compared a group of 60 Japanese women, who sought help from the menopause clinic at Tohoku University School of Medicine, with a control group matched for residence, age and past gynecological history. All the women were asked to complete a postal questionnaire.

About 80% responded in both groups. The help-seeking group had a lower degree of self-esteem that was statistically significant, and felt more anxiety about the future. Women in this group more often had an unemployed husband (16% as against 4%). From this study it was concluded that problems associated with the menopause appear more pronounced in women living in urban areas than in the women living in rural areas. This is not a surprising finding since it is well known that Japanese people tend to be psychologically very stable when living in close-knit, homogeneous environments.

CONCLUSIONS

Although anecdotal reports on the climacteric syndrome have been available for centuries, reliable epidemiological studies on the prevalence of climacteric symptoms and complaints are scarce, even in the West. There is consequently an urgent need for comparable data from the whole range of cultures and subcultures that color this world. This is necessary not only because science is under an obligation to map accurately the impact of the menopause as a universal phenomenon, but also because different cultures could learn from each other as a result.

According to Potts (personal communication) a subculture exists in Thailand in which women celebrate the moment they believe they have become postmenopausal. They receive presents and are the center of interest for the day. Perhaps this is the right way to approach the climacteric. Marcha Flint once wrote an article entitled 'The menopause, reward or punishment?' In many cultures the state of being postmenopausal is unfortunately still regarded as a punishment. If we could change attitudes so that it came to be seen as a reward instead, we could begin to view the menopause in its proper perspective – as a physical phenomenon that is sometimes accompanied by symptoms or complaints and sometimes followed by the effect of estrogen deficiency. Nowadays, treatments and prophylaxis are available for all of these problems and these can improve the quality of life for women everywhere, whatever the culture in which they live and grow old.

REFERENCES

1. Jaszmann, L., Lith, N. D. van and Zaat, J. C. A. (1969). The perimenopausal symptoms: the statistical analysis of a survey. *Med. Gynaecol. Sociol.*, **4**, 268
2. Keep, P. A. van and Kellerhals, J. (1974). The influence of social and cultural factors on symptom formation. *Psychother. Psychosom.*, **23**, 251
3. Flint, M. P. (1979). Transcultural influences in perimenopause. In Haspels, A. A. van and Musaph, H. (eds.) *Psychosomatics in Perimenopause*. pp. 41-56. (Lancaster: MTP Press)
4. Maoz, B. (1973). The perception of menopause in five ethnic groups in Israel. *MD thesis*, Leiden
5. Wilbush, J. (1980). The female climacteric. *D.Phil. thesis*, Oxford
6. McKinlay, S. M. and Jefferys, M. (1974). The menopausal syndrome. *Br. J. Prev. Soc. Med. (UK)*, **28**, 108-15
7. Thompson, B., Hart, A. S. and Durno, D. (1973). Menopausal age and symptomatology in a general practice. *J. Biosoc. Sci.*, **5**, 71-82
8. Crawford, M. P. and Hooper, D. (1973). Menopause, ageing and family. *Soc. Sci. Med.*, **7**, 339-72.
9. Severne, L. Psycho-social aspects of the menopause. In Haspels, A. A. and Musaph, H. (eds.). *Psychosomatics in Perimenopause*
10. Sharma, V. K. and Saxena, M. S. L. (1981). Climacteric symptoms: a study in the Indian context. *Maturitas*, **3**, 1
11. Flint, M. P. (1975). The menopause: reward or punishment? *Psychosomatics*, **16**, 161-3
12. Moore, B. (1981). Climacteric symptoms in an African community. *Maturitas*, **3**, 25
13. Agoestina, T. and Keep, P. A. van (1985). The climacteric in Bandung, Indonesia. *Maturitas* (In press)

Chapter 14

Climacteric expressions in a crosscultural study

Y. Beyene

The menopause is a universal physiological phenomenon. In the West the associated biological transition, the climacteric is assumed to have inevitable physiological and behavioral effects. The relationship between the biophysical and behavioral factors of the climacteric has been obscured by the tendency of Western biomedicine to conceive and define the climacteric as a disease episode rather than as a natural process.

Moreover, in the youth-oriented culture of the West, such as the United States, the menopause is a symbolic milestone on the way to old age. Thus the dominant view in Western culture associates the postmenopausal rôle with lowered status and emotional and physical distress[1-5].

Some writers[6-8] have questioned the universality of the consequences claimed for the climacteric by Western biomedicine, and suggested that the experience of this phase of life is conditioned by the cultural context that shapes the pattern of a woman's rôle. They view culture as an organized system that gives meanings to reality, thus giving each natural phenomenon a particular meaning and significance[9].

Since meanings vary from culture to culture, different meanings will be attached to menopause. Thus in some societies women experience few, if any, of the physiological and psychological symptoms of which Western women commonly complain in connection with the climacteric[1, 10, 12]. These differences are often attributed to the fact that the menopause precipitates a positive rôle change for women in many non-Western cultures[1, 2, 11]. A change from high to low status is assumed to correlate with circumstances in which the postmenopause is experienced as negative and disabling. Where the postmenopause is associated with freedom from the cultural taboos associated with childbearing years, women's attitudes are reported as being positive or indifferent to this event and symptomatic complaints to be fewer. On the other hand, if the climacteric is principally a hormonal event, one would expect that women throughout the world would experience symptoms in the same way.

This chapter reports the result of a 3-year extended ethnographic study that investigated this expectation through comparing the climacteric experiences of women in two different cultures where there is no hormonal therapy for the physical and emotional changes said to occur.

DESIGN AND METHODOLOGY

The two cultures studied were rural Mayan Indians living in Yucatan, Mexico and rural Greek women living on the island of Evia, Greece. Their selection was based on two criteria: differences from dominant Western cultural values concerning women and aging and accessibility as a result of prior contact by the researcher.

The field work was conducted utilizing a systematic ethnographic approach. This involved informal and formal interviews and direct observation and participation in everyday activities of women for 12 months in each of the cultures. Since the subject matter of the study was personal as well as cultural information, one-third of the research time was spent in establishing good rapport and social ties with the women in the villages. I presented myself as someone who wanted to study the lives of women. Thus women in both cultures took an interest in teaching me how to cook and allowed me to participate in their everyday activities. One hundred and seven Mayan and 96 Greek women were studied in three categories: premenopausal, perimenopausal and postmenopausal. They were interviewed regarding general life history including pregnancy, health, experience and attitudes towards menstruation, menopause and aging. In addition unstructured interviews were conducted with key informants such as older women, traditional healers, midwives (among the Mayans) and medical personnel in the health services and clinics that served the villagers.

FINDINGS

The comparison of the data from these two groups indicates some similarities and marked differences between women in the two cultures. The women seem to share similar cultural values with respect to beliefs and practices regarding menstruation and childbearing but show differences in their experiences with menopause, childbearing patterns, diet, and the ecological niche they inhabit. There are also genetic differences between the Greek and Mayan women.

Similarities

Here are some of the similarities: the data indicate that women in both cultures are concerned much more with menstruation and factors related to childbirth than with menopause. Both Mayan women and Greeks have elaborated taboos and restrictions related to menstruation and child-bearing. For example, rural Greek women believe that menstruation is a curse resulting from 'Eve's sin'. Thus among Greek peasants a menstruating woman and a woman who just gave birth are not allowed to participate in religious activities because they are considered 'unclean' and contaminating. Mayans believe that a menstruating woman can cause disaster and induce sickness in a newborn baby. Moreover, in both cultures, citrus fruit, cold drinks, and bathing are forbidden during menstruation because they are believed to stop the menstrual flow. Both groups use a variety of herbs to treat menstrual irregularities and different illnesses.

Women in both cultures perceive the postmenopause as a life stage free of taboos and restrictions, and offering increased freedom to participate in many activities. For example, Greek women can participate fully in church activities and Mayan women move freely without anxiety about inducing sickness in others. Since the risk of pregnancy is no longer present both groups reported that they felt more relaxed about sexual activities, improving sexual relationship with their husbands. The women also stated that they felt relieved from the fear of unwanted pregnancies, as well as from the monthly menstrual flow, which was considered bothersome. In Greek culture, age and appropriate life stage are very important. For example, a woman would feel very embarrassed if she gave birth to a child at the same time her daughter or daughter-in-law did so. Moreover, it is embarrassing for her grown-up son to see his mother pregnant, since it reveals the sexuality of the mother.

The data also indicate that in both cultures, the roles of 'good' mother, housekeeper, and hard worker are highly valued. In both societies old age is associated with increased power and respect. Particularly for a woman, her status increases with age, as her sons marry and establish their own families. The mother-in-law, both in Mayan and Greek culture, occupies the most authoritative position as the head of the extended family households of her married sons. Apart from the points mentioned the menopause does not bring changes in her household rôles. Particularly for Mayan women, the rôle of grandparent does not necessarily come at the same time as the menopause. Mayan women continue bearing children after becoming grandparents; this is not unusual, given the early age for marriage.

Moreover, older women are believed to possess special healing skills. Therefore, in both Mayan and Greek villages the older woman of the family is the first to be consulted when a family member gets sick, particularly her grandchildren. In both cultures it is believed that, for the older woman, the role of healing is part of her nurturing rôles as a mother and as a carrier of old traditions.

Differences

The data also indicate marked differences between the Mayan and Greek women in relation to the climacteric experience, diet, childbearing patterns and their respective ecological niches.

The mean age for menarche in both cultures is approximately the same; 13 for Mayan women and 14 for Greek women. However, the mean age at menopause is 42 for the Mayans and 47 for the Greeks. When we look at the age categories for age at menopause, the difference in age at menopause between the two groups is quite striking. The Mayan women cluster in the age categories of 36–45 and the Greek women cluster in the age categories of 41–55.

Moreover, Mayan women do not associate the menopause with any physical or emotional symptoms. The only recognized physiological event associated with the menopause is the cessation of menstruation. Among the Mayan women menopause is welcomed and expressed with such phrases as 'being happy', 'free like a young girl again', 'content and good health'. No Mayan woman reported having hot flashes or cold sweats or other symptoms of discomfort associated with the climacteric. Anxiety, negative attitudes, health concerns and stress for Mayan women are associated with the childbearing years, not with the climacteric. For Mayan women the menopause is not a negatively perceived event. Women are pleased to get rid of their periods, thus premenopausal women in the study look forward to the menopause. Menopause is considered by Mayan village women as the beginning of a very tranquil and calm stage in a woman's life.

On the other hand, the climacteric experiences among rural Greek women seem to bear more resemblance to the experiences of Western women. Even though the postmenopausal women reported being relieved from the taboos and restrictions of childbearing years at menopause, overall it is perceived negatively by the premenopausal women. The premenopausal women expressed anxiety and anticipated possible health problems with the menopause, and were not looking forward to its onset. There is respect and status gain for older women in Greek culture, but getting old is perceived by some Greek women as tantamount to dropping out of the main stream of life. Thus some Greek women, particularly the premenopausal group, associated the menopause with growing old, diminution of energy, and a general down-hill course in life. In striking contrast to the Mayan women, Greek premenopausal women reported anxiety and a negative affect in association with menopause.

The Greek perimenopausal and postmenopausal women reported hot flashes and some cold sweats similar to Western women. However, Greek women differ from American women in their perception and management of hot flashes. These Greek women in my study *do not* perceive hot flashes as a disease symptom, and do not seek medical intervention. While they have a variety of herbs to treat menstrual pain and discomfort, there are none for hot flashes. They felt that it is a natural phenomenon causing a temporary discomfort that would stop with no intervention. Their explanation for hot flashes is that the retained menstrual blood in a woman's body boils up so that a perimenopausal woman has a sensation of heat. Even though symptoms such as irritability, melancholia, and emotional problems are not expected in the normal process of the perimenopause, these symptoms were reported in association with 'off-time' menopause, i.e. when the menopause occurs before the age of 40.

Another striking difference between the two cultures is diet. The Mayan diet consists of corn, beans, tomatoes, *chaya* (a green leafy plant), some radishes, squash, *camote* (sweet potatoes), very little animal protein, and no milk products. Greeks, on the other hand, have a wide variety of nutrients: wheat, cheese, milk, eggs, olives, a variety of wild greens, legumes, plenty of meat, fish, fruit, and wine. My information from medical personnel serving the Mayan villages indicated that the Mayans have a high incidence of vitamin deficiency and anemia.

Women in the two cultures also differ in their patterns of childbearing. For Mayan women pregnancy is viewed as a stressful experience. Since they do not use any birth control methods, many were pregnant at regular 2-year intervals. The average number of pregnancies for women in the Mayan sample was seven, with an average of 4.7 children surviving the first year of life. They marry early and continue having children until the menopause. They all breast-feed their children until these reach 1½–2 years of age. It is rare for Mayan women to have a steady menstrual cycle since successive pregnancies and long periods of amenorrhea due to lactation are so common. For example, one woman in the study said that she had not had her period for 15 years because she was either pregnant or lactating.

Unlike the Mayan women, the Greek women have few pregnancies; they marry in their late 20s or early 30s; use birth control methods, and plan their family size. The average number of pregnancies for women in the Greek sample was 2.9 with an average of 2.3 children surviving the first year of life. They breast-feed only 6–9 months and they tend to have steady menstrual cycles.

Moreover, the two cultures differ in their environment and subsistence economy. The Mayans live in a semitropical environment, a lowland with poor soil, and use a slash-and-burn technique of farming. The climate in Yucatan is generally humid and hot. On the other hand the Greeks live in a rugged mountainous area and the climate in Greece varies from season to season. Even though the land in general cannot be called fertile, the plots used by the Greeks for farming have more topsoil than those used by the Mayans and produce a greater variety of foods than do the Mayans. Although both groups are agrarian, the nature of the political economy and the levels of technological development are different.

CONCLUSIONS

This comparison suggests that the existence or lack of physiological symptoms of the climacteric cannot be explained in terms of rôle changes at middle age or by the removal of cultural taboos. Thus, the differences that emerged between the Mayan and Greek women cannot be imputed solely to social and cultural factors. If climacteric hot flashes are physiological, hormonally induced phenomena, factors that could affect hormonal production in a woman's body must be considered. Although the Mayan and Greek women have some similarity in their cultural values regarding their beliefs and practices concerning menstruation, childbearing, and women's rôles, they showed striking differences in diet and fertility pattern. There are also genetic differences between these groups. Even though there are no supportive data at this time, it is possible that the above-mentioned differences could be some of the factors involved in the variation in the age at onset of menopause as well as climacteric experiences.

Diet

It has been documented that nutrition plays a role in reproduction – affecting conception, fetal mortality, the health of the newborn, and the length of postpartum amenorrhea. Not only is menarche related to nutritional status; menstrual activity also continues to be affected by nutritional factors throughout a woman's reproductive life[13-15].

Differences in hormone production between populations have been partly accounted for by differences in diet. It has also been reported that diet affects ovarian function and adrenal activity, and that adrenal activity could be increased by a high-protein diet. Thus dietary factors, such as dietary fat intake, are reported to influence the hormone profile in women[16-17]. However, the process whereby these factors affect age at menopause and presence or absence of climacteric symptoms is unknown.

Diet does vary dramatically between Mayan and Greek women. The cultural practices of nutritional intake, and ecological as well as economic limitations, are major factors in the differences in diet between these two cultures. If diet is known to affect growth and development and hormone production, it is possible that malnutrition can be identified as one of the factors for the relatively early menopause for Mayan women. However, the effect of the Mayan diet on climacteric symptoms is unknown and needs further investigation.

Information from physicians providing services in these villages indicates that in both cultures osteoporosis does not appear to be a problem. This could be due to the mineral contents of the nutrients that these people eat and their daily activities. Even though the Mayan diet is deficient in protein, people get an adequate supply of calcium derived from their tortillas and from their drinking water. For example, the use of lime water to soak maize before grinding it into *masa* for tortillas, a practice common to the Mayan and other Latin American peoples, is proven to provide needed calcium in the diet. A Mexican gets more than 500 mg of calcium per day from tortillas alone[18]. Moreover, the Mayan diet includes *chaya*, a leafy green plant that is known to be a rich source of calcium and vitamin A. Mayans also have calcium in their drinking water because of the abundant lime in their soil. The Greeks, on the other hand, have calcium from their use of milk and cheese. In the West, physicians prescribe both high dietary intake of calcium and physical exercise as ways of preventing osteoporosis[19, 20]. In addition to their dietary calcium intake, both Mayan and Greek village women of all ages maintain a high level of physical activity. They habitually perform rigorous work at home and in the fields and walk long distances.

Fertility patterns

Another striking difference between the Mayan and Greek women is their fertility patterns. As discussed before, Mayan women marry early, have successive pregnancies, and experience long periods of amenorrhea (because of prolonged lactation coupled with malnutrition). Therefore it is rare for Mayan women to have a steady menstrual cycle. This raises questions about the extent to which successive childbearing and prolonged amenorrhea affect the production of reproductive hormones and the degree to which the latter may affect age at menopause and the presence or absence of hot flashes.

Genetic

There are also genetic differences between these two groups. Genetic factors affect rate of growth and development and age at menarche[21]. Correlations are found between twin sisters, mother–daughter, and sister–sister regarding age at menarche and patterns of menstrual flow[22-24]. However, we do not know to what extent genetic factors affect the menopause.

SUMMARY

This study focused on the experience of the menopause, its cultural significance and meaning, and physiological manifestation, in rural Mayan and Greek women. The lack of physiological symptoms, such as hot flashes, among the Mayan women cannot be accounted for by biological or cultural factors alone. Like other human developmental events, the perimenopause is a biocultural experience, and factors such as diet and childbearing patterns that can affect the production and equilibrium of hormones in a woman's body must also be considered.

The research indicates that the perception and experience of the climacteric vary crossculturally. The data suggest the interrelation of several variables that may account for differences in the age at menopause and the physiological, psychological and cultural manifestations of the climacteric in different cultures.

Acknowledgement

This research was funded by NIA, grant number AGO2622.

REFERENCES

1. Flint, M. (1975). The menopause: reward or punishment? *Psychosomatics*, **16**, 161–3
2. Griffin, J. (1977). A cross-cultural investigation of behavioral changes at menopause. *Soc. Sci. J.*, **14**(2), 49–55
3. Fessler, L. (1950). Psychopathology of climacteric depression. *Psychoanalyt. Q.*, **19**, 28–42
4. Hoskins, R. (1944). Psychological treatment of the menopause. *J. Clin. Endocrinol.*, **4**, 605–10
5. Deutsch, H. (1945). *The Psychology of Women.* (New York: Grune & Stratton)
6. Ehrenreich, B. and English, D. (1973). *Complaints and Disorders. The Sexual Politics of Sickness.* (New York: The Feminist Press)
7. Rothman, B. (1979). Women, health and medicine. In Freeman, J. (ed.) *Women: A Feminist Perspective.* pp. 27–40. (Palo Alto, California: Mayfield)
8. Seaman, B. and Seaman, G. (1977). *Women and the Crisis in Sex Hormones.* (New York: Rawson)
9. Van Keep, P. A. and Kellerchals, J. (1974). The influence of social and cultural factors on symptom formation. *Psychother.*, **23**, 251
10. Dowty, N., Maoz, B., Antonovsky, A. and Wijsenbeek, H. (1970). Climacterium in three cultural contexts. *Trop. Geog. Med.*, **22**, 77–86
11. Griffin, J. (1982). Cultural models for coping with menopause. In Voda, A., Dinnerstein, M. and O'Donnell, S. (eds.) *Changing Perspective on Menopause.* pp. 248–62. (Austin: University of Texas Press)
12. Maoz, B., Antonovsky, A., Apter, A., Wijsenbeek, H. and Datan, N. (1977). The perception of menopause in five ethnic groups in Israel. *Acta Obstet. Gynecol. Scand.*, **65** (Suppl.), 35–40
13. Frisch, R. (1980). Fatness, puberty and fertility. *Nat. Hist.*, **89**, 16–27
14. Eveleth, P. and Tanner, J. (1976). *World Wide Variation in Human Growth.* (Cambridge: Cambridge University Press)
15. Hill, P., Garbaczewski, L., Helman, P., Huskisson, J., Sporangisa, E. and Wynder, E. (1980). Diet, lifestyle, and menstrual activity. *Am. J. Clin. Nutr.*, **33**, 1192–8
16. Hill, P., Chan, P., Cohen, L., Wynder, E. and Kuno, K. (1977). Diet and endocrine-related cancer. *Cancer*, **39**, 1820–6

17. Macmahon, B., Cole, P., Brown, J., Aoki, K., Lin, T., Morgan, R. and Woo, N.-C. (1974). Urine estrogen profiles of Asian and North American women. *Int. J. Cancer*, **14**, 161-7
18. Cravioto, R., Anderson, R., Lockhart, E., Miranda, F. and Harris, R. (1945). Nutritive value of the tortilla. *Science*, **102**, 91-3
19. Nordin, C. (1982). Bone loss at menopause. *Menopause Update*, 1(1), 5-9
20. Bachmann, G. (1984). Evaluation of the climacteric women - an overview. *Midpoint*, **1**(1), 9-13
21. Golub, S. (1983). Menarche: the beginning of menstrual life. In Golub, S. (ed.) *Lifting the Curse of Menstruation*. pp. 17-36. (New York: Haworth Press)
22. Shields, J. (1962). *Monozygotic Twins*. (London: Oxford University Press)
23. Tanner, J. (1978). *Foetus into Man*. (Cambridge, Mass.: Harvard University Press)
24. Chern, M., Gatewood, L. and Anderson, V. (1980). The inheritance of menstrual traits. In *The Menstrual Cycle*, vol. 1. (New York: Springer)

Chapter 15

Climacteric in a Newfoundland fishing village

D. L. Davis

THE PROBLEM

What is menopause? How has it affected you? What effect, if any, has it had on other people you know? How did you learn about it? These are three seemingly straightforward questions designed to collect information on women's experience of the climacteric. Medical studies have tended to favor the 'precision' of symptom reports, attitude scales, clinical accounts, and hormonal assays[1]. Social research instruments developed on the basis of clinical and medical perspectives consist mainly of quantitative surveys, with multiple-choice answer options, which are ideally administered to large, representative samples of women. Such cost-efficient methods have shaped the social and medical science view of women's experiences of middle aging. Precision research dominates climacteric research in Western as well as non-Western cultures.

The major limitation of precision research, or directed response, is the focus on symptoms and assumption that the questioner and respondent share similar frames of reference. Yet symptoms are a very small dimension of women's experience of the climacteric and it is difficult to isolate symptomatologies from the cultural influences which may dominate their generation and expression. Even anthropologists, specialists in the holistic approach, in their eagerness to provide quantitative data relevant to clinical practitioners, have tended to describe the climacteric and menopause as a physiological, symptom-ridden aspects of middle age. Easily measured factors such as depression, role change, age, and attitudes are held to influence this time of life[2]. This focus of attention on the 'pieces' of culture results in a tendency to overlook broader interpretations of more qualitative aspects of experience.

The strength of anthropology lies in its qualitative as well as quantitative research strategies. Total immersion in a culture, intimate, daily, long-term, personal interaction with people has traditionally been the hallmark of the anthropological method. Anthropologists regard the people they work with as collaborators rather than 'human subjects' or 'data producing objects'[3].

Through participant observation the anthropologist must acquire and learn to operate within the idioms, beliefs and lore, which organize and shape behavior and experience in local society[4]. In villages, all residents know each other and community-wide knowledge is readily accessible to every villager. Anthropologists know a lot about villages, and villages are small enough to be particularly amenable to anthropological techniques because anthropologists work with whole systems[3].

Table 15.1 Local responses to open-ended inquiries about experience of menopause

Question	Response
What is menopause?	(a) Menopause, what's that, my dear?
	(b) It's your nerves on the change, only a bother to some, though.
	(c) It's your blood, dear – the final cleaning out, gets us all some terrible.
How has it affected you? What effect if any has it had on other people you know	(a) Problems? No me pretty, now's best I ever was.
	(b) To tell the truth, my dear, Cassie, over in Burnt Cove, suffered some bad. Every time she left the house, she took thread cross her throat – would choke some awful. She was house bound on the change for years.
	(c) Which change, my dear? The last change? Why, I sailed right through it, no problems at all . . . not like some others round here. (Quote from Cassie, Burnt Cove)
Where did you learn about menopause?	(a) Couldn't tell my dear, I just knows.
	(b) My mother.
	(c) Did ya hear 'bout the bloody horse's urine, me lovie. That's in those pills Effie's been taken.

This chapter is based on just such intimate, first-hand observations of day-to-day life in a southwest coast Newfoundland fishing village. (Fieldwork was conducted from October 1977 to December 1978. Research was funded through a 2-year traineeship from the US National Institute of Child Health and Development administered by the University of North Carolina Population Center.) Table 15.1 illustrates unstandard answers to standard, open-ended questions commonly asked to record women's experiences of the menopause, the climacteric and middle age. The answers make little sense to one not versed in the idioms of local culture; yet they reveal a great deal that is relevant to the village women's experience of aging. Three 'keys' to understanding how local idioms, beliefs and lore can shape climacteric behavior and experience in Grey Rock Harbour are: (1) the generality of expression; (2) the relationship of individual behavior to community ethos; and (3) the particularistic, localized nature of oral communication patterns. In order to properly discern how these basic factors may function, it is first necessary to consider the meaning of perception, stereotypes and localism as they relate to the nature of community life and a sense of belonging.

Living in a small, bounded, homogeneous community, daily inter-acting with its members, and appreciating them as whole persons with multiple roles, complex pasts and a shared future, is essential to under-standing the climacteric as a symbolic social process through which ethos and identity are maintained. Observation of the relationship between idiocentric, situational, particularistic events and processes, on the one hand, and community lore or the creation and shaping of tradition, on the other, can provide insight to cultural dynamics of middle aging. Using data from the southwest coast fishing village of Grey Rock Harbour, I will show how the climacteric has more local viability as a social and symbolic activity than as a biomedical phenomenon.

BACKGROUND

Perception and meaning are facets of both individual and community interaction. All cultures organize and interpret events and experiences. The process of acquiring a vocabulary of bodily experience is a partially shared one[1]. Anthropologists have long recognized that their methods consist of two distinct levels of meaning – the etic or view of those from the outside looking in, and the emic or what people themselves perceive as reality[2]. The process of making symptoms/complaints, middle age, or any other experiential phenomena, intelligible can be done etically by the physician or medical specialists or emically by the individual woman or her peers. It is the latter perspective that is the primary concern of the following analysis of shared stereotypes and the development of local lore.

Stereotypes are collective phenomena. They are standardized mental pictures held in common by a group. In Grey Rock Habour, local stereo-types, or folk models, of middle age are generated by both situation-specific and community-wide events and processes. The term, folk models[2], describes the notions, concepts, and ideas shared by every member of a society, which are relevant, actually or potentially, to the conduct of life. (Margaret Lock[5] has conducted a study on the formation of folk models of menopause among medical practitioners.) Folk know-ledge is intersubjective or public[6]. Despite the paradoxical qualities of climacteric life[7], this stock of folk knowledge governs daily experience and is presented in more or less coherent frameworks such as 'blood' and 'nerves'. These conceptual structures are not set and fixed. They are continually created and re-created on the basis of a relatively low number of theoretical principles.

Folk models of 'middle aging' in Grey Rock Harbour cannot be understood apart from the nature of the local community, the character of personal interaction and a sense of belonging. In small, out-of-the-way local communities, people become aware of their culture and experience its distinctiveness through the evaluation of everyday practices. These practices become value-laden for their distinctiveness from mass society[8]. Personal interaction is shaped by the fact that people see whatever specific thing they are doing, whatever activity they are engaged in, as somehow addressing the whole complex of their life[8]. The personal characteristics of the members are public knowledge. Such knowledge provides the currency of social interaction. People do not engage with each other for the limited purposes attributable to a specialized 'role'; rather they come across each other all the time, engaging as whole persons. All knowledge about people is judged to be relevant to those with whom they interact[8-10]. The sense of belonging in a community means being (1) a repository of its traditions and values, (2) a performer of its hallowed skills, and (3) an expert in its idioms and idiosyncracies[8]. Local communities are characterized by a dialectic of individual and collective identity. People develop local vocabularies for expressing their uniqueness and attachments; a vocabulary which is so fluid that it can serve and mask conflicting phenomena[10]. In Grey Rock Harbour I will show how idioms surrounding the individual and collective experience of middle aging among women create a legitimate rhetoric which strengthens both cultural continuity and a sense of belonging.

SUBJECT

The outport fishing village of Grey Rock Harbour is situated on the southwest coast of Newfoundland. About 800 inhabitants live in colorful painted houses posed on cliffsides overlooking the sea – somewhat resembling houses in the inside of a bowl. One area of the village is clearly visible from any other area of the village. All houses have picture windows which look over the harbor. Fishing always has dominated, and continues to dominate, the community. Men wear distinctive fisherman's attire. Local language is dominated by fishing terms. Everyday and seasonal life is focused on fluctuations in the fishery. Most boats are family-owned and the fishing strategies are similar for all villagers. (Grey Rock Harbour is characterized by an inshore fishery. The majority of men fish in day trips from open dories or motor boats.) Endogamy has created a population of villagers who are interrelated and families who have resided in the village for over seven generations[11].

To the outsider the homogeneity of village life may appear to be stifling. All inhabitants are Anglican. Houses are of essentially four different modes of construction – all equal in interior design and space. There are no social class differentiations or significant differences in material consumption. All purchases of clothing and household goods are made through the Simpson-Sear's catalogue. This makes the insides of houses and dress of men, women and children quite uniform. Women's hairstyles are all similar and they all wear the same 'Labrador style' coats, almost year-round. Household routines are highly regimented, Saturdays and Wednesdays bread is set, and laundry is hung outside to dry on Monday morning. Mornings are for cooking and cleaning, afternoons for visiting, and evenings for staying at home or attending numerous village-wide recreational activities such as ladies' church and lodge functions[12].

Although likeness is valued and being different discouraged, the community has not remained static or changeless through time. Historically Newfoundland outport communities were characterized by acute poverty and isolation. Confederation with Canada in 1949 greatly increased the quality of village life. In the late 1960s a road was built into the village, bringing with it all the conveniences of modern life. Those who can remember life before the road are aware of the dramatic change it has made in their lifestyle. Contact with the outside has enhanced the sense of community.

Grey Rock Harbour is a physically bounded, occupational community with no schisms based on religion or social class or other special interests. (Not all Newfoundland villages are homogeneous. Some are characterized by schisms based on religion, ethnicity, occupation or social class.) Family and fishing are the major focus in the lives of men and women alike. Villagers strongly believe that 'we all go up or we all go down together'.

PRESENTATION OF DATA

Responses to questions shown in Table 15.1 cannot be adequately understood apart from the contexts of local life, which include: (1) the generality of expression; (2) the practice of selective forgetting and relationship of the individual to the community ethos; and (3) the localized nature of the oral communication of relevant knowledge. A closer look at the unstandard responses to each of the standard climacteric inquiries illustrates the important role that local stereotypes and lore can play in shaping women's experience of middle aging.

What is menopause?

An oral tradition, while less subject to critical reflection, is more flexible than a written tradition and open to numerous reinterpretations in light of specific contexts[6]. Responses to the question, what is menopause? illustrates this point. (The word menopause as used here is meant to be synonymous with climacteric, rather than refer to last menses. The women could not be expected to be familiar with the term 'the climacteric'. Because women did not understand the word 'menopause' they were then asked about 'the change of life, when you've had your last period'.) Because they do not recognize the term 'menopause' or 'climacteric', nor do they have equivalent folk terms, they realize that menstruation ceases and this process is, more or less, accompanied by infertility. The closest terms to menopause or climacteric are 'the change' or the 'change of life'. However, 'the change', in local idiom, may refer to any female complaint including menarche, dysmenorrhoea, postpartum bleeding or depression, the menopause, or even postmenopausal cyclical mood changes. More importantly, 'the change' is also used by both men and women to describe the dramatic process of social change that occurred when the road was built.

Communication patterns are contextual rather than discrete. Although the collective life of community members can be categorized as 'before the road' and 'after the road' the lives of individuals are not experienced in discrete categories[11]. The question – which change, my dear? – not only illustrates the intimate nature of outport society, but also the lack of age grading among women and consequent lack of terminology to express it. There are no significant family role changes that can be said to characterize middle-aged women as a group. There is no equating youth, as opposed to middle age, with beauty or sexual desirability. With the introduction of birth control menopause has lost its contraceptive significance[11, 12].

The vast range of idiocentric, experiential phenomena are incorporated in the more general, all-purpose, terms of nerves and blood[7]. The reference to nerves and blood as explanatory categories in Grey Rock Harbour is universal. Such terms do not limit the range of experience, but they do place diverse states of being into mutually intelligible and actionable categories. The range of individualism is limited and contained within the communal vocabulary so that the essential coherence and ideological integrity of the community are not diminished. The blood and nerves terms entail body/mind and event status. In village life they act as extremely effective tools for 'state-of-self' disclosure[11].

How has the change affected you or others you know

The two responses concerning Caissie's experience at middle age not only represent the problems of collecting reliable data on symptoms but also illustrate the complex local rules governing state-of-self disclosure. The ambiguity of the two individuals' responses is influenced by at least three factors: (1) the informant's relationship with the questioner; (2) the local strategies of communicating relevant health complaints; and (3) the cultural ideal of the good woman.

The woman who told me of Cassie's complaints was a woman I knew quite well. She had just explained to me her own extensive problems with her nerves at middle age; related her own case of nerves to the 'good woman' theme; and then, in all humbleness, referred to Cassie who had suffered even more than herself. When I questioned Cassie, I hardly knew her. Her responses to all my questions were perfunctory and un-elaborated. She denied having problems because she did not want me to judge her as a 'weak' woman. Symptom revelation in Grey Rock Harbour is an extremely complex matter. Common courtesy requires that symptoms be revealed in stages – going from the general complaints of blood and nerves to more specific complaints. If one person does not care to discuss another's health complaints she will let the remark pass at the nerves and blood stage. The personal revelation of specific complaints implies a close intimate relationship and the understanding that any request for help will be met[13]. In addition, a woman's reputation as a good woman rests on her communication of complaints and their subsequent interpretation by the community women as justified or unjustified. The first woman freely repeated Cassie's troubles because she thought they were justified. Cassie would not tell me because she could not be sure whether I would evaluate her by local or by some other standards. All this cannot be understood apart from impression management in the community and the folk model of nerves, the medium through which all other symptoms are expressed.

The folk ideal of the 'good woman', is a woman who has worked hard all her life, sacrificed for her husband and children and stoically endured all the trials of poverty and hardship that characterized life before the road[14]. Nerves can be worn away by stress and suffering. Those women who suffered most in the past were more likely to use up their nerves and experience health difficulties in later life[7]. Women who grew to maturity 'before the road' are regarded as folk heroines[15] in the village. They are the embodiment of all that is noble in women and the strength of character that underlies adaptation in a cruel and demanding fishery. One of the things women fear most is being labelled a 'weak woman' or a whiner, complaining about the 'least little thing'. If a woman can successfully (most of them do) relate her health complaints to hardships that she has endured in the past then she can use them in impression management. Cassie would not honestly tell me about her climacteric problems because she had not yet had the opportunity to lay the ground work to present herself as the 'good woman'. As I came to know her better she was able to supply the proper context to her suffering, and freely admitted it to me. The relationship between nerves, suffering, idealization of the past and impression maintenance is so strong that even women who do not have nerves complain of them[14].

Thus, in the local frame of reference, any inquiry into state of health, via elicitation of symptoms or complaints, is understood as an indirect inquiry as to whether or not that individual merits belonging to a community with a hallowed tradition of suffering and self-sacrifice.

How does one learn about the change?

One can become very frustrated trying to obtain information on a directed question of this kind. Given the personalistic character of village life, the nature of collective knowledge, and the lack of formal education, women feel that they just know things. They either do not actually recall the learning process or are all too ready to give standard answers such as 'from the television' or 'from my mother'. However, these answers provide limited insight into the real nature of oral communication and information transmission in village life. The statement about mare's urine represents the collective process of information processing in the local community.

A woman in the community who had had a hysterectomy was undergoing estrogen treatment to control her hot flashes. She showed me her prescription and asked me what it was. I told her about estrogens originally being prepared from blood serum of horses. The woman thought this was very funny. This encounter took place just before the 12 days of Christmas. During these days individuals visit each other's houses, all drink and partake of a constantly replenished buffet of sweets and drinks, passing a couple of hours in one house and moving on to another until well into the morning. Such occasions would be characterized by groups of women numbering five to ten, of all ages, chatting together in the parlor, and with men drinking heavily in the kitchen. A theme reiterated over and over from house to house during the entire 12 days of Christmas was the woman who was taking the 'Bloody! mares' urine'. (Men were also involved in this joking process, their language not quite so polite.) I was responsible for the rumor but it obtained a life of its own. My 'serum means blood' explanations were patiently listened to but urine was a 'Bloody bit' funnier – a far superior topic for social joking. Thus, the Bloody mare's urine became a piece of local lore, and much to my chagrin provided another weapon in the arsenal of anti-medical sentiment[13]. Fortunately the woman continued to take her medication because it worked, and enjoyed all the good humor that happened at her (or my) expense.

The insular nature of village life shapes knowledge. The village 20 miles away will not have a menopause/horse's urine joking tradition. Just as friendship cliques develop an ingroup knowledge or argot, the humor and oral mode of communication and learning that characterizes Harbour folk is continually shaped by a long heritage of shared experience.

Wright[16], in her Navajo study, supports the notion that the experience of climacteric symptoms is fundamentally a biological phenomenon. Gross and social differences among cultures are unlikely to affect the number of symptoms an individual woman may experience. Yet the differences in interpretation and expectations may be unique in differing cultural contexts. In Grey Rock Harbour uniqueness is subsumed under the community ethos and shared folk models. The highly generalized bio-social folk models, like nerves and blood, the hard worker and the good woman, constitute a means of labeling one's fellow-villagers according to a shared code, so that each person is publicly and consensually invested stereotypically with certain characteristic qualities. In this respect, lore accompanying the process of middle aging – which remains minimally differentiated from other periods of the life cycle and incorporates diverse physical, psychological and social phenomena – forms a means of organizing knowledge and of symbolically associating every individual with the community as a whole.

ANALYSIS OF DATA

Flint[2] takes anthropology to task for its descriptive and anecdotal nature. Kaufert[17] warns us about the expediency of keeping menopause-dependent events conceptually separate from potentially coinciding events, and criticizes anthropology for its focus on menopause as a rite of passage. This study has relied on descriptive and anecdotal accounts of middle aging. Rather than focus on the identification of menopause-dependent events, I have preferred to view middle aging as a process – not an event. In my holistically oriented analysis of local life I have made little attempt to separate the womens' experience of the climacteric from coinciding events. Finally, although women in Grey Rock Harbour do not undergo any rite of passage at the end of their childbearing careers, the village itself is experiencing rebirth into the modern industrial age. This is another factor which coincidentally influences Harbour women's experience of middle aging.

In Grey Rock Harbour, menopause and the climacteric are considered to be normal and unremarkable. They do not warrant an event status. Small community observations and descriptions help to demonstrate how women's experience of middle aging is embedded in sociocultural phenomena. In the local view it is the general quality of one's nerves and blood, rather than any specific events or complaints, that shape a woman's experience of middle aging. The folk models of nerves and blood provide a background of meaning for her experience. Whatever the diversity of experience, the meaning is expressed in proximity to a symbolic ideal of the good woman or hard worker.

Why is the ideal of the good woman so important? Why are middle-aged women so adept at impression maintenance? Why is status maintenance at middle age so important? How do nerves and blood symbolically reflect community processes? The change in Grey Rock Harbour is not so much an anxiety of aging as an anxiety of localism. Culture change rather than the change of life is the central issue. Threats of unemployment, out-migration, and a deteriorating fishery cause anxiety. The Harbour folk are worried; can their way of life last? People respond to the threat of change with ideological continuity. Change becomes masked by a rhetoric of continuity and evocation of past values and that stabilizes identity in the face of culture change. In local communities whose traditional and valued way of life is threatened, commonplace events may become meta-phorical statements of the culture in which they occur[8].

In Grey Rock Harbour, middle-aged women more than any other element of society represent a tie with the past. They are the social models for all that is best in outport life. They are guardians of the collective ethos[14]. A pervasive theme in Harbour life is 'we all come up together, or we don't come up at all'. Being different is frowned upon. Being better than anyone else is not acceptable, nor is bragging about one's accomplishments. There is little outlet for individual expression, especially for Harbour women. However one cannot be responsible for one's body. Physical individuality is recognized and expressed in indirect contexts through the medium of blood and nerves. Women are characterized in the community according to the state of their nerves and blood. Health is a topic of daily conversation and communication, yet it poses no threat to the collective image.

CONCLUSION

The holistic view of the climacteric as embedded in culture and cultural processes adds to our knowledge of the complex issues that can be raised by crosscultural variation of any facet of human behavior. Certainly the gene pools, traditional diet, obesity, parity, poverty, and lack of medical services help to shape a woman's climacteric experience[1]. The ideal method of climacteric research would be to combine medical/lab/questionnaire and anthropological/participant observation methods.

It is the characteristic of anthropology to approach broader interpretations and more abstract analysis from the direction of exceedingly small matters[18]. This analysis of 'cultural localism'[8] has focused on explaining how the every day, mundane facets of women's experience of the climacteric may relate to the wider realm of village life.

SUMMARY

Women's experience of the climacteric in a Newfoundland fishing village is analysed from the holistic perspective of anthropology. Special attention is focused on the relationship between emic stereotypes and idioms of middle aging and a sense of belonging to the local community.

REFERENCES

1. Koeske, R. (1982). Toward a biosocial paradigm for menopause research: lessons and contributions from the behavioral sciences. In Voda, A. *et al.* (eds.) *Changing Perspectives on Menopause.* pp. 3–23. (Austin: University of Texas Press)
2. Flint, M. (1982). Anthropological perspectives of the menopause and middle age. *Maturitas,* **4,** 173–80
3. Mead, M. (1980). On the viability of villages. In Reining, P. and Lenkerd, B. (eds.) *Village Viability in Contemporary Society.* pp. 19–32. (Boulder: American Association for the Advancement of Science Selected Symposium 34)
4. Cohen, A. (1978). Ethnographic method in the real community. *Sociol. Rur.,* **23**(1), 1–22
5. Lock, M. (1982). Models and practice in medicine: menopause as a syndrome of life transition? *Culture, Med. Psychiatry,* **6**(3), 261–80
6. Holy, L. and Stuchlik, M. (1980). The structure of folk models. In Holy, L. and Stucklik, M. (eds.) *The Structure of Folk Models.* pp. 1–34. (New York: Academic Press)
7. Davis, D. (1982). Women's status and experience of menopause in a Newfoundland fishing village. *Maturitas,* **4,** 207–16
8. Cohen, A. (1982). Belonging: the experience of culture. In Cohen, A. (ed.) *Belonging, Identity and Social Organization in British Rural Cultures.* pp. 1–20. (Manchester: Manchester University Press)
9. Cohen, A. (1979). The Whalsay croft: traditional work and customary identity in modern times. In Wallman, S. (ed.) *Social Anthropology of Work.* pp. 249–67. (London: Academic Press)
10. Cohen, A. (1982). A sense of time, a sense of place: the meaning of close social association in Whalsay Shetland. In Cohen, A. (ed.) *Belonging: Identity and Social Organization in British Rural Cultures.* pp. 21–49. (Manchester: Manchester University Press)
11. Davis, D. (1983) Blood and nerves: an ethnographic focus on menopause. Memorial University of Newfoundland Institute of Social and Economic Research, St John's
12. Davis, D. (1983). The family and social change in a Newfoundland outport. *Culture,* **3**(1), 19–32
13. Davis, D. (1984). Medical misinformation: communication difficulties between Newfoundland women and their physicians. *Soc. Sci. Med.,* **18**(3), 273–8
14. Davis, D. (1983). Woman the worrier: confronting feminist and biomedical archetypes of stress. *Women's Studies,* **10**(2), 135–46
15. Davis, D. (1985). 'Shore skippers' and 'grass widows': active and passive roles for women in a Newfoundland fishery. In Nadel, D. and Davis, D. (eds.) *Women in Fishing Economies.* Memorial University of Newfoundland Institute of Social and Economic Research, St John's (In press)
16. Wright, A. (1983). A cross-cultural comparison of menopausal symptoms. *Med. Anthropol.,* **7**(3), 20–35
17. Kaufert, P. (1982). Anthropology and the menopause: the development of a theoretical framework. *Maturitas,* **4,** 181–93
18. Geertz, C. (1973). *The Interpretation of Cultures.* (New York: Basic Books)

Chapter 16

A survey of perimenopausal symptoms in Nigeria

O. Bajulaiye and P. M. Sarrel

INTRODUCTION

The climacteric experience of Black African women has received little attention in the medical literature. In fact, because almost all menopause surveys have been of almost entirely non-Black populations, little is known about Black women's climacteric experience or of the meanings and significance of this turning point in their life cycles.

This is a report of a study of 250 Black women individually interviewed in Lagos, Nigeria between February and April 1984. None of the women had had any previous gynecological treatment or hormone replacement therapy. All the interviews were done by a single investigator who used a questionnaire developed in collaboration with the director of the Menopause Program at Yale University. Attention focused on vasomotor, neuropsychiatric and psychosexual issues.

The aim of this study was to identify the prevalence of climacteric symptoms in Nigerian women and to alert the medical profession to the fact that the menopause poses a major medical issue, especially in Africa where most women do not recognize this fact.

MATERIALS AND METHODS

Between February and April 1984, 250 Nigerian women were randomly selected and interviewed with a structured questionnaire. The study population was contacted through the Young Women's Christian Association and the Market Women Association. Some patients from the Lagos

University Teaching Hospital in Lagos are also included. However, less than 10% of the women sought attention for treatment of climacteric symptoms. The survey therefore should be considered to be one of a general population and not of a menopause clinic population.

All interviews were done by a medical doctor, a Nigerian (O.B.). The study was done in part to fulfill the requirements for the Masters of Public Health Degree from the Yale University School of Medicine.

None of the women had received ovarian hormone replacement therapy at any time. None of the women had had a hysterectomy or oophorectomy.

The questionnaire included general questions about age, marital status, social class, pregnancies, medication, general health and partner's health, height, weight, blood pressure and diet. Gynecological questions related to operative procedures, previous history of gynecological disease and use of oral contraceptives or of any other hormonal preparation.

Climacteric-related questions cluster into three categories: vasomotor changes, neuropsychiatric changes and changes that have to do with sexuality. The original study design included taking blood samples for hormonal assay. However, the occurrence of a political revolution in the months just prior to this investigation precluded the blood sampling as permission could not be obtained in time.

FINDINGS

Demographic data

The demographic data are summarized in Tables 16.1 and 16.2.

The women were categorized by menstrual age. 'Premenopause' connotes women who had regular menses. 'Perimenopause' connotes women who have menstruated within the past year, but whose menses have become irregular apparently due to decreased ovarian function. 'Postmenopause' were women who were at least 1 year from the time of their last menstrual flow (Table 16.1(d)).

Age of perimenopause and menopause

Thirty-one per cent of women aged 45–49 were postmenopause, as were 98.5% of women aged 50 or older. The mean age of menopause was between 49 and 50.

Attitude about menopause

As summarized in Fig. 16.1, 45% of women regularly menstruating had a positive attitude towards menopause while 28% in the 1–3-year post-

Table 16.1 Demographic data of the Nigerian women, Lagos, Nigeria, 1984 ($n = 250$; age range = 38–65 years)

(a) Age distribution

Age (years)	No.	Percentage
Under 45	64	25.0
45–49	77	30.8
50–54	59	23.6
Above 54	50	20.6
Total	250	100.0

(b) Marital status

Status	No.	Percentage
Married	206	82.4
Unmarried	12	4.8
Divorced	14	5.6
Other	18	7.2
Total	250	100.0

(c) Social class

Status	No.	Percentage
Lower	63	24.4
Middle	130	52.8
Upper	57	22.8
Total	250	100.0

(d) Menstrual age

Status	No.		Percentage
Premenopause	56	=	22.4
Perimenopause	66	=	26.4
Postmenopause			
1–3 years ago	58	=	23.2
4–6 years ago	30	=	12.0
7–9 years ago	26	=	10.4
above 9 years ago	14	=	5.6
Total	250		100.0

menopause group had a positive attitude. Negative attitudes were found in 68.5% of the women with dyspareunia, 70% of the women with depression and 75% of the women with hot flashes.

Table 16.2 Demographic data of the Nigerian women, Lagos, Nigeria, 1984 (frequency distribution (percentages) of calendar age for each of the defined menstrual age groups; $n = 250$). $C_1 = 1-3$ yrs; $C_2 = 4-6$ yrs; $C_3 = 7-9$ yrs; $C_4 =$ over 9 yrs

Menstrual age groups	Calendar age				
	Under 45	45–49	50–54	Above 54	Total row (%)
Premenopause	93	7	0	0	100
Perimenopause	15	83	2	0	100
Postmenopause C_1	3	31	61	5	100
Postmenopause C_2	0	0	77	23	100
Postmenopause C_3	0	0	0	100	100
Postmenopause C_4	0	0	0	100	100
Total column (N)	64	77	59	50	250

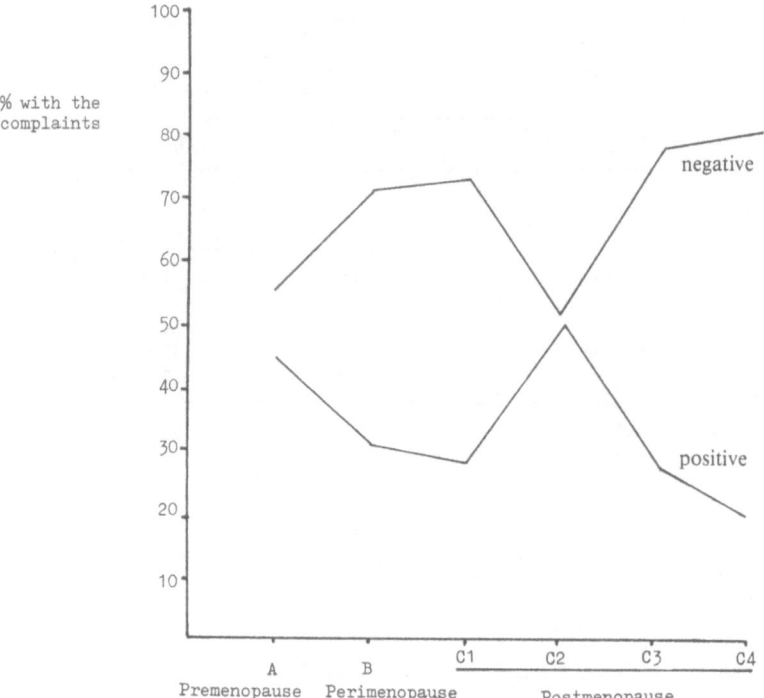

Figure 16.1 Frequency of positive and negative attitudes about menopause, Lagos, Nigeria, 1984

Changes that have to do with sexuality

Breast changes

Figure 16.2 shows that 5% of regularly menstruating women complained of breast changes (shrinkage, loss of firmness, irregularity of shape); 14%

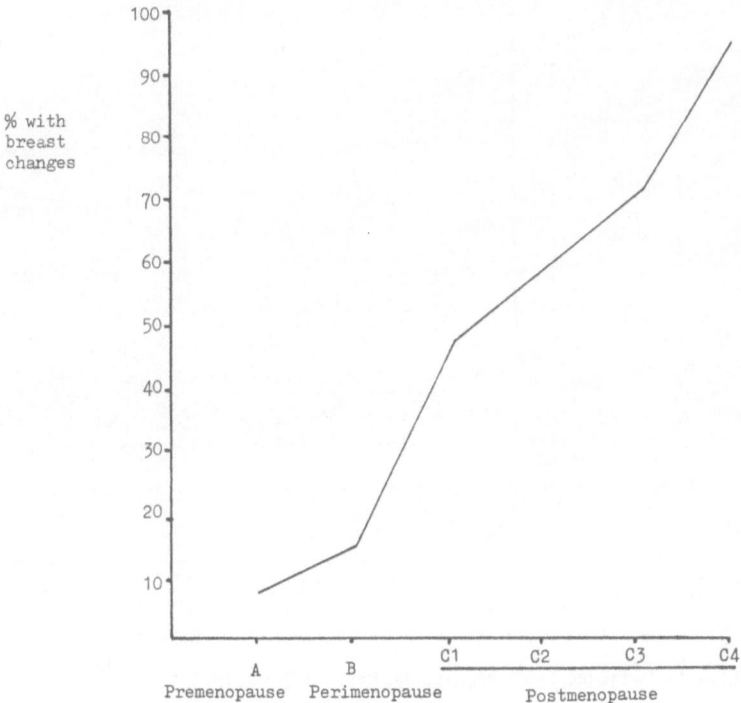

Figure 16.2 Frequency of breast changes, Lagos, Nigeria, 1984

of perimenopausal women had this complaint and 44% of women 1-3 years after cessation of menses. Ninety-two per cent of women who were more than 9 years after menopause complained of the breast changes as an indicator of loss of feminine attractiveness.

Dyspareunia

Figure 16.3 shows that 9% of women still menstruating complained of pain with intercourse. Seventeen per cent of the perimenopause women and 31% of the women within 1-3 years after the menopause had this complaint. By 9 years after menopause the incidence of dyspareunia dropped to 21%. However, by that time almost 70% of the women had become sexually inactive. Of those with dyspareunia, 48% complained of vaginal dryness; 57% of loss of sexual desire; 41% of change in sexual desire of their partner and 41% of a change in sexual response of their partner. Fifty-two per cent (28/54) of the women with dyspareunia did not experience vaginal dryness. Their pain was almost entirely pain at the vaginal opening with penetration.

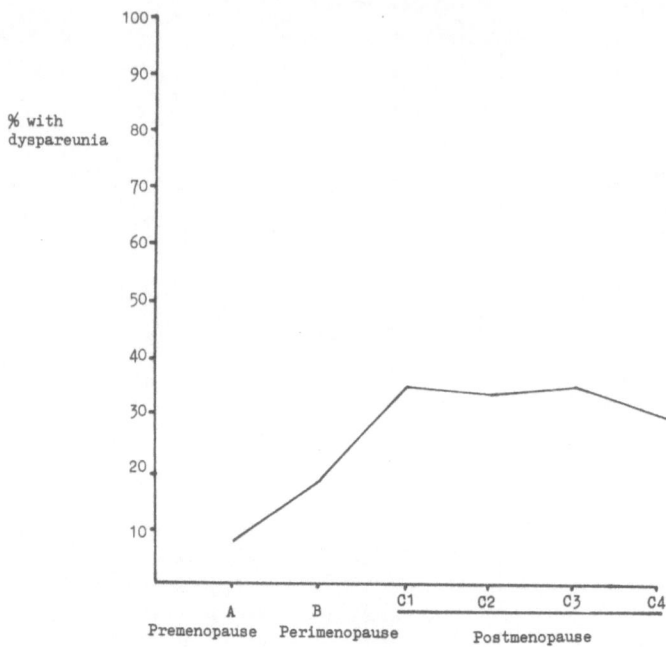

Figure 16.3   Frequency of dyspareunia, Lagos, Nigeria, 1984

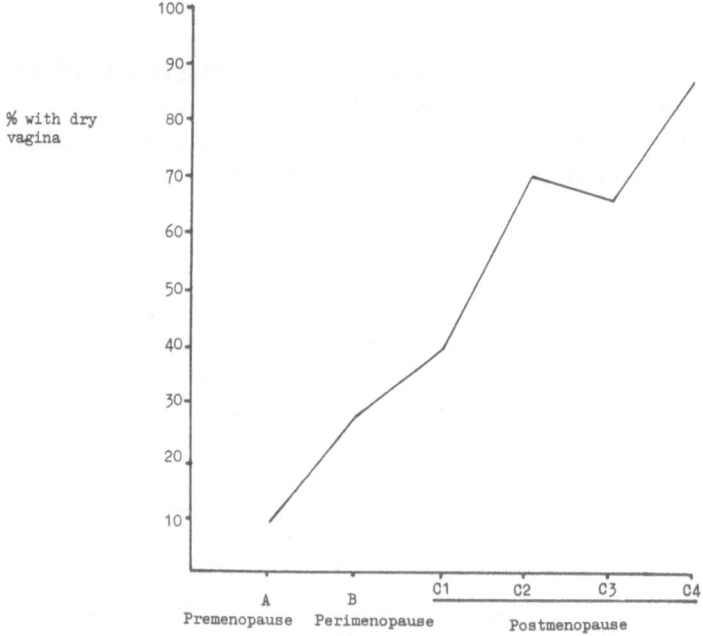

Figure 16.4   Frequency of dry vagina, Lagos, Nigeria, 1984

Dry vagina

Figure 16.4 shows that 9% of premenopausal women complained of dry vagina; 40% at 1–3 years after menopause and 67% by 4–6 years after menopause. None of the women had received medication for treatment of vaginal dryness and most of the women believed that no such treatment was available.

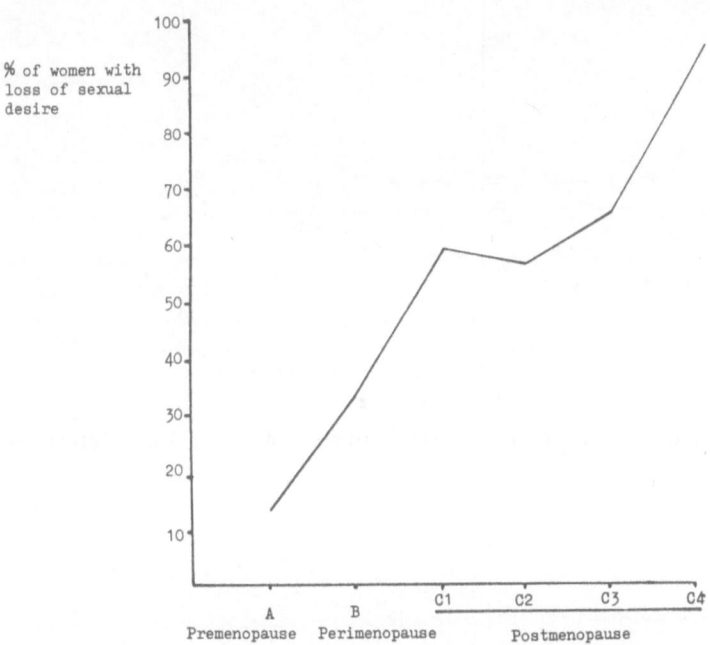

Figure 16.5   Frequency of loss of sexual desire, Lagos, Nigeria, 1984

Loss of sexual desire

Figure 16.5 indicates the loss of sexual desire with increasing menopausal age.

Most of the women associated their loss of desire to old age. Unfortunately, no data were obtained about orgasmic response and whether or not this capacity changed at the menopause. The investigator felt he could not comfortably ask the women about orgasm as it was not a subject ordinarily discussed between men and women in the Nigerian culture.

Changes in the sexual partner

Figures 16.6 and 16.7 indicate how the women reported that their male partners experienced decrease in sexual desire and sexual response with increasing menstrual age.

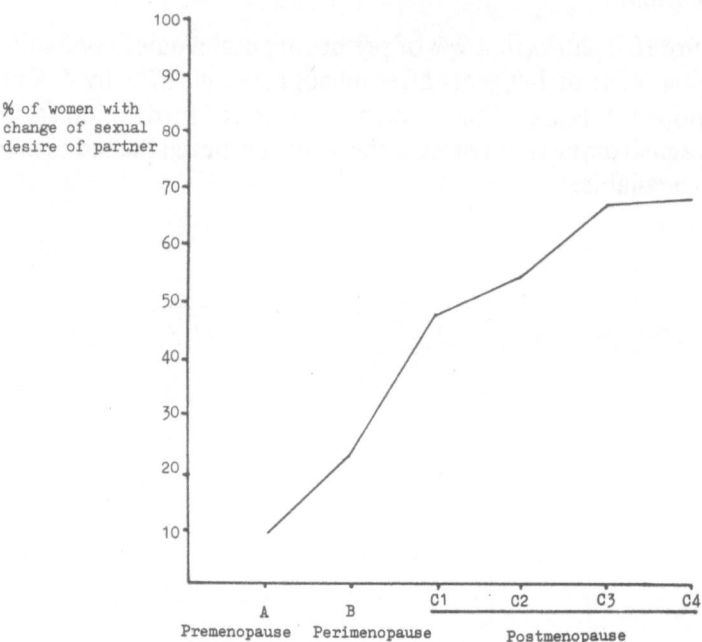

Figure 16.6 Frequency of change in sexual desire of partner, Lagos, Nigeria, 1984

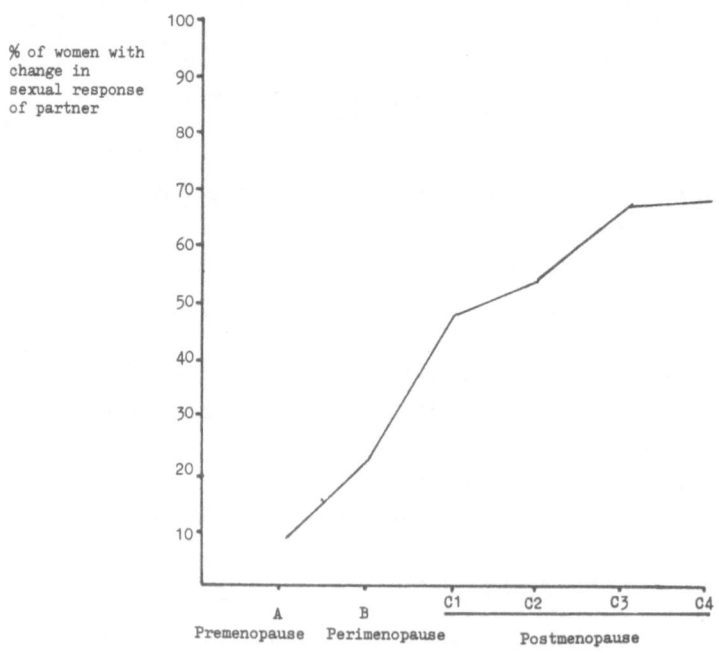

Figure 16.7 Frequency of change in sexual response of partner, Lagos, Nigeria, 1984

Vasomotor symptoms

Figure 16.8 shows the percentage of women with hot flashes in each menstrual age group. Seventy-two per cent of the women who had hot flashes also experienced excessive sweating. Differences in incidence of hot flashes were found in the different social classes: lower class 43%; middle class 40% and upper class 23%.

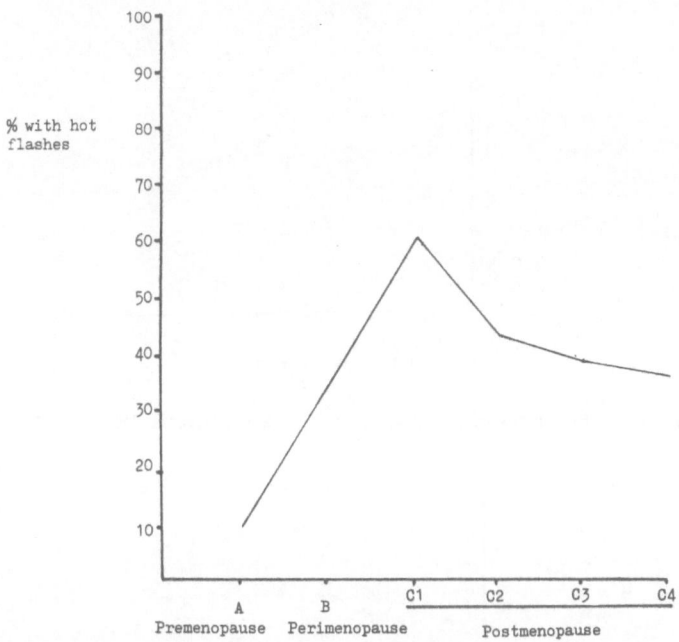

Figure 16.8 Frequency of hot flashes, Lagos, Nigeria, 1984

Neuropsychiatric symptoms

Irritability

The women were asked if they had noticed anything different about how it felt to be touched. Those who had noticed that they avoided being touched were regarded to have developed a state of increased irritability. Touch-avoidance was reported by 1% of the premenopausal women, 15% of the perimenopausal women and 46% of the women who were within 1-3 years of menopause. The incidence of this symptom declined with passing years and dropped to 8% in the women 9 or more years after menopause. Sixty-six per cent of the women who complained of touch-avoidance also complained of numbness in their fingers and toes.

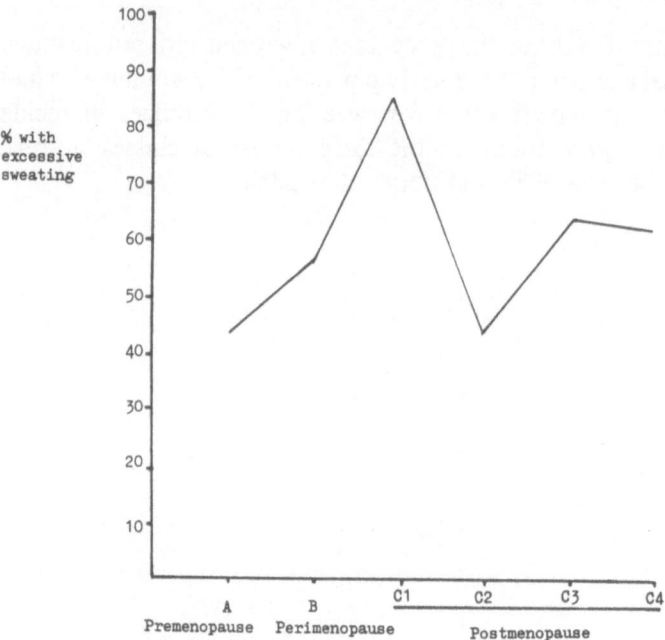

Figure 16.9 Frequency of excessive sweating, Lagos, Nigeria, 1984

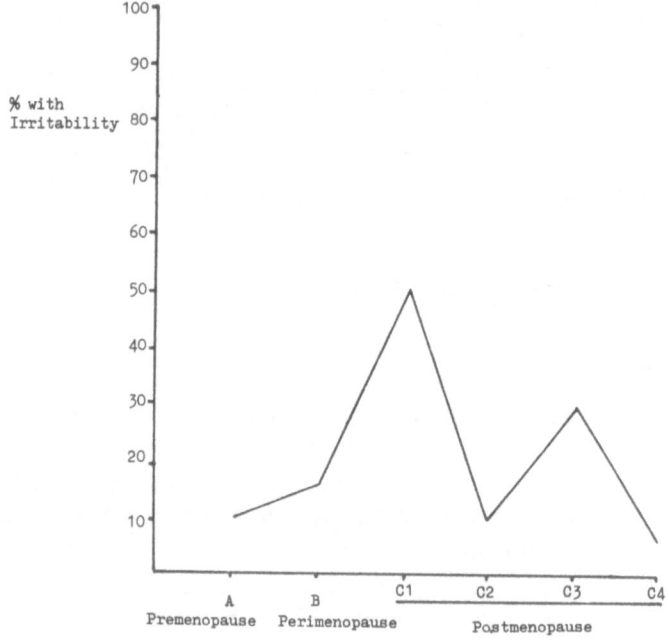

Figure 16.10 Frequency of irritability, Lagos, Nigeria, 1984

Numbness

As indicated by Figure 16.11, numbness was another neurological complaint associated with menopausal changes.

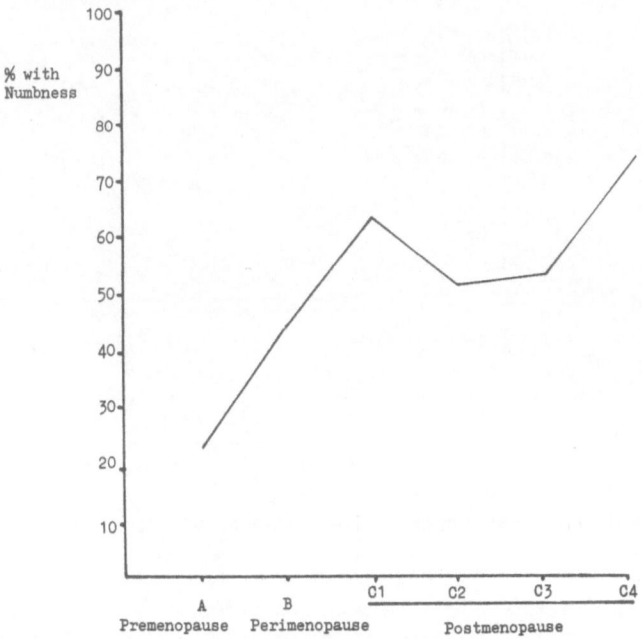

Figure 16.11   Frequency of numbness, Lagos, Nigeria, 1984

Insomnia

Figure 16.12 shows the insomnia findings. The women were asked about frequent awakening, difficulty going to sleep and early awakening. Frequent awakening was the type of insomnia experienced by most of the women who suffered from disturbed sleep.

Headache and dizziness

The frequency of these symptoms is illustrated by Fig. 16.13. A pattern similar to the incidence of insomnia was found.

Depression

Depression was defined as lowered spirit and sadness. Thirty-four per cent of all the women experienced some degree of depression during the

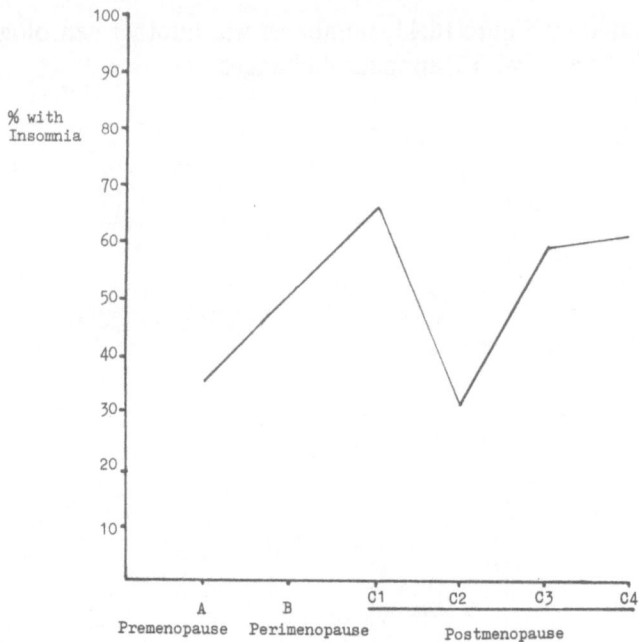

Figure 16.12 Frequency of insomnia, Lagos, Nigeria, 1984

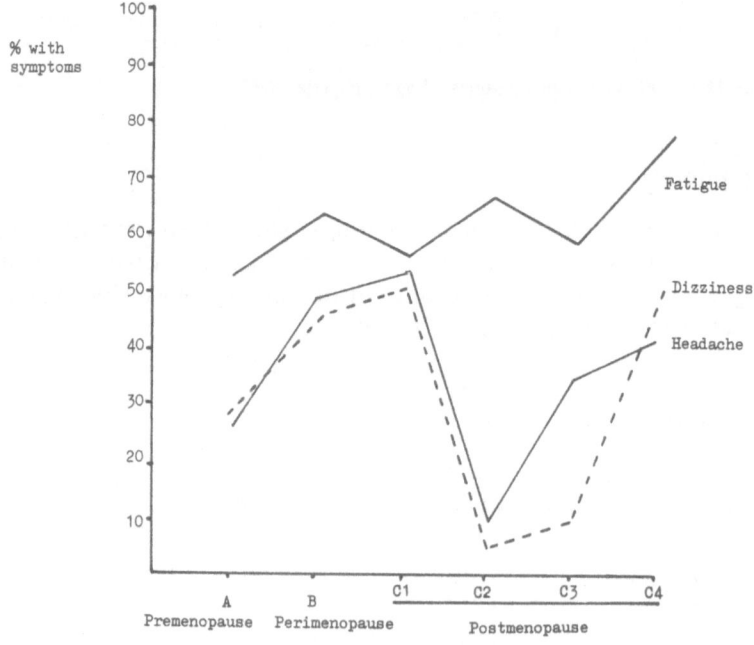

Figure 16.13 Frequency of fatigue, headache and dizziness, Lagos, Nigeria, 1984

time periods studied. The percentage of those who were depressed was highest in the middle social class (38%), followed by 29% of the upper-class women and 26% of the lower social class.

DISCUSSION

This study is one of very few menopause surveys of African women[1-3]. We believe it is the first study done in Nigeria. It is also unusual in being a study of an entirely Black, non-patient population as review of the major published epidemiologic studies indicates the women surveyed were almost entirely Caucasian[4-6]. It appears from this survey that the pattern of symptom formation in Nigerians in Lagos is similar to that of women elsewhere. Nevertheless, none of the women had received hormone replacement therapy and few of the women themselves were aware that medical treatment existed for their problems.

Attitude toward menopause in different cultures has been regarded as a determinant of symptomatology[6-8]. In this survey, attitudes toward menopause appeared to be determined to a large extent by the degree of signs and symptoms experienced. Most negative were the women in the 1-3-year postmenopause group who were having the most vasomotor, psychosexual and neuropsychiatric symptoms. The lower social class women had the most severe symptoms, e.g. the incidence of hot flashes in the lower socioeconomic class was almost twice that of the women in the upper socioeconomic class. A similar finding was reported in studies of western European women[9,10].

The mean age of menopause in this study is 1-2 years younger than commonly reported in other surveys[6,11].

It is clear from this study that menopause has detrimental effects on sexuality, for both the women and their marital partners. The decrease in sexual activity is in keeping with the studies of Pfeiffer et al.[12], Bottiglioni and DeAloysio[13] and Hallstrom[14]. Both male and female loss of sexual desire and sexual dysfunction contribute to a decline in activity, so that by 9 years after menopause only 30% of married couples continue to maintain a regularity to their sex lives together. In parts of Nigeria, menopause marks a point at which a husband marries a second younger wife with whom an entire new family is procreated. This cultural pattern contributes significantly to the population increase. It is interesting to consider that attention to the sexuality of the couple at mid-life could help the problem of population explosion in a country where there are already more than 80 million people and resources are limited.

It was not possible to gain as complete a picture of sexuality as has been reported by others. For example, Leiblum et al.[15] have described the problem of vulva and vaginal atrophy as contributing to decreased activity. As none of the women in this study population received hormones, atrophy may well have been prevalent. However, no pelvic examinations were done as the population was not a patient group.

Sarrel and Whitehead have described sex problems at menopause in the desire, excitement and orgasm phases of the sex response cycle[16]. In addition, Sarrel has described the impact of female biological change on the male partner's sexual interest and response[17]. The present findings also indicate sexuality change in the husbands at the time of the wife's menopause. It was not possible, however, to interview the men and trace further the specifics of female change which impacted on the men. Neither was it possible to obtain detailed information about orgasm or clitoral response or other sexually intimate matters, as such topics are rarely discussed in such a way in the Nigerian culture. Because pelvic examinations were not included in the study, it was not possible to determine to what degree vaginismus contributed to dyspareunia. In the Sarrel and Whitehead study, 50% of the women with dyspareunia had demonstrable vaginismus[16].

Vasomotor symptoms were present in 10% of the women still menstruating regularly. Hot flashes therefore are relatively common in this country, which lies between latitudes 4 degrees and 14 degrees north of the equator. Humidity, which can be as high as 95% for long periods of time, is also a factor, especially in the south and west. The frequency of hot flashes does rise, however, to a peak of 60.3% in the 1–3 years postmenopause women, and 55.7% of the 9 years postmenopause women are still experiencing these symptoms.

Among the neuropsychiatric symptoms, attention is drawn to the signs of altered peripheral sensory nerve function. The symptoms include numbness and tingling, aversion to touch and clothing intolerance. As previously reported[16, 17], these symptoms affected approximately 30% of women seen in the King's College Hospital Menopause Clinic and the Yale Menopause Program. Jaszmann[6] and Bungay[4] have described a similar frequency of neurological symptoms. The symptoms may reflect a change in peripheral nerve function as a primary change (the work of Kow and Pfaff[18] and of Rauramo[19] is relevant in this regard), or may be secondary to ischemia as peripheral blood vessels react to the hypo-estrogenic state. The blood flow enhancing effects of estrogen have been shown by Semmens and Wagner in their studies of vaginal change before and after estrogen replacement[20]. More recently, Sarrel has shown similar effects on vulva blood flow using a laser Doppler instrument to measure change[21]. In the Nigerian women the maximal incidence of neurologic symptoms reached 46.5% in the women 1–3 years postmenopause. Change in neurologic function may bear significance to change in sexual function, and also to impairment of functional capacity both at work and in the home.

In conclusion, we find a high incidence of menopausal signs and symptoms among Nigerian women in Lagos documenting a need to direct attention to these issues as a major medical concern, especially since neither the women themselves nor their husbands recognize the potential for health information and health care to be of help.

REFERENCES

1. Abramson, J. B. *et al*. (1960). Age at menopause of urban Zulu women. *Science*, **132**, 356–7
2. Maoz, B. *et al*. (1977). The perception of menopause in five ethnic groups in Israel. *Acta Obstet. Gynecol. Scand*. (Suppl.), **65**, 69–76
3. Utian, W. H. (1972). The true clinical features of post-menopause and oophorectomy and the response to oestrogen therapy. *S. Afr. Med. J.*, **46**, 732
4. Bungay, G. R. *et al*. (1980). Study of symptoms in middle life with special reference to the menopause. *Br. Med. J.*, **281**, 181–3
5. Gray, R. H. (1976). The menopause-epidemiological and demographic considerations. In Beard, R. J. (ed.) *The Menopause*. pp. 25–40. (Lancaster: MTP Press)
6. Jaszmann, L. J. B. (1976). Epidemiology of the climacteric syndrome. In Campbell, S. (ed.) *The Management of the Menopause and Post-menopausal Years*. pp. 11–23. (Lancaster: MTP Press)
7. Flint, M. P. and Garcia, M. (1979). Culture and the climacteric. *J. Biol. Sci.* (Suppl.), **6**, 197–215
8. Maoz, B. *et al*. (1970). Female attitudes to menopause. *Soc. Psychol.*, **5**(1), 35
9. Van Keep, P. A. and Kellerhals, M. (1975). The impact of sociocultural factors on symptom formation. *Psychother. Psychosom.*, **23**, 251
10. Van Keep, P. A. (1974). *The Menopause: a study of the attitudes of women in Belgium, France, Gt. Britain and West Germany*. (Geneva: International Health Foundation)
11. McKinlay, S. *et al*. (1972). An investigation of the age at menopause. *J. Biol. Sci.*, **4**, 161–73
12. Pfeiffer, E., Verwoerdt, A. and Davis, G. C. (1972). Sexual behavior in middle life. *Am. J. Psychiatry*, **128**, 1262–7
13. Bottiglioni, F. and DeAloysio, D. (1982). Female sexual activity as a function of climacteric conditions and age. *Maturitas*, **4**, 27–32
14. Hallstrom, T. (1977). Sexuality in the Climacteric. In Greenblatt, R. B. and Studd, J. (eds.) *Clin. Obst. Gynecol.: The Menopause*, Vol. 4, pp. 227–39. (London: Saunders)
15. Leiblum, S. *et al*. (1983). Vaginal atrophy in the post-menopausal woman – the importance of sexual activity and hormones. *J. Am. Med. Assoc.*, **249**, 2195–8
16. Sarrel, P. and Whitehead, M. (1985). Sex and menopause: defining the issues. *Maturitas*
17. Sarrel, P. (1982). Sex problems after menopause: a study of fifty married couples treated in a sex counseling program. *Maturitas*, **4**, 231
18. Kow, L. M. and Pfaff, D. W. (1973). Effects of estrogen treatment on the size of receptive field and response threshold of pudendal nerve in the female rat. *Neuroendocrinol.*, **13**, 299–313
19. Rauramo, L. (1972). Aging and estrogen. In Van Keep, P. and Lauritzen, N. (eds.) *Progr. Hormone Res.* p. 121. (Basel: Karger)
20. Semmens, J. and Wagner, G. C. (1982). Estrogen deprivation and vaginal function in post-menopausal women. *J. Am. Med. Assoc.*, **248**, 445–8
21. Sarrel, P. (1984). The use of the laser Doppler to measure vulva blood flow during sexual fantasy. Paper presented to the Xth Annual Meeting of The International Academy of Sex Research (submitted)

Chapter 17

The cultural climacteric in crosscultural perspective

Brian M. du Toit

> Although we surely ought to document regularities in human behavior and perception, we need equal appreciation for the diversity of aging experiences humans can create (ref. 1, p. 31)

The material presented here, as well as the discussion which follows, assume a clearcut dichotomy between two major components of human existence. This dichotomy is emphasized by disciplinary specialization and focus. I am speaking of the contrast between the physiological-anatomical and the sociocultural-behavioral. This dichotomy has long been recognized and is assumed in the writings of Brown, Wilbush and others, while it is explicit in the writings of Kaufert. This chapter recognizes a growing list of contributors to the field of climacteric studies; however, it will place emphasis on the sociocultural aspects. Thus, while hormonal and cellular changes mark the female climacteric, these may or may not be recognized by a particular people at a particular time. This *clinical climacteric* is marked by the slow-down of ovarian functions, by related hormonal imbalances, and finally by the cessation of menstruation - a clinical event called menopause. There is, however, also a *cultural climacteric*. This is marked by role changes brought on by age and family, by the social recognition of having achieved a certain stage in the life cycle, and by rights and privileges allowed such a person. These may or may not coincide with the physiological and biological changes and the ultimate cessation of menstruation.

INTRODUCTION

In a previous study we argued[2] that in traditional societies menstruation was not the regular event experienced by modern women. Thus, what people in traditional societies recognized was frequently not menopause (in the clinical sense) but the completion of the reproductive years (in a socio-jural sense). What was seen and terminologically distinguished was not a woman whose ovaries had failed but one who had completed her childbearing role and had entered her postreproductive phase by voluntarily accepting a socially defined postreproductive status even before this was necessitated by her physiological condition. She was not necessarily of the chronological age nor the clinical condition that we would designate as postmenopausal.

Because this frequently referred to a sociocultural status, we also find that researchers frequently use terms like 'passed their climacteric'[3], 'past childbearing'[4] or 'passed the menopause'[5] indiscriminately. Van Arsdale[6] writes about the traditional Asmat (New Guinea) society he studied. He states that 'only 12.3 percent is over 45, or clearly "old"' but he then says that the menopause signals the onset of 'old age' in women. We know that many women stop menstruating by 45 but as many stop at 55. I would venture that these authors were dealing with the sociocultural status of women who had completed their childbearing role – women thus who had returned to a socially defined non-reproductive status.

The position to be taken in this discussion is that there in fact exists a cultural climacteric and that it is a justifiable subject for research and study. A growing number of researchers are contributing to this field. Constructive recent studies include refs 2, 6–11. While consideration of the cultural climacteric cannot ignore physiological changes, it must be viewed and interpreted in terms of other sociocultural phenomena. These latter include the sociological life cycle, life course and life events, roles associated with marriage and motherhood, and status ascribed and achieved in these contexts. Chronologically (and clinically) we recognize a life cycle from birth, through maturation, aging and death. Culturally, however, a group of people might recognize a large number of stages depending on such things as circumcision, ritual purity versus pollution, marriage, the birth of the first child, marriage of own children and so forth. Not only do each of these imply changes in status and the role to be performed, but they may also involve changes in name, dress, and behavior.

The hypothesis which will present a central theme to this discussion, might be phrased in the following words:

Hypothesis
A woman who is believed to have completed her childbearing years is released from restrictions which had been placed on her when she

entered the reproductive state. Stated differently: the lifting of restrictions associated with the female reproductive function is based on socially defined criteria.

Two corollaries can be derived:

Corollary 1: A woman past childbearing returns to a socially defined nonreproductive state. In this state roles are not dependent upon the clinical climacteric.
Corollary 2: In the traditional world a woman past childbearing gains in prestige and status, and thus experiences an expansion of roles. The cultural climacteric is thus liberating.

To test this we should discuss the concepts in crosscultural perspective using as wide a frame of reference as possible. We also need to clarify the concept of liberation, i.e. the freeing of a woman from restrictions (social and ritual) and the expansion of optative features in her role-playing as well as status ascription. Angrist[13] uses a very useful concept, namely 'sex role constellation'. According to this we would consider a variety of numerous and changing roles as these find expression in different contexts and locations. These certainly apply to the climacteric woman.

The concept of liberation implies, of course, that there is no stigma attached to the new life phase being entered; that restrictions which governed the earlier life phase are now relaxed; it implies that roles in the new life phase are valued and useful, providing prestige; that women in the new life phase experience an expansion of status and roles; in short, that they are liberated from earlier restrictive and constrictive conditions. Each of these will be discussed in the light of crosscultural evidence. While there is a new awareness concerning the crosscultural perspective, 'crosscultural data on the menopause' are extremely limited[7, 14]. There is furthermore a need for these kinds of studies. *Lancet* (12 July 1982) remarked editorially that 'information from developing countries in particular is scanty; there are virtually no data on such basic matters as the age distribution of the menopause; and little is known about the sociocultural significance of the menopause in different settings'. One welcome addition in this context is the recently published volume edited by Brown and Kerns[15].

NO STIGMA

It is common in traditional societies to find not only a lack of stigma attached to age but in fact an increase in prestige. This pertains equally to the cultural climacteric. Speaking of the Black Carib, Kerns[9] states: 'Infertility and old age are so closely connected in Black Carib thought that they frequently use one for the other . . . of course no real stigma attaches to menopause'. This is also true in Mexico where women welcome it because they will no longer be able to bear children[16]. All through Africa age is respected, and in China it is a compliment to be addressed as 'aged dame' and young women frequently are heard wishing that they were old[17].

But age is very relative. The end of the childbearing years does not necessarily agree with clinical menopause. Most researchers now agree that the age of menopause, around 50, has not changed significantly in centuries. When we thus read that women's status changes after they have completed their childbearing years we are usually dealing not with menopause, but with a sociocultural (and environmental) influence which causes a woman to have her last child between the ages of 30 and 45. Usually, having completed this phase of her life, she is considered old. Roberts and Sinclair[18], discussing the menstrual cycle among women in Jamaica, explain that the cycle terminates at ages over 45, 'that is after the completion of their childbearing period' (pp. 92-3). Also in Colombia[19] old age is transferred to the period of the 40s, and relatively few people reach 'old age' in Peru[20].

Age 35 in women seems to have been considered a critical transitional age. Speaking of the Bontoc Igorot of the Philippines, Jenks[21] states that 'by 30 she is getting old', while Held[22] for the Waropen of New Guinea sees 35 as the critical age[23]. Data for some of the American Indians mention the same ages. 'A woman is old on the plains at the age of 35 years, and seldom healthy.' The reproductive age was from 18 to 35[24]; see related ages given by Dorsey[25]. This also pertained to the Inuit in the Canadian Arctic[26].

African ethnographies suggest much the same picture in terms of statuses which are recognized. Thus the Nyamwezi recognize the female life cycle as consisting of a baby, young girl, young woman and old woman[27]. The status 'old woman' among the Dorobo is achieved 'when they begin to look old'[28]. None of these authors refer to the cessation of menstruation nor do any of the ethnographers who use the term 'menopause'. By the use of this term they refer to a woman who is old, who no longer experiences pregnancies, or who no longer has sexual intercourse[29-31]. In fact, women of this age are frequently expected to refrain from sexual intercourse. Such women may be grandmothers, women whose children have reached marriageable age, a woman whose eldest child is circumcized (at puberty) and so forth (see discussion in ref. 32). Women past childbearing age could no longer pollute hunters or their gear[33]. But these references should not suggest that these conditions are restricted to traditional societies. During the 1930s French doctors advised that 'postmenopausal women abstain from sexual activity' and this was also true in Germany[34].

Our own current research among Indian South Africans has failed to produce a culturally recognized status of 'postmenopausal woman'. Thus the woman who is released from *purdah* in Indian society, or the woman who is terminologically recognized as having entered the status of older woman, may or may not menstruate – it is beside the point. Tamil-speaking informants recognize the *peri pombla* or 'big woman' in her 40s and 50s (usually a young grandmother in contrast to the *kalevi* or 'old woman'). If these people are related to the speaker they might be addressed as *ama* (mother) or *aya* (grandmother) respectively. Gujarati-speakers speak of a *dosima* or old lady, based on age only. All of these categories of women are expected to be past the age of sexual involvement. Discussion in research of a possible pregnancy at age 43 is invariably met with dismay and a statement that it would cause great embarrassment. Part of this derives from a woman having grown children, and especially sons, because her status is enhanced by having a daughter-in-law.

Not being sexually active assures that there will be no pregnancies, and when this is associated with early anovulation, the status change from 'woman' to 'neutral' is recognized early. Thus Khmer women at this stage crop their hair close to the scalp showing that they renounce worldly concerns and it also 'neutralizes their sex'[35]. At this stage women are said to be without sexual allure[36], or may be said to 'look like men'[37], or are 'often called men'[39]. Women who were beyond the childbearing age were said to be ritually neutral and could thus participate in religious and ritual activities. Not only did their status change, but also their role in society.

RELAXATION OF RESTRICTIONS

Most societies in the world mark the attainment of menarche with some ritual accentuating the girls' potential for childbearing. Having completed the childbearing stage of their lives, these same women return to a liberated state in which they may once again enter the cattle byre, appear in public without a veil, or sit in the company of men. (Hammond-Tooke[40] reflects the position in numerous African societies when he remarks that among the Bhaca 'women after menopause and girls before the age of puberty are allowed free entry to the cattle-kraal . . .' (pp. 69–70).)

Black Carib women in their mid-40s have 'borne their last children and at about this age they begin to take a more active part in ritual affairs. They enjoy greater freedom of movement, association, and activity as fertility declines and they pass the age of childbearing'[41]. Also in Algeria the childbearing years are correlated with the sexually active years when women are secluded. Those who have passed the childbearing years are seen on the street without veils[42]. This is essentially the same for Pakistani women for whom there is a relaxation of the constraints of *purdah*[43]. (See also Modak[44] with reference to India.) The same freeing from restrictions and freedom of movement is also found in Taiwan[45], Korea[46], and Yugoslavia[47].

EXPANSION OF STATUS AND ROLE

Freedom from restrictions, social as well as ritual, is not necessarily equivalent to an increase in status and access to new spheres of authority. The latter features are, however, found in association with the climacteric in numerous societies. By 'graduating from sex and childbearing' a woman also graduates from the restrictions of the female role. In a legal sense she becomes a 'man'.

This expansion of roles is clear among the Mundurucu. In the meetings of men, which are usually closed to adult women, men will in fact make room for such a liberated woman to sit among them[48]; the liberated Zapotec woman may go anywhere alone and attend fiestas[49]; for the first time since menarche a Gypsy woman is not subject to the strict *mokadi* regulations[50]; and in Ethiopia a woman may mark her attainment of venerated elder status with a rite of *Kasa*, for it is assumed such an elder, man or woman, is 'too old to sin any longer'[51]. Speaking of a Serbian community, Halpern[52] points out that women of 40 have reached the status of respected elder which also gives them prestige and authority. Much the same status change is found among Puerto Rican women[53], and Iteso women[4] past the childbearing age; among Sotho women who have 'passed their climacteric'[3] and among 'postmenopausal' women in Central America[60]. (This is true for most of Africa. See Basden[54], Herrick[55], Wagner[29], Nukunya[5], and Baxter and Butt[58]. It also applies to the Malagasy area[59].) Such older women may in fact become involved in cults and secret societies 'in search of a new sphere of authority'[61]. (Current research among Indian South Africans has demonstrated the increased involvement of grandmothers who are past the stage of having more children in religion and ritual. These women are recognized as ritually pure, as having time to participate in prayers and ritual, and as having religious wisdom and insight.) In an overall sense it could be suggested that as the economic or reproductive roles of men or women decrease, so the ritual roles and access to supernatural forces will increase. In most societies the respect with which the aged are treated is a direct incidence of this shift of power.

THE USEFUL NEW ROLE

It is uncommon for women who are no longer childbearers to lose their domestic roles. They usually continue to serve as babysitters for grandchildren, and still do light household chores. They are usually seen as experienced or even experts at childrearing; as having the wisdom of age combined with the practical experience; and as having more time and patience.

Amos and Harrell[33] point out that because of this role continuity women in many societies 'managed to weather the aging process better than men'. The senior citizens, as we like to call them, are not isolated from their families but continue to be a vital part, giving and receiving support. (Shanas[62] and Bart[63] have both discussed the significance of role continuity as it finds expression in the extended family.) In Malaysia women in this new status are treated with 'polite deference'[64], as are women in Burma[65], Poland[66], and the Andean region of South America[67]. In Thailand we find much the same position as postmenopausal women retire from active household management but spend their time caring for grandchildren, and helping with general chores such as cooking. At this age they are freer in their behavior and manner, breaking many taboos and prohibitions[68, 69].

Rituals are frequently part and parcel of status acquisition. We do not necessarily have a ritual to mark the beginning and the end of a particular status. Thus marriage is marked by a ritual; its termination normally is not. Becoming a student is not ritually marked; graduation has all the trappings of ritual. The interesting fact is that while the attainment of the reproductive phase of life, and the status associated with it, is commonly marked by ritual, its termination is not. In Van Gennep's terminology, the attainment of fertility is a *rite de passage*, Hardly anywhere in the world is the menopause marked by such a ritual. The single example which we have come across pertains to the Meo of Northern Thailand.

> Each village has what is called a playground where the younger people assemble after a hard day's work in the field and pair off. Sex is available and happy. They also have a menopause ceremony for the older women. When a woman goes through the menopause she has a celebration if she can afford it. It is the only culture which I know of which celebrates the menopause in a positive manner. The woman gains some of the social attributes of a man. For instance, she is allowed to plant the first rice in the fields, which previously only men could do. This ceremony is a great celebration for all the family and the whole village is invited to it; it involves killing a good many ducks and pigs and is obviously expensive. Also, caution has to be exercised. One woman went through this ceremony and then her husband died – she remarried which manifestly proved that she was a woman again. This meant the new husband had to pay back her original family for all the animals that had been killed for the ceremony. Another woman had a child after the ceremony and she had to repay many ducks and pigs[70]!

Interesting as this example may seem it is obvious that we are once again dealing with the inaccurate use of the term 'menopause'. If a woman had in fact gone through the menopause we would not expect either a renewed menses nor a pregnancy. We would suggest that this in fact refers to the termination of reproduction, i.e. the achieving of 'old women' status, rather than clinical menopause.

These comments bring us to the ritual and religious realm. Hardly anywhere is this better expressed than in those communities where Muslims dominate.

The Middle East, or more specifically Islamic societies, are particularly conservative. Female religious activities mostly take place at home while men practice public worship. The latter activity is shared by post-menopausal women[71]. In daily life women are strictly controlled, first by their fathers and brothers and later by their husbands. But once they have passed the childbearing years they are considered to be 'without sexual allure' and are permitted greater freedom[36, 72]. Speaking of Iranian nomads, Tapper[73] states: 'For women, leadership is only possible after menopause, when their status approximates that of men. This happens both because of the old woman's presumed loss of sexuality and because of her freedom from many of her former domestic responsibilities, including childbearing'. While her status may improve outside the home she dreads the loss of the 'wife-and-mother' role in the home. 'Out of panic, they sometimes try to have just one more child, who will rejuvenate them in their husbands' eyes more effectively than a face lift[74]. (If the cessation of the menstrual flow marks menopause and thus old age, and if this had a negative connotation, then one might expect some people to aim at continuing the flow which would produce an extension of youth. The Chorti Indians in Guatemala use certain plant remedies which relieve hemorrhages. In large doses this same herb induces the menstrual flow. 'They are often drunk by older women to induce the flow after menopause'[75].) The Egyptian sociologist Hamed Ammar[76] documents the freedom which an old woman enjoys and the fact that she may pass a group of men without covering her face. These restrictions and their relaxation are based squarely on injunctions found in the Koran. Women who are menstruating are not pure (*tahir*) and may not enter the mosque, nor may they handle the sacred writings. Certain fasting periods are also affected, as is the pilgrimage to Mecca. Those who are pregnant or postmenopausal may participate in these rituals. (Section 3:25 in the Koran promises men in heaven 'companions pure and holy'. The word used is *motohara*, derived from *tahir* referred to in the text and with an -a (feminine) ending.) Saudi Arabia in fact has a question on the official immigration forms asking whether or not an applicant has reached the menopause.

WOMEN AS MOTHERS

Almost universally we find reference to old age coinciding with changes in the mother role and the cessation of sexual activity. These two, are, of course, separable. One of the best examples in this connection is the so-called 'ghost marriage' among the Nuer, a pastoral people in the Sudan. In this case an influential older woman who has no children, or who wishes to have an heir, may marry a girl. The older woman finances the marriage transaction complete with bride-wealth as if she were a man. The younger woman may be visited by lovers and bear children. These serve to establish the older woman as their 'father' for purposes of inheritance and social status[77]. It is important to recognize that we are dealing here with the social recognition of a certain status. Gender is incidental to the role played (and ritual performed) and the status thus achieved. As an old woman, classified as sexless, may adopt a child, so an older woman can 'produce' a child without her sexual involvement entering into the role.

NEGATIVE VIEWS

Less common is the tendency to view the later climacteric years in a negative way. This may in fact be related to the western European syndrome associated with fear of the loss of youth and the loss of status attached to it. Grunberger[78] and Schalk[79] respectively comment on the 'twilight of eugenic superfluity' and the 'fortyish matron' when writing about the German woman. Also in the United States and some other western European countries we find the fear of status loss which accompanies the maturing of the family, the 'empty nest syndrome' and tensions created by a role change forced on women in the absence of the extended family.

Bart, in a number of very stimulating studies has addressed this issue[6, 14, 63, 80, 81]. She suggests that the presumed causal relationship between menopause and mental depression is spurious. Rather, depression results from a situation where a woman either cannot continue rewarding roles, or her role receives negative value. An example is her role after the children leave home – men experience the same depression when after retirement there is no role continuity. Bart, speaking of the United States, says: 'Black women had a lower rate of depression than white women. The patterns of black female-role behavior rarely result in depression in middle-age. Often, the 'granny' or 'aunty' lives with the family and cares for the children while the children's mother works; thus, the older woman suffers no maternal role loss[63]. Much the same positive experience due to generational interchange is reported from Italy[82]. (This position is also true among Indian South Africans where the *Kutum* (extended family) still is fairly strong. When a woman has grandchildren her whole orientation changes. She now starts to dote on them and cares for them almost day and night. As increasing numbers of younger women are working the grandmother, often in her late 30s or early 40s, takes over as matriarch in the 'big house'.)

A question which has not yet been studied is the total constellation of women's roles, i.e. what components other than mother and sex partner are of critical importance in different cultures. Dougherty[83] raises a very important question when she asks: 'what transitions occur cross-culturally for childless women (customarily 10–20% of women and a higher proportion in some groups) and women who have no children that survive to adulthood?'. What happens to women who adopt children? Is adoption equal to natural parentage and does adoption substitute in cases where parents do not have naturally born offspring? Counts[84] points out that adoption is quite common and widespread in the Pacific, 'and in West New Britain people continue to adopt children up into their seventies'. Does the social and legal role of parenthood substitute for the biological one? My own research among New Guinea highlanders, and currently among urban Indians in South Africa, tends to offer a positive reply. In the case of childlessness adoption is repeatedly mentioned as a viable alternative and one which would satisfy a very critical and demanding mother-in-law.

It is quite common in traditional societies to find a great deal of ritual and status associated with motherhood. This is related no doubt to the need for offspring to strengthen the kin group numerically, to generate bride-wealth, and to give continuity to the family. Thus, premarital women among the Homa nomadic pastoralists care for the cattle, a role which is also assigned to spinsters and divorcees. The postmenopausal woman, however, does not resume these duties even though she has lost the reproductive functions, since she gains new authority free from ritual restrictions[85]. (See also Mitchell *et al*[86] for Guyana, and Holleman[87] for the Shona of Zimbabwe.) Even though she does not return to cattle herding, she is freed from restrictions which mark women who are married and can have children. 'Having a child . . . changes the status of a woman in all classes of Indian society', says Roy[88]. She goes on to discuss the Bengali woman in her middle age but ties it directly to the aspects of motherhood and childbearing. Large families are common but among urban and better-educated women fewer children are valued. Thus a woman may stop reproducing before she is even close to the age of menopause. But after her last child she is made to believe by society that she is entering the time of waning sexual and reproductive capacity, even though in reality she may not be. If she has her last child in her mid-thirties, she may only remain absorbed in rearing it till she is forty. In this respect, the Bengali proverb 'A woman is old by the time she is twenty' has some truth in it[88].

CONCLUSION

The hypothesis which guided this discussion was based on the understanding that there is a cultural climacteric to be distinguished from a clinical climacteric. It also implied that when authors in the past wrote about 'menopause' they did not necessarily imply the cessation of the menstrual flow. Menopause then was frequently used as synonymous with postreproductive, postchildbearing or old. The latter are all socio-cultural concepts which imply a specific status within the society and a particular role associated with that status. These are sociobehavioral concepts and must be analyzed and explained within the sociobehavioral context.

Specifically our hypothesis stated that a woman in her postrepro-ductive state (however that may be defined) is released from restrictions. These women then *return* to a nonreproductive state with the status and role associated with this state. Such a woman experiences an expansion of roles which is liberating.

The data from a very wide geographical range confirm both the hypothesis and the corollaries.

Acknowledgements

This chapter was written while in the research field in Africa, away from my office and library. I therefore very sincerely appreciate constructive comments on an earlier draft of this paper by Judith K. Brown.

REFERENCES

1. Karp, D. A. and Yoels, W. C. (1982). *Experiencing the Life Cycle: a social psychology of aging.* (Springfield, Ill.: Charles C. Thomas)
2. Du Toit, B. M. and Suggs, D. (1983). Menopause: a sociocultural definition. *Florida J. Anthropol.*, **8**(2), Part 1, 1–23
3. Ashton, H. (1967). *The Basuto.* p. 100. (London: Oxford University Press)
4. Lawrence, J. C. D. (1957). *The Iteso.* p. 124. (London: Oxford University Press)
5. Nukunya, J. K. (1969). *Kinship and Marriage among the Anlo Ewe.* p. 153. (New York: Humanities Press)
6. Van Arsdale, P. W. (1981). The elderly Asmat of New Guinea. In Amoss, P. T. and Harrell, S. (eds.) *Other Ways of Growing Old: anthropological perspectives.* p. 118. (Stanford: Stanford University Press)
6a. Bart, P. (1969). *Why Women's Status Changes in Middle Age: the turns of the social Ferris wheel.* Sociological Symposium, Fall
7. Griffen, J. (1978). A cross-cultural investigation of behavioral changes at menopause. In Blumhagen, K. O. and Johnson, W. D. (eds.) *Women's Studies.* (London: Western Social Science Education)
8. Kaufert, P. A. (1982). Anthropology and the menopause: the development of a theoretical framework. *Maturitas*, **4**, 181–93
9. Kerns, V. (1980). Aging and mutual support relations among the Black Carib. In Fry, C. L. (ed.) *Aging in Culture and Society.* p. 116. (New York: J. F. Bergin)
10. Kerns, V. (1980). Menopause and the post-reproductive years. *National Women's Anthropology Newsletter*, vol. 4, Nos. 2 and 3
11. Brown, J. K. (1982). A cross cultural exploration of the end of the childbearing years. In Voda, A. M., Dinnerstein, M. and O'Donnell, S. R. (eds.) *Changing Perspectives on Menopause.* (Austin: University of Texas Press)

12. Flint, M. (1982). Anthropological perspectives of the menopause and middle age. *Maturitas*, **4**
13. Angrist, S. S. (1972). The study of sex roles. In Bardwick, J. M. (ed.) *Readings on the Psychology of Women*. (New York: Harper & Row)
14. Bart, P. (1977). The loneliness of the long-distance mother. In Stein, P. J., Richman, J. and Hannon, N. (eds.) *The Family*. (London: Addison-Wesley)
15. Brown, J. K. and Kerns, V. (eds.) (1984). *In Her Prime*. (South Hadley: Bergin and Garvey)
16. Lewis, O. (1963). *Life in a Mexican Village - Tepoztlàn Restudied*. p. 411. (Chicago: University of Illinois Press)
17. Creel, H. G. (1937). *The Birth of China*. p. 353. (New York: Reynal and Hitchcock)
18. Roberts, G. W. and Sinclair, S. A. (1978). *Women in Jamaica*. p. 92. (Millwood, NJ: KTO Press)
19. Reichel-Dolmatoff, G. and Reichel-Dolmatoff, A. (1966). *The People of Aritama: the cultural personality of a Colombian Mestizo village*. p. 335. (Chicago: University of Chicago Press)
20. Stein, W. W. (1961). *Hualcan: Life in the Highlands of Peru*. p. 164. (Ithaca, NY: Cornell University Press)
21. Jenks, A. E. (1905). *The Bontoc Igorot*. p. 44. (Manila: Bureau of Public Printing)
22. Held, G. J. (1957). *The Papuas of Waropen*. p. 38. (The Hague: Martinus Nijhoff)
23. Viljoen, S. (1936). *The Economics of Primitive Peoples*. p. 71. (London: P. S. King & Son)
24. Denig, E. T. (1930). *Indian Tribes of the Upper Missouri. The Assininboin*. (Ed. J. N. B. Hewitt). Annual Report of the Bureau of American Ethnology 1928-1929. p. 513. (Washington: Smithsonian Institution)
25. Dorsey, J. O. (1884). *Omaha Sociology*. Third annual report of the Bureau of American Ethnology, 1881-1882. p. 267. (Washington: Smithsonian Institution)
26. McElroy, A. (1975). Canadian Arctic modernization and change in female Inuit role identification. *Am. Ethnol.*, **2**, 662-86
27. Abrahams, R. G. (1967). *The Peoples of Greater Unyamwezi, Tanzania*. Part XVII, p. 67. (London: International African Institute)
28. Huntingford, G. W. B. (1969). *The Southern Nilo-Hamites*, Part VIII, p. 62. (London: International African Institute)
29. Wagner, G. (1960). The Abaluyia of Kavirondo (Kenya). In Forde, D. (ed.) *African Worlds: studies in the cosmological ideas and social values of African peoples*. pp. 38 and 42. (Oxford: Oxford University Press)
30. Winter, E. H. (no date). *Bwamba*. p. 174. (Cambridge: W. Heffer and Sons)
31. Schapera, I. (1941). *Married Life in an African Tribe*. p. 194. (Evanston: Northwestern University Press)
32. Ware, H. (1979). Social influences on fertility at later ages of reproduction. In Parkes, A. S., Herbertson, M. A. and Cole, J. (eds.) *Fertility in Middle Age*. Supplement No. 6 of *J. Biosoc. Sci.* (London: Spottiswoode Ballantyne)
33. Amos, P. T. and Harrell, S. (1981). *Introduction. Other ways of growing old: Anthropological perspectives*. p. 231, p. 8. (Stanford: Stanford University Press)
34. Stearns, P. N. (1976). *Old Age in European Society*. pp. 106 and 141. (New York: Holmes & Meier)
35. Ebihara, M. M. (1968). Svay, A Khmer village in Cambodia. Doctoral dissertation, Columbia University, p. 501
36. Crapanzano, V. (1980). *Tuhami: portrait of a Moroccan*. p. 31. (Chicago: Chicago University Press)
37. Warner, W. L. (1958). *A Black Civilization*. p. 132. (New York: Harper & Bros.)
39. Kidd, D. (1904). *The Essential Kafir*. p. 230. (London: Adam and Charles Black)
40. Hammond-Tooke, W. D. (1962). *Bhaca Society*. (London: Oxford University Press)
41. Kerns, V. (1983). *Women and the Ancestors: Black Carib kinship and ritual*. p. 191. (London: University of Illinois Press)
42. Walpole, N. C. *et al.* (1965). *US Army Area Handbook for Algeria*. p. 128. (Washington, DC: Foreign Area Studies Division, US Government Printers)
43. Pastner, C. McC. (1978). The status of women and property on a Baluchistan oasis in Pakistan. In Beck, L. and Kedie, N. (eds.) *Women in the Muslim World*. p. 445. (London: Harvard University Press)

44. Modak, M. R. (1945). *The Land and the People of India*. p. 98. (Philadelphia: J. B. Lippincot and Co.)
45. Gallin, B. (1966). *Hsin Hsing, Taiwan: A Chinese Village in Change*. p. 215. (Berkeley: University of California Press)
46. Osgood, C. (1951). *The Koreans and their Culture*. p. 114. (New York: Ronald Press)
47. McDonald, G. C. *et al.* (1973). *Area Handbook for Yugoslavia*. p. 127. (Washington, DC: Foreign Area Studies Division, US Government Printers)
48. Murphy, Y. and Murphy, R. F. (1974). *Women of the Forest*. p. 105. (New York: Columbia University Press)
49. Chinas, B. L. (1973). *The Isthmus Zapotecs: women's roles in cultural context*. p. 60. (New York: Holt, Rinehart and Winston)
50. Trigg, E. B. (1973). *Gypsy Demons and Divinities*. p. 54. (Secaucus, NJ: Citadel Press)
51. Gamst, F. C. (1969). *The Qemant: a pagan-Hebraic peasantry of Ethiopia*. p. 111. (New York: Holt, Rinehart and Winston)
52. Halpern, J. M. (1958). *A Serbian Village*. p. 203. (New York: Columbia University Press)
53. Steward, J. H. *et al.* (1956). *The People of Puerto Rico*. p. 223. (Urbana: University of Illinois Press)
54. Basden, G. T. (1966). *Among the Ibos of Nigeria*. p. 96. (London: Frank Cass)
55. Herrick, A. B. (1969). *Area Handbook for Uganda*. p. 111. (Washington, DC: Foreign Area Studies Division, US Government Printers)
58. Baxter, P. J. W. and Butt, A. (1953). *The Azande and Related Peoples of the Anglo-Egyptian Sudan and Belgian Congo*. p. 115. (London: International African Institute)
59. Nelson, H. D. *et al.* (1973). *Area Handbook for the Malagasy Republic*. p. 87. (Washington, DC: Foreign Area Studies Division, US Government Printers)
60. Cosminsky, S. and Scrimshaw, M. (1982). Sex roles and subsistence: a comparative analysis of three central American communities. In Loveland, C. A. and Loveland, F. O. (eds.) *Sex Roles and Social Change in Native Lower Central American Societies*. p. 44. (Chicago: University of Illinois Press)
61. Lewis, J. M. (1974). Patterns of protest among Non-Western women. In Prince, R. and Banner, D. (eds.) *Configurations*. p. 99. (Toronto: C. D. Heath)
62. Shanas, E. (1977). Family-kin networks and aging in cross-cultural perspective. In Stein, P. J., Richman, J. and Hannon, N. (eds.) *The Family*. (London: Addison-Wesley)
63. Bart, P. (1972). Depression in middle-aged women. In Bardwick, J. M. (ed.) *Readings on the Psychology of Women*. p. 140. (New York: Harper and Row)
64. Maday, B. C. *et al.* (1965). *Area Handbook for Malaysia and Singapore*. p. 150. (Washington, DC: Foreign Area Studies Division, US Government Printers)
65. Henderson, J. *et al.* (1971). *Area Handbook for Burma*. p. 74. (Washington, DC: Foreign Area Studies Division, US Government Printers)
66. Benet, S. (1951). *Song, Dance and Customs of Peasant Poland*. p. 228. (London: Willmer)
67. Bourge, S. C. and Kay, B. W. (1981). *Women of the Andes*. p. 105. (Ann Arbor: University of Michigan Press)
68. Blanchard, W. (1958). *Thailand: its people, its society, its culture*. p. 437. (Connecticut: Human Relations Area Files)
69. De Young, J. (1955). *Village Life in modern Thailand*. p. 66. (Berkeley: University of California Press)
70. Potts, M. (1979). Discussion on sterilization and abortion in middle age. In Parkes, A. S. *et al.* (eds.). Fertility in middle age. Supplement No. 6, *J. Biosoc. Sci.* p. 162
71. Saunders, M. O. (1980). Women's role in a Muslim house town (Mirria, Republic of Niger). In Bourguignon, E. (ed.) *A World of Women*. p. 64. (New York: Praeger)
72. Maher, V. (1978). Women and social change in Morocco. In Beck, L. and Keddie, M. (eds.) *Women in the Muslim World*. (London: Harvard University Press)
73. Tapper, N. (1978). The women's subsociety among the Shahsevan Nomads of Iran. In Beck, L. and Keddie, N. (eds.) *Women in the Muslim World*. p. 377. (London: Harvard University Press)
74. Minai, N. (1981). *Women in Islam: tradition and transition in the Middle East*. p. 194. (New York: Seaview Books)
75. Wisdom, C. (1940). *The Chorti Indians of Guatemala*. p. 289. (Chicago: University of Chicago Press)

76. Ammar, H. (1954). *Growing up in an Egyptian Village*. p. 49. (London: Routledge and Kegan Paul)
77. Evans-Pritchard, E. E. (1951). *Kinship and Marriage among the Nuer*. (Oxford: Clarendon)
78. Grunberger, R. (1971). *A Social History of the Third Reich*. p. 262. (London: Cox and Wyman)
79. Schalk, A. (1971). *The Germans*. p. 341. (Englewood-Cliffs, NJ: Prentice-Hall)
80. Bart, P. (1970). Mother Portnoy's complaint. *Transactions*, vol. 8
81. Bart, P. (1976). Portnoy's mother's complaint: depression in middle-aged women. In Koltun, E. (ed.) *The Jewish Woman: new perspectives*. (New York: Schocken Books)
82. Silverman, S. F. (1975). The life crisis as a clue to social function: the case of Italy. In Reiter, R. R. (ed.) *Toward an Anthropology of Women*. p. 313. (London: Monthly Review Press)
83. Dougherty, M. C. (1982). Comment on Judith K. Brown, 'Cross-Cultural Perspectives on Middle-aged Women'. *Current Anthropol.*, 23(2), 149
84. Counts, D. A. (1982). Comment on J. K. Brown, 'Cross-Cultural Perspectives on Middle-aged Women'. *Current Anthropol.*, 23(2), 149
85. Elam, Y. (1973). *The Social and Sexual Roles of Homa Women*. p. 219. (Manchester: Manchester University Press)
86. Mitchell, W. B. *et al.* (1969). *Area Handbook for Guyana*. p. 82. (Washington, DC: Foreign Area Studies Division, US Government Printers)
87. Holleman, J. F. (1969). *Shona Customary Law, with Reference to Kinship, Marriage, the Family and Estate*. p. 205. (Manchester: Manchester University Press)
88. Roy, M. (1975). *Bengali Women*. p. 125. (Chicago: University of Chicago Press)

Section 4

How do hormones work?

Chapter 18

Presentation of estrogens to target tissues

V. H. T. James, R. C. Bonney and M. J. Reed

INTRODUCTION

The menopause is associated with a marked reduction in estrogen production that results from the cessation of estrogen formation by the ovaries. The decrease in estrogen production can give rise to minor symptoms of estrogen deficiency or can result in more serious complications such as osteoporosis. As well as being at risk from conditions associated with an estrogen deficiency, postmenopausal women also have an increased risk of developing breast or endometrial cancer and estrogens have been implicated in the development of these disorders. Studies we are carrying out, some of which are reviewed in this chapter, are an attempt to reveal the factors which regulate the formation and metabolism of estrogens in postmenopausal women, and also the availability of estrogens to target tissues.

CONVERSION OF ANDROSTENEDIONE TO ESTRONE

In vivo studies have established that in postmenopausal women estrone is derived from the peripheral conversion of androstenedione, which is secreted mainly by the adrenal gland and partly by the ovary[1]. The efficiency with which androstenedione is converted to estrone, by the aromatase enzyme complex, is related to age[2], although the mechanism responsible for the increased conversion by postmenopausal women is not known. The conversion of androstenedione to estrone is also influenced by body weight[1] and a major site in which aromatization takes place is adipose tissue[3], although conversion has been demonstrated in other tissues[4,5]. Results of *in vitro* studies[6] have shown that the ability of samples of adipose tissue, obtained at surgery, to convert androstenedione to estrone is similar in tissues obtained from obese and normal-weight women. Thus the increased efficiency with which androstenedione is converted to estrone in obese subjects probably reflects the increased mass of adipose tissue available in which aromatization can occur.

More recently interest has been directed to the possibility that the activity of the aromatase enzyme complex may be regulated by glucocorticoids. Simpson *et al.*[7] originally demonstrated that aromatase activity could be stimulated *in vitro* using the synthetic glucocorticoids, and particularly by dexamethasone. As well as confirming these results, studies in our department[8] showed that aromatase activity could be stimulated by concentrations of cortisol similar to the free or biologically active cortisol concentration in plasma. The results from these *in vitro* studies therefore suggested that cortisol could have a physiologic role in controlling aromatase activity. It had been previously found that the production rate of cortisol is elevated in obese women[9] and there is some evidence[10] for an increase in the free fraction of cortisol in older women. If glucocorticoids do have such a physiologic role these observations would be consistent with the increased efficiency of aromatization in older and obese women. While the role of stress in the development of malignant diseases remains controversial[11] there is some evidence that women who develop breast cancer may have been exposed to an increased number of stress-related events in their lives. If so, it is possible that stress which results in an increase in secretion of ACTH could increase tissue exposure to estrogens, not only by increasing the amount of substrate (adrenal androstenedione) for conversion to estrone but also by enhancing aromatase activity.

Because of the potential importance of glucocorticoids in regulating aromatase activity, we have carried out a number of studies to examine if there are any correlations between aromatase activity measured in samples of adipose tissue by an *in vitro* technique and plasma or tissue concentrations of cortisol. *In vivo* investigations have also been carried out in which the conversion of androstenedione to estrone was measured after the administration of dexamethasone.

Aromatase activity was measured in adipose tissue obtained from two women with Cushing's disease, a condition in which plasma levels of cortisol are chronically raised. One patient demonstrated normal aromatase activity, and in the other, activity was elevated. Further studies in which aromatase activity in adipose tissue was compared with the plasma free concentration of cortisol revealed a statistically significant correlation[12]. However, when aromatase activity was related to the concentration of cortisol in subcutaneous or breast adipose tissue a negative correlation was found.

The effect of glucocorticoids on the *in vivo* conversion of androstene-dione to estrone has also been studied using infusions of non-labeled and isotopically labeled steroids. Non-labeled androstenedione (204 μg/h for 9 h) was infused into three perimenopausal women after they had taken dexamethasone (2 mg/day) for 1 week. Blood samples were taken during the infusion to monitor changes in plasma levels of androstenedione and product steroids. Plasma levels of androstenedione increased rapidly after the start of the infusion and plasma levels of estrone sulphate and estrone also increased (Fig. 18.1). For one subject a significant increase

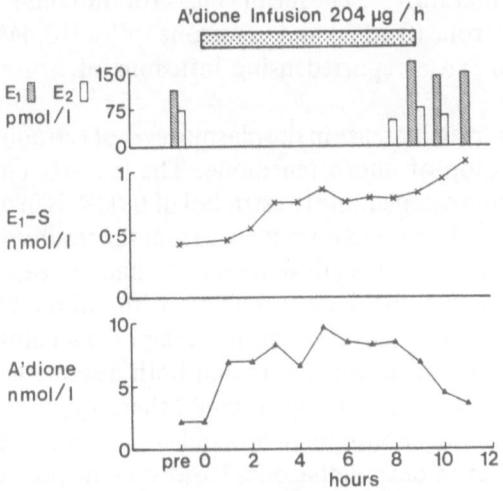

Figure 18.1 Plasma levels of estrone (E1), estradiol (E2), estrone sulfate (E1S) and androstenedione (A'dione) before and during infusion of androstenedione

in the plasma level of estradiol was detected. Metabolic clearance rates for androstenedione (MCR-A) were calculated from the incremental steady-state concentration of androstenedione divided by the rate of infusion of androstenedione (Table 18.1). The mean value for MCR-A of 2436 l/24 h obtained using infusion of non-labeled androstenedione is

Table 18.1 Metabolic clearance rate androstenedione (MCR-A) and transfer constants for the conversion of androstenedione to estrone ($[\rho]^{AE1}$) and the conversion of androstenedione to estrone sulfate ($[\rho]^{AE1S}$)

Subject	MCR-A (l/24 h)	$[\rho]^{AE1}$ (%)	$[\rho]^{AE1S}$ (%)
1	3140	0.49	0.28
2	1953	1.70	0.60
3	2215	0.20	0.43
Mean $\pm$ SE	2436 $\pm$ 361	0.80 $\pm$ 0.46	0.44 $\pm$ 0.09

similar to values measured using isotopically labeled androstenedione[13]. Transfer constants for the conversion of androstenedione to estrone and to estrone sulfate are also shown in Table 18.1. Transfer constants were calculated from the ratio of product to precursor steroid concentrations in plasma at the end of the infusion period multiplied by the ratio of product to precursor metabolic clearance rates. The MCR-A measured for each subject was used in this calculation and for the MCR estrone sulfate, the mean value of 106 1/24 h obtained after infusion of non-labeled estrone sulfate[14]. The MCR-E_1 used to calculate transfer constants for the conversion of androstenedione to estrone of 1610 1/24 h was taken from the literature[15]. The mean values for the conversion of androstenedione to estrone (0.80%) and to estrone sulfate (0.44%) are in good agreement with those reported using infusions of isotopically labeled steroids.

For one woman an increase in the plasma level of estradiol was detected during the infusion of androstenedione. The transfer constant for the conversion of androstenedione to estradiol of 0.08% is in agreement with reported values[13]. There was no evidence from the results of these investigations, however, that taking dexamethasone had increased the extent of conversion of androstenedione to estrone with values being similar to those reported for women who had not taken dexamethasone.

In vitro studies had shown clearly that both dexamethasone and cortisol stimulate aromatase activity. It could therefore be argued that the suppression of endogenous glucocorticoid production may balance any stimulatory effect of dexamethasone. However, the dose of dexamethasone used for these studies is equivalent to about four times the daily production rate of cortisol[16], and so the inhibition of cortisol production is unlikely to account for the failure of stimulation.

The results of the initial study were confirmed in postmenopausal women by measuring the conversion of androstenedione to estrone using a double isotope technique[17] before and after taking dexamethasone. The mean value for the conversion of androstenedione to estrone before dexamethasone was 1.05%, and after 1.05%. In a further study no increase in the conversion of androstenedione to estrone was observed after ACTH stimulation. The results from these studies are consistent with the results of a previous study[17] in which plasma levels of cortisol were measured at 2-hourly intervals for 24 h and related to the conversion of androstenedione to estrone. As shown in Fig. 18.2 a negative correlation was found.

Thus, although it remains possible that glucocorticoids may stimulate aromatase activity in specific tissues, there is no evidence from our studies to suggest that glucocorticoids influence the overall conversion of androstenedione to estrone *in vivo*. A possible reason for the discrepancy between the ability to stimulate aromatase activity *in vitro* and *in vivo*

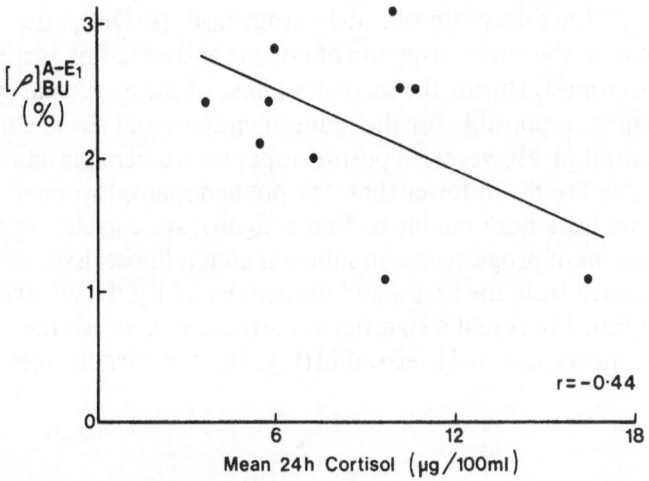

Figure 18.2 Correlation between transfer constants for the conversion of androstenedione to estrone ($[\rho]_{BU}^{A-E_1}$) and mean 24 h plasma concentrations of cortisol

may be that *in vivo* stimulation of cortisol secretion will be accompanied by an increase in adrenal androgen production. 5α-reduced androgen metabolites are potent inhibitors of aromatase activity and it is also possible that a metabolite of dexamethasone could inhibit aromatase activity.

We are also currently investigating the ability of other steroids to regulate aromatase activity. However, we have so far found no significant correlations between aromatase activity measured *in vitro* and tissue concentrations of testosterone or progesterone. For progesterone, higher tissue concentrations are associated with reduced aromatase activity. Naftolin *et al.*[18] have previously shown that progesterone decreased aromatase activity in the central nervous system. Tseng *et al.*[19] found that aromatase activity is lower in endometrial samples from women during the secretory phase of the menstrual cycle than during the proliferative phase. However, Tseng[20] has shown that progesterone can stimulate aromatase activity in endometrial stromal cells but not glandular cells, demonstrating that the factors that regulate aromatase activity vary for different cell types, and also that *in vivo* and *in vitro* studies may give apparently conflicting results.

CONVERSION OF ESTRONE TO ESTRADIOL

While the conversion of androstenedione to estrone is a key step in the synthesis of estrogen by the postmenopausal women, it is now generally considered that the role of estrone is that of a prehormone for the formation of the biologically active estrogen, estradiol. The activity of estradiol 17β-hydroxy steroid dehydrogenase (E_2DH), the enzyme responsible for the interconversion of estrone and estradiol, is stimulated by progesterone[21]. During the secretory phase of the menstrual cycle this mechanism is responsible for the reduced endometrial tissue concentrations of estradiol. However, in postmenopausal women, plasma levels of progesterone are much lower than for premenopausal women[6].

So far we have been unable to find a significant correlation between concentrations of progesterone in subcutaneous adipose tissue or adipose tissue obtained from the breast and the activity of E_2DH. *In vivo* studies have also failed to reveal a significant correlation between the extent to which estrone is converted to estradiol (Fig. 18.3) or estradiol metabolized

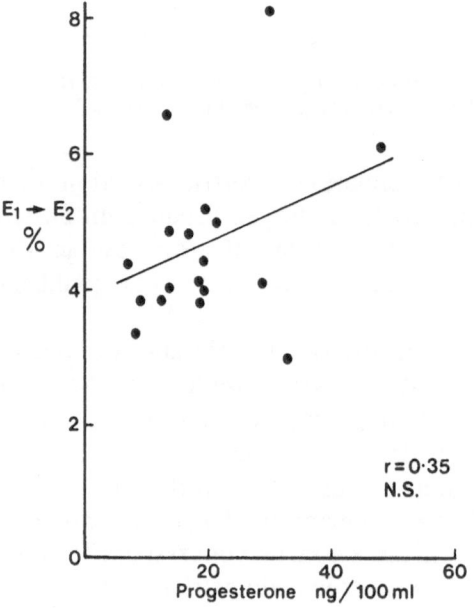

Figure 18.3 Relationship between transfer constants for the conversion of estrone to estradiol and plasma levels of progesterone for postmenopausal women

to estrone and plasma levels of progesterone. In contrast to these results from our *in vivo* studies, a significant negative correlation was found between the extent to which estradiol was converted to estrone and plasma levels of dehydroepiandrosterone sulfate (DHA-S). *In vitro* studies have confirmed the ability of DHA-S and its metabolites, dehydroepiandrosterone (DHA) and 5-androstenediol (5-Adiol) to inhibit E_2DH activity in samples of endometrial tissue[22]. The androgens also have the ability to inhibit E_2DH activity in breast tumor tissue (Fig. 18.4). In breast tumor tissue E_2DH activity is reduced by about 60% in the presence of DHA-S and DHA and 5-Adiol was only slightly less effective and reduced the

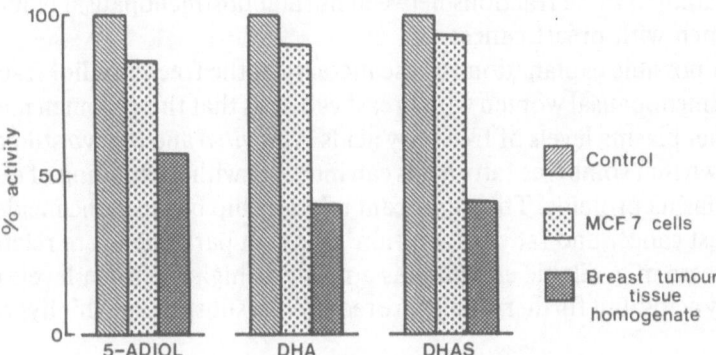

Figure 18.4 Inhibition of estradiol 17β-hydroxysteroid dehydrogenase activity in breast tumor tissue and MCF-7 cells by 5-androstenediol (5-Adiol), dehydroepiandrosterone (DHA) and dehydroepiandrosterone sulfate (DHAS)

activity of E_2DH by 44%. This degree of inhibition of E_2DH activity by these androgens in breast tumor tissue is similar to that found for the same androgens in human endometrial tissue[22]. In contrast, the effect in MCF-7 cells was much less pronounced and only minimal inhibition was demonstrated (Fig. 18.4).

AVAILABILITY OF PLASMA ESTRADIOL

The enzymes responsible for the conversion of androstenedione to estrone and for estrone to estradiol have been shown to be present in breast and endometrial tissues[23, 24]. However, the contribution that local estrogen formation makes to the cellular concentration may be relatively small[25]. Thus, estrogens formed at other sites, such as adipose tissue, and transported via the blood will have an important role in determining the exposure of target tissue to estrogen. Any factor that influences the distribution of estrogen in plasma will therefore influence the presentation of estrogens to target tissues. Until recently it had been generally accepted that only the small 1-2% of estradiol present in plasma in an unbound state is able to diffuse across cell membranes and interact with cellular receptors. It has now been suggested that the fraction of steroid bound to albumin[26] and/or sex hormone binding globulin[27] may also be available to tissues, although further studies are required to resolve the question of the availability of these plasma fractions to tissues. In postmenopausal women with breast cancer the free estradiol fraction is increased compared with the free fraction in normal postmenopausal women[28, 29] although the reason for this increase is not known. We have also measured the fraction of estradiol bound to albumin or SHBG in normal and breast cancer patients, but have not so far found any significant differences in either these fractions or concentration of estradiol in these fractions between normal postmenopausal women and women with breast cancer.

A possible explanation for the increase in the free estradiol fraction in postmenopausal women with breast cancer is that these women may have higher plasma levels of free fatty acids[30]. *In vitro* and *in vivo* studies have shown that some free fatty acids can interfere with the binding of estradiol to plasma proteins. The significant relationship between the incidence of breast cancer and fat consumption[31] may, in part, therefore relate to an increase in available estradiol as a result of higher plasma levels of free fatty acids, but further studies are required to substantiate this hypothesis.

ESTROGEN METABOLISM

The presentation of estrogens to target tissues will also be influenced by their rate and route of metabolism. The metabolic clearance rates of estrogens are elevated in postmenopausal women with breast or endometrial cancer[32, 33]. A significant correlation was found between the free estradiol fraction in plasma and metabolic clearance rate for estradiol in normal and postmenopausal women with breast or endometrial cancer[34]. If, as previously discussed, lipids are responsible for the increased free estradiol fraction found in cancer patients, this could also offer a possible explanation for the increased clearance rates of estradiol in postmenopausal women with breast or endometrial cancer.

Differences in estradiol metabolism have also been reported between normal and breast cancer patients. In women with breast cancer 16-hydroxylation of estradiol is increased[35]. The binding affinities of the products, estriol and 16α-hydroxy estrone, to SHBG are 3% and < 0.5%, of that of estradiol[36]. Therefore, estradiol metabolism via 16-hydroxylation could result in increased tissue exposure to estrogens. There is evidence that a diet high in fat results in increased 16-hydroxylation of estradiol[37]. Thus, diet may ultimately be shown to be a major factor in determining the degree of target tissue exposure to estrogens.

Acknowledgement

This work was supported by a grant from the Cancer Research Campaign.

REFERENCES

1. Siiteri, P. K. and MacDonald, P. C. (1973). Role of extraglandular estrogen in human endocrinology. In Greep, R. O. and Astwood, E. B. (eds.) *Handbook of Physiology.* pp. 615-29. (Washington, DC: American Physiological Society)
2. Hemsell, D. L., Grodin, J. M., Brenner, P. F., Siiteri, P. K. and MacDonald, P. C. (1974). Plasma precursors of estrogen. II. Correlation of the extent of conversion of plasma androstenedione to estrone with age. *J. Clin. Endocrinol. Metab.*, **38**, 476

3. Nimrod, A. and Ryan, K. J. (1975). Aromatization of androgens by human abdominal and breast fat tissue. *J. Clin. Endocrinol. Metab.*, **40**, 367

4. Frost, P. G., Reed, M. J. and James, V. H. T. (1980). The aromatization of androstenedione by human adipose and liver tissue. *J. Steroid Biochem.*, **13**, 1427

5. Longcope, C., Pratt, J. H., Schneider, S. H. and Fineberg, S. E. (1978). Aromatization of androgens by muscle and adipose tissue *in vivo. J. Clin. Endocrinol. Metab.*, **46**, 146

6. James, V. H. T., Reed, M. J. and Folkerd, E. J. (1981). Studies of oestrogen metabolism in postmenopausal women with cancer. *J. Steroid Biochem.*, **15**, 235

7. Simpson, E. R., Ackerman, G. E., Smith, M. E. and Mendelson, C. R. (1981). Estrogen formation in stromal cells of adipose tissue of women: induction by glucocorticoids. *Proc. Natl. Acad. Sci. USA*, **78**, 5690

8. Folkerd, E. J. and James, V. H. T. (1983). Aromatization of steroids in peripheral tissues. *J. Steroid Biochem.*, **19**, 687

9. Mlynark, P., Gillies, R. R., Murphy, B. and Pattee, C. J. (1962). Cortisol production rated in obesity. *J. Clin. Endocrinol. Metab.*, **22**, 587

10. Jones, M. K., Dyer, G. I., Ramsay, I. D. and Collins, W. P. (1981). Studies on apparent free cortisol and testosterone plasma from patients with breast tumours. *Postgrad. Med. J.*, **57**, 89

11. Cooper, C. L. (1982). Psychosocial stress and cancer. *Bull. Br. Psychol. Soc.*, **35**, 456

12. James, V. H. T., Folkerd, E. J., Bonney, R. C., Beranek, P. A. and Reed, M. J. (1982). Factors influencing estrogen production and metabolism in postmenopausal women with endocrine cancer. *J. Endocrinol. Invest.*, **5**, 335

13. Longcope, C., Kato, T. and Horton, R. (1969). Conversion of blood androgens to oestrogens in normal adult men and women. *J. Clin. Invest.*, **48**, 2191

14. Reed, M. J., Noel, C. T., Jones, D. L., Jacobs, H. S., Scanlon, M. J. and James, V. H. T. (1985). The use of nonradiolabelled steroid infusions to investigate the origin of oestrone sulphate in postmenopausal women. *J. Steroid Biochem.* (In press)

15. Longcope, C. (1971). Metabolic clearance and blood production rates of oestrogens in postmenopausal women. *Am. J. Obstet. Gynecol.*, **111**, 778

16. Slater, J. D. H., Heffron, P. F., Vernet, A. and Nabarro, J. D. N. (1959). Clinical and metabolic effects of dexamethasone. *Lancet*, **1**, 173

17. Reed, M. J., Hutton, J. D., Baxendale, P. M., James, V. H. T., Jacobs, H. S. and Fisher, R. P. (1979). The conversion of androstenedione to oestrone and production of oestrone in women with endometrial cancer. *J. Steroid Biochem.*, **11**, 905

18. Naftolin, F., Ryan, K. J., Davies, J. J. and Reddy, V. V. (1975). The formation of oestrogens by central neuroendocrine tissue. *Rec. Prog. Horm. Res.*, **31**, 295

19. Tseng, L., Mazella, J., Mann, W. J. and Chumas, J. (1982). Estrogen synthesis in normal and malignant human endometrium. *J. Clin. Endocrinol. Metab.*, **55**, 1029

20. Tseng, L. (1984). Effect of oestradiol and progesterone on human endometrial aromatase activity in primary cell culture. *J. Clin. Endocrinol. Metab.*, **115**, 833

21. Tseng, L. and Gurpide, E. (1975). Induction of endometrial estradiol dehydrogenase by progestins. *Endocrinology*, **97**, 825

22. Bonney, R. C., Reed, M. J. and James, V. H. T. (1983). Inhibition of 17β-hydroxysteroid dehydrogenase activity in human endometrium by adrenal androgens. *J. Steroid Biochem.*, **18**, 59

23. Li, K., Chandra, D. P., Foo, T., Adams, J. B. and MacDonald, D. (1976). Steroid metabolism by human mammary carcinoma. *Steroids*, **28**, 561

24. Tilson-Mallett, N., Santner, S. J., Feil, P. D. and Santen, R. J. (1984). Biological significance of aromatase activity in human breast tumours. *J. Clin. Endocrinol. Metab.*, **57**, 1125

25. Bradlow, H. L. (1982). A reassessment of the role of breast tumour aromatization. *Cancer Res.*, **42**, 3362

26. Pardridge, W. M., Mietus, L. J., Frumar, A. M., Davidson, B. J. and Judd, H. L. (1980). Effects of human serum on transport of testosterone and estradiol into rat brain. *Am. J. Physiol.*, **239**, E103

27. Siiteri, P. K., Murai, J. T., Hammond, G. L., Nisker, J. A., Raymoure, W. J. and Kahn, R. W. (1982). The serum transport of steroid hormones. *Rec. Prog. Horm. Res.*, **38**, 457

28. Moore, J. W., Clarke, G. M. G., Bulbrook, R. D., Hayward, J. T., Hammond, G. L. and Siiteri, P. K. (1982). Serum concentrations of total and non-protein bound estradiol in patients with breast cancer and in normal controls. *Int. J. Cancer*, **29**, 17
29. Reed, M. J., Cheng, R. W., Dudley, H. A. F. and James, V. H. T. (1983). Plasma levels of oestrone, oestrone sulphate and oestradiol and percentage of unbound oestradiol in postmenopausal women with and without breast cancer. *Cancer Res.*, **43**, 3940
30. Basu, T. K. and Williams, D. C. (1975). Plasma and body lipids in patients with carcinoma of the breast. *Oncology*, **31**, 172
31. Armstrong, B. and Doll, R. (1975). Environmental factors and cancer incidence and mortality in different countries with special reference to dietary practices. *Int. J. Cancer*, **15**, 617
32. Kirschner, M. A., Cohen, F. B. and Ryan, C. (1978). Androgen-oestrogen production rates in postmenopausal women with breast cancer. *Cancer Res.*, **38**, 4029
33. Reed, M. J., Beranek, P. A., Ghilchik, M. W. and James, V. H. T. (1985). Estrogen production and metabolism in normal postmenopausal women and postmenopausal women with breast or endometrial cancer. (In press)
34. Reed, M. J., Beranek, P. A., Cheng, R. W., Ghilchik, M. W. and James, V. H. T. (1985). The distribution of oestradiol in plasma from postmenopausal women with or without breast cancer: relationships with metabolic clearance rates of oestradiol. *Int. J. Cancer*, **35**, 457
35. Fishman, J., Schneider, J., Hershcope, R. J. and Bradlow, H. L. (1984). Increased estrogen-16α-hydroxylase activity in women with breast and endometrial cancer. *J. Steroid Biochem.*, **20**, 1077
36. Fishman, J. and Martucci, C. (1980). Biological properties of 16α-hydroxyoestrone: implications in estrogen physiology and pathophysiology. *J. Clin. Endocrinol. Metab.*, **51**, 611
37. Musey, P. I., Collins, D. C., Gould, K. G. and Preedy, J. R. K. (1983). Oxidation of oestradiol by the chimpanzee: effect of high fat diet. *Fed. Proc.*, **42**, 554 (abstr. 1536)

Chapter 19

Recent progess in the study of the mechanism of action of progesterone

F. Logeat, R. Pamphile, M. Applanat, M. T. Vu Hai and E. Milgrom

Two approaches are used in the study of the mechanisms of action of hormones. One involves the analysis of the modifications which are imprinted in the target cells by the administration of hormones. In the case of steroids, which act mainly through modifications of protein synthesis, this involves the study of specific gene products. The other approach aims at understanding the fate of the hormone in the target cell, i.e. its interaction with specific receptors. To analyze the mechanisms of action of progesterone in the mammalian uterus we have used as a model system the rabbit endometrium and studied in this classical target organ[1] on the one hand the regulation of the expression of a specific gene (the uteroglobin gene) and on the other hand the structure, the biosynthesis and the intracellular localization of the progesterone receptor.

HORMONAL CONTROL OF THE UTEROGLOBIN GENE

Uteroglobin[2], also called blastokinin[3], is a protein synthesized by the rabbit endometrium and secreted into the uterine lumen. Its concentration is physiologically increased by progesterone; it is thus present in pregnant, pseudopregnant or progesterone-treated rabbits.

The role of uteroglobin is not clearly understood, it binds progesterone and some metabolites of progesterone[4]; it also may play a role in the immunological tolerance of the embryo[5]. Uteroglobin is made of two identical subunits of 71 amino acids each. The messenger RNA for uteroglobin has been characterized[6]. The cDNA[7] and the gene[8] have been cloned and sequenced[9]. The gene consists of three exons which correspond to different functional domains of the protein: the first exon encodes in part the signal peptide, the second exon encompasses the steroid binding region, the third exon corresponds to the region of the protein by which the two subunits are held together[9, 10].

Radioimmunoassay of uteroglobin and mRNA hybridization to a specific cDNA allowed study of the hormonal regulation of uteroglobin and its messenger RNA[11]. It was observed that the increase of uteroglobin mRNA follows very rapidly the administration of progesterone, thus probably being a primary effect of the hormone. Moreover, progesterone was also shown to have a non-transcriptional effect which further amplified protein synthesis[12]. Estrogen at high concentration inhibited the latter effect of progesterone.

Uteroglobin is present at low concentration in the lung. Its synthesis and that of its mRNA are constitutive[13]. Progesterone or combinations of estrogen and progesterone have no effect, although the progesterone receptor is present in the lung. This situation offers an interesting model to understand how hormonal regulation and cellular differentiation interplay in the expression of genes.

The interaction between the cloned uteroglobin gene and the purified progesterone receptor has been studied[9]. The presence of high-affinity sites (putative regulatory regions) was observed upstream from the gene and in the 5' part of the gene.

STRUCTURE, BIOSYNTHESIS AND INTRACELLULAR LOCALIZATION OF THE PROGESTERONE RECEPTOR

The steroid-binding properties, the hormonal regulation and the physiological variations of the progesterone receptor have been extensively studied (review in ref. 14). However, little is known about its structure, biosynthesis and intracellular localization. Preparation of the polyclonal[15] and monoclonal[16] antibodies against the rabbit uterine receptor has allowed us to directly analyze these problems.

Using the 'Western blot' method it has been possible to study the receptor in crude cellular extracts, thus avoiding any purification step which could lead to the loss or alteration of receptor subunits. These experiments showed the receptor to consist, in both cytosol and nuclei, of a single 110 000 dalton subunit; smaller forms, and especially the 79 000 dalton form, being due to the action of endogenous proteolytic enzymes[17, 18].

The progesterone receptor mRNA was characterized by translation in a reticulocyte lysate and immunoprecipitation with monoclonal and polyclonal antireceptor antibodies[17]. A 110 000 dalton radioactive protein was found to be the translation product of receptor messenger RNA. Thus, the receptor does not undergo major changes after its synthesis since the molecular weight of the translation product and that of the final protein are very similar if not identical.

Translation of poly (A+) RNAs from uteri of estrogen-treated and non-treated rabbits showed that the induction of progesterone receptor by estrogen is due to an increase of messenger concentration.

The monoclonal antibodies were used to purify the progesterone receptor in a single step[18]. A high-capacity immunosorbent was synthesized by cross-linking a monoclonal antibody to protein A-Sepharose through its Fc fragment. The monoclonal antibody was also selected for its property of releasing the antigen at pH 10.5–11, i.e. in conditions where the receptor remains stable for extensive periods of time. It was possible, using this method, to purify both steroid–receptor complexes and aporeceptor (receptor devoid of bound ligand).

The monoclonal antibodies could also be used for the immunocyto-chemical detection of receptor[19]. It was possible to use paraffin-embedded, fixed tissue. The receptor was found inside the nuclei even in the absence of the hormone. A similar situation has been described by King and Greene for the estrogen receptor[20]. The hormone thus does not provoke the translocation of the receptor from the cytoplasm to the nucleus but does induce a change in the affinity of the receptor towards chromatin. In the absence of the hormone the receptor is loosely attached to the nucleus and can be easily solubilized if the tissue is homogenized. Activated steroid–receptor complexes become strongly bound to chromatin and can only be extracted by high salt.

Another observation made by the immunocytochemical method was the existence of a heterogeneity in receptor distribution among cells of the same histological type. This suggests that at a given time only a fraction of the cells may be hormonally responsive.

REFERENCES

1. Clauberg, C. (1933). In Springer, J. (ed.) *Die Weiblichen Sexual Hormone*. pp. 88–100. (Berlin: Springer Verlag)
2. Beier, H. M. (1968). Uteroglobin: a hormone-sensitive endometrial protein involved in blastocyst development. *Biochim. Biophys. Acta*, **160**, 289–91
3. Krishnan, R. S. and Daniel, J. C. (1967). 'Blastokinin' inducer and regulator of blastocyst development in the rabbit uterus. *Science*, **158**, 490–2
4. Fridlansky, F. and Milgrom, E. (1976). Interaction of uteroglobin with progesterone 5-alpha pregnane 3,20 dione and estrogens. *Endocrinology*, **99**, 1244–51
5. Mukherjee, A. B., Ulane, R. E. and Agrawal, A. K. (1982). Role of uteroglobin and transglutaminase in masking the antigenicity of implanting rabbit embryos. *Am. J. Reprod. Immunol.*, **2**, 135–41
6. Atger, M. and Milgrom, E. (1977). Progesterone induced messenger RNA. Translation, purification and preliminary characterization of uteroglobin mRNA. *J. Biol. Chem.*, **252**, 5412–18
7. Atger, M., Perricaudet, M., Tiollais, P. and Milgrom, E. (1980) Bacterial cloning of the rabbit uteroglobin structural gene. *Biochem. Biophys. Res. Commun.*, **93**, 1082–8

8. Atger, M., Atger, P., Tiollais, P. and Milgrom, E. (1981). Cloning of rabbit genomic fragments containing the uteroglobin gene. *J. Biol. Chem.*, **256**, 5970-2
9. Bailly, A., Atger, M., Atger, P., Cerbon, M. A., Alizon, M., Vu Hai, M. T., Logeat, F. and Milgrom, E. (1983). The rabbit uteroglobin gene. Structure and interaction with the progesterone receptor. *J. Biol. Chem.*, **258**, 10384-9
10. Mornon, J. P., Fridlansky, F., Bailly, A. and Milgrom, E. (1980). X-ray crystallographic analysis of a progesterone binding protein. The C222, crystal form of oxidized uteroglobin at 2.2 Å resolution. *J. Mol. Biol.*, **137**, 415-29
11. Loosfelt, H., Fridlansky, F., Savouret, J. F., Atger, M. and Milgrom, E. (1981). Mechanism of action of progesterone in the rabbit endometrium. Induction of uteroglobin and its messenger RNA. *J. Biol. Chem.*, **56**, 3465-70
12. Loosfelt, H., Fridlansky, F., Atger, M. and Milgrom, E. (1981). A possible non-transcriptional effect of progesterone. *J. Steroid Biochem.*, **15**, 107-10
13. Savouret, J. F., Loosfelt, H., Atger, M. and Milgrom, E. (1980). Differential hormonal control of a messenger RNA in two tissues; uteroglobin mRNA in the lung and the endometrium. *J. Biol. Chem.*, **255**, 4131-6
14. Vu Hai, M. T., Logeat, F., Warembourg, M. and Milgrom, E. (1977). Hormonal control of progesterone receptors. *Ann. NY Acad. Sci.*, **286**, 199-209
15. Logeat, F., Vu Hai, M. T. and Milgrom, E. (1981). Antibodies to rabbit progesterone receptor: cross-reaction with human receptor. *Proc. Natl. Acad. Sci. USA*, **78**, 1426-30
16. Logeat, F., Vu Hai, M. T., Fournier, A., Legrain, P., Buttin, G. and Milgrom, E. (1983). Monoclonal antibodies to rabbit progesterone receptor. Cross-reaction with other mammalian progesterone receptors. *Proc. Natl. Acad. Sci. USA*, **80**, 6456-9
17. Loosfelt, H., Logeat, F., Vu Hai, M. T. and Milgrom, E. (1984). The rabbit progesterone receptor. Evidence for a single steroid-binding subunit and characterization of receptor mRNA. *J. Biol. Chem.*, **259**, 14196-202
18. Logeat, F., Pamphile, R., Loosfelt, H., Jolivet, A., Fournier, A. and Milgrom, E. (1984). One-step immunoaffinity purification of active progesterone receptor. Further evidence in favor of the existence of a single steroid binding subunit. *Biochemistry*, **24**, 1029-35
19. Perrot-Applanat, M., Logeat, F., Groyer-Picard, M. T. and Milgrom, E. (1984). Immunocytochemical study of mammalian progesterone receptor using monoclonal antibodies. *Endocrinology*, **116**, 1473-84
20. King, W. J. and Greene, G. L. (1984). Monoclonal antibodies localize estrogen receptor in the nuclei of target cells. *Nature*, **307**, 745-9

Chapter 20

Ovarian hormone action in the brain: implications for the menopause

B. S. McEwen

Concerning the various bodily consequences of the decline of ovarian hormone levels in the menopause, it is only recently that the brain has gained attention as an organ which suffers from the withdrawal and absence of the ovarian steroids. Behavioral, followed by neurochemical and neuroanatomical, studies over the past 20 years have established that the central nervous system (CNS) is an important target for ovarian hormones as well as adrenal steroids and other hormones, and that the steroid hormones have many important effects on the structure and function of the brain. All of this information has been gained from experiments on laboratory animals, and it is the purpose of this communication to outline some of the most salient information.

Before discussing hormones it is important to point out that our concepts of chemical communication within the CNS have changed radically during recent years. We formerly viewed chemical transmission as a simple one-way communication involving the release of excitatory or inhibitory neurotransmitters and their action on *postsynaptic* receptors on the dendrites of adjacent cells. Now we know that there are additional factors such as *presynaptic* receptors which respond to a variety of chemical signals from the same or adjacent neurons, or to circulating hormones, and increase or decrease the release of neurotransmitters. In addition, dendrites, long regarded as recipients of chemical signals, sometimes produce and release transmitters which affect themselves as well as adjacent pre- and postsynaptic events. Finally, hormones, chemical signals from *outside* the brain, have both direct pre- and postsynaptic actions as well as indirect influences which modify the ways in which neurons carry out their functions.

Ovarian steroids have both direct and indirect actions which influence nerve cell function. Direct electrical effects, with onset latencies of milliseconds to a few minutes, have been reported using electrophysiological recording techniques. Direct interactions with membrane, membrane receptors and enzymes have been reported for estrogens, especially the catecholestrogens; and these interactions modify neurotransmitter receptor binding and enzyme activity, although in the experiments conducted thus far the hormones are effective only at supraphysiological concentrations. At the same time as they may exert direct effects, steroid hormones' major mode of action is via intracellular receptors, sites of high affinity and specificity located in or near the cell nucleus. These receptors interact with DNA in the genome and increase, or decrease, the production of specific messenger RNAs which code for specific proteins.

The brain has receptor sites of this type for the ovarian hormones, estradiol and progesterone; they are located in discrete groups of nerve cells throughout the hypothalamus and 'limbic' brain. (The 'limbic' system controls vegetative functions and governs emotions.) Some, but not all, of the estrogen and progestin receptors are found in the same cells; we know this because in many of the estrogen-sensitive areas of hypothalamus and preoptic area, estradiol treatment induces an increase in progestin receptor content. This induction is undoubtedly at the root of the well-known synergism between estradiol and progesterone and also the reason that concurrent administration of progesterone with estradiol can modify and even inhibit estrogen action. We now know that the interaction of ovarian steroids with these intracellular steroid receptors alters the levels of a number of enzymes and neurotransmitter receptors. In one instance we know that this interaction alters the production of a specific messenger RNA, and we believe that many other effects involve the same type of mechanism. Each of these effects is localized to specific groups of estrogen-sensitive neurons. For example, estradiol treatment induces an increase in the enzyme for acetylcholine formation in a group of neurons in the basal forebrain, which innervate cortical and subcortical structures and are implicated in cognitive function. Estradiol also depresses the formation of the rate-limiting enzyme for the formation of dopamine in the basal hypothalamus; dopamine in this part of the brain is involved in control of prolactin release and the control of ovulation. Estrogens also depress the activity of monoamine oxidase (MAO), an enzyme which degrades catecholamines and serotonin. Blockade of MAO by drugs leads to antidepressant effects on mood, and it is therefore interesting in the context of changes in mood during the menstrual cycle and during and after menopause that not only does estradiol *decrease*

MAO in a few regions of the 'limbic' brain and hypothalamus, but also progesterone can rapidly reverse the effects of estradiol and *elevate* MAO activity. Estradiol also elevates the levels of receptors for acetylcholine, serotonin and noradrenaline in discrete areas of the brain. Thus, the neurotransmitter sensitivity of nerve cells in some brain regions is increased by estrogen treatment, along with hormone-dependent changes in the ability of nerve cells to synthesize and degrade neurotransmitters.

What is interesting about all of these effects is that some of them are sex-specific, in that the male brain does not show the same responses to estradiol as the female brain. This is not such a peculiar comparison as it may seem, because the male brain makes use of estradiol as a product of the metabolism of testosterone and contains estrogen receptors which are distributed much as in the female brain. Sex differences in hormone action are reflections of underlying differences between males and females in behavior, cognitive function and the incidence and characteristics of nervous and mental disorders. They must be borne in mind as important variables in the response to drugs. We know, for example, that estrogens exacerbate the symptoms of Parkinson's disease and reduce the symptoms of tardive dyskinesia. Both of these effects of estradiol can be explained by invoking a mode of action which is 'anti-dopaminergic'.

What are we to make of this information in relation to the menopause? Ovarian hormones such as estradiol play an important role in the development of the brain as well as influencing adult brain function. From this and the fact that these hormones influence the capability of certain neurons to conduct their business of chemical neurotransmission, it stands to reason that the withdrawal of ovarian hormones at the menopause would lead to an altered state of brain function. Why there are individual differences in the response to this withdrawal is a great puzzle, just as it is puzzling that there are individual variations in premenstrual and post-partum symptomatology when ovarian hormone levels are also changed. As a researcher on animal models I cannot throw any light on these problems, but I can suggest that the use of estrogen therapy for osteoporosis and other maladies of the post- or perimenopausal period presents an ideal opportunity for careful observations of mood, neurological status and cognitive abilities.

FURTHER READING

McEwen, B. S., Biegon, A., Fischette, C. T., Luine, V. N., Parsons, B. and Rainbow, T. C. (1984). Toward a neurochemical basis of steroid hormone action. In Martini, L. and Ganong, W. F. (eds.) *Frontiers in Neuroendocrinology*. pp. 153–76. (New York: Raven Press)

Bedard, P., Langelier, P. and Villeneuve, A. (1977). Oestrogens and extrapyramidal system. *Lancet*, **2**, 1367–8

Section 5

Hot flashes

Chapter 21

An animal model for pharmacologic evaluation of the menopausal hot flush

J. W. Simpkins and M. J. Katovich

1. CRITERIA FOR ANIMAL MODELS FOR HUMAN DISEASES

Animal models are extremely important in our efforts to understand human diseases. For obvious ethical reasons, human experimentation is limited in its scope and is heavily dependent upon inferences drawn from case reports, retrospective studies and prospective evaluations using limited sample sizes and strict limits on invasive procedures. Efforts to study the mechanism of diseases and the initial evaluation of their therapy usually require animal experimentation. These animal evaluations allow for the control of a variety of variables, the required sampling of tissues believed to be involved in the disease process and the use of appropriate sample sizes. In this respect, animal experimentation can serve as an indispensable tool for the ultimate resolution of the mechanism of human disease and, as a result, for the development of an appropriate therapy.

The usefulness of an animal model depends upon several basic criteria. First, the animal must be relatively inexpensive, readily available and not require elaborate maintenance conditions. Hence the animal model would be available to investigators interested in a variety of aspects of the disease and who could apply their methodologies to its understanding. Second, the animal species should be genetically homogeneous, a characteristic which reduces the inherent variability of biological data. A persistent problem in many clinical studies is the high variability of the endpoints used in the evaluation of disease states. Finally, the anatomy and physiology of the tissues, organs and/or organ systems involved in the disease should be well understood in the animal model. The basis of our understanding of pathophysiology is the extent to which we understand the normal function of a system.

Given the basic criteria, the most appropriate animal models are those in which the human disease appears spontaneously. Thus, for example, animal models are available in which hypertension, atherosclerosis, obesity, diabetes mellitus or a variety of tumors develop spontaneously. More often, however, diseases are induced in animals in an attempt to mimic the human syndrome. Numerous disease states can be induced by a variety of experimental manipulations. Induced animals model are available for diabetes mellitus, hypertension, obesity, tumors, Parkinson's disease, Altzheimer's disease, etc. While the appropriateness of each of these models is the subject of continuing investigation, there is little question that these animal models have contributed enormously to our understanding of a variety of disease states.

We describe in this report the basis for a preliminary evaluation of an animal model using the rat for the menopausal hot flush. Our primary purpose in developing this animal model was to evaluate the hormonal and endocrine factors which contribute to flushes and to provide a means of effectively testing alternative therapies for the vasomotor syndrome.

2. THE MENOPAUSAL SYNDROME AS A GONADAL STEROID WITHDRAWAL PHENOMENON

The perimenopausal period refers to the time of involution of the ovaries and the various responses of the body to the loss of ovarian steroid secretion[1,2]. The menopause defines the specific event of the cessation of menses which accompanies the loss of cyclic secretion of ovarian steroids[3,4]. In response to the loss of ovarian estrogens and progestins, several 'extragenital' symptoms appear in most women. These symptoms most often express themselves as hot flushes, perspiration, muscle and joint pain, fatigue, headaches and irritability[3,4]. Their intensity and frequency vary among women and symptoms do not occur at all in about 25% of menopausal women.

The most frequent and characteristic extragenital symptom of the menopause is the hot flush, an episodic disturbance of thermoregulation characterized by a sensation of heat followed by a sudden spreading flush and perspiration. Of women who experience hot flushes, 82% report that the symptoms last for more than 1 year while 26% experience hot flushes for more than 5 years[5]. Like the other symptoms of the menopause, hot flushes vary in frequency and intensity among women to such an extent that some never experience hot flushes while others report 20 or more flushing episodes per day[5, 6]. Flushes can be provoked by warm ambient temperature, hot drinks, alcoholic beverages or mental stress[7-10].

A flushing episode is composed of many physiological alterations which are transient and temporally organized. Prior to the hot flush, women report the sensation of heat or burning and the perception of intracranial pressure[11]. This perception may last for up to 4 min, and signals an imminent flush. It has been suggested that the premonition of a hot flush is the consequence of CNS neuronal alteration associated with changes in the brain 'set-point' for body temperature regulation[6, 8, 12, 13]. Additionally, a transient phase of tachycardia precedes the elevation in skin temperature[10], a surge in secretion of luteinizing hormone (LH) accompanies the flush[12-14] and a fall in core body temperature follows the onset of the skin temperature increase[6-8, 12-16]. While initial evaluations failed to observe correlation between the hot flush and serum norepinephrine (NE), epinephrine or dopamine (DA)[12], subsequent studies have shown that epinephrine concentrations increase in concert with the skin temperature increase during hot flushes[17]. Additionally, the adrenal steroids cortisol, progesterone, dehydroepiandrosterone and androstenedione show phasic hypersecretion associated with the hot flush[14] and serum levels of β-endorphin increase during flushing episodes[18]. Since most serum β-endorphin originates from adrenocorticotropes in the anterior pituitary gland and is co-secreted with adrenocorticotropin (ACTH[19]) it is likely that ACTH release is stimulated during the hot flush. This synchronized increase in LH, ACTH, β-endorphin, adrenal steroids and adrenal catecholamines with the hot flush indicates that the hot flush may be associated with the activation of a CNS stress mechanism or that the hot flush may cause a stress response and the associated hormonal changes.

The hot flush appears to reflect a disorder in the brain thermoregulatory mechanism. This conclusion is supported by several pieces of indirect evidence. First, the perception of an impending flush is likely a cognitive response to the resetting of the brain thermostat. Second, enhanced heart rate[10] and an increase in metabolic rate[20] occur before vasodilation and the resulting heat loss. These two changes likely reflect the initial phases of the brain activation of the heat loss mechanism. Third, the concurrent release of LH and β-endorphin during the hot flush likely reflect the activation of CNS sympathetic, noradrenergic neurons and the resulting release of luteinizing hormone-releasing hormone (LHRH)[21] and corticotropin-releasing factor (CRF)[22]. Fourth, patients with diencephalic epilepsy have several flushing episodes per day[23, 24]. Thus, it appears that a brain mechanism initiates the hot flush and the accompanying physiological alterations.

Inasmuch as hot flushes occur after ovariectomy or with the natural cessation of ovarian function at the menopause, the loss of gonadal steroid or physiological responses to ovarian steroid decline are likely causative in the hot flush. The most dramatic hormonal alteration associated with the menopause is the decline in circulating levels of 17-β-estradiol (E_2) and progesterone and the associated elevations in the gonadotropins, LH and follicle stimulating hormone (FSH)[6, 25-32]. Best documented is the precipitous decline in levels of E_2, primarily because the controls for these studies are typically women at the mid-follicular stage of their menstrual cycle. However, when compared to mid-luteal phase concentrations of progesterone the decline in serum progesterone after the menopause is equivalent to that of E_2[33-35]. Thus, deficiencies in both of the major gonadal steroids accompany the loss of gonadal function in menopausal women. Interestingly, serum levels of estrone do not show a decline at the menopause, likely because this estrogen is produced systemically from the conversion of adrenal androgens[36, 37]. However, circulating estrone alone is ineffective in preventing the appearance of estrogen-deficient symptoms after the menopause.

A problem which has not been fully resolved is the relationship between serum estradiol levels and the symptomatology of the menopause. Comparisons of total estradiol levels in symptomatic and asymptomatic patients have failed to document differences[29-32]. Similarly, the rate of fall in total estrogens after ovariectomy does not differ in symptomatic and asymptomatic women[29]. Recently, however, Judd and colleagues[26, 27] have observed slightly higher free estradiol levels in women who are asymptomatic after the menopause when compared to women who experience hot flushes. These results suggest that the measurements of total circulating estrogens are inappropriate in assessing a correlation between steroids and the occurrence of flushes, since that fraction of estradiol which is available for transport into the brain is the portion not bound to plasma protein (i.e. the free estradiol fraction). Additional studies will be needed to verify this point.

It appears that the attempts to dissociate symptomatic from asymptomatic women based upon absolute gonadal steroid concentrations may be a misdirected effort. The decline in gonadal steroids after ovariectomy or at the menopause likely creates an endocrine milieu which is conducive for skin temperature instability. Whether hot flushes are expressed or not during this gonadal steroid-deprived state then depends upon factors which are independent of ovarian secretions. These factors may include circulating sex hormone binding globulin levels (which would result in changes in free estradiol levels), brain sensitivity to gonadal steroids, adrenal cortical hormone levels, differences in the responsiveness of the peripheral vasculature to circulating catecholamines or other vasoactive factors, difference in the responsiveness of the brain to non-steroidal signals, etc. Thus, sex steroid may exert a stabilizing influence on the brain mechanism which controls skin blood flow. During steroid deficiency this control mechanism may be very sensitive to a variety of stimuli which precipitate hot flushes.

The hot flush appears to be a steroid hormone withdrawal phenomenon. Thus, symptoms appear abruptly in women after ovariectomy and the accompanying rapid decline in serum gonadal steroid levels[29] and gradually in women during the perimenopausal period when circulation gonadal steroid hormone levels decline more slowly[28, 33, 35]. Interestingly, brain exposure to gonadal steroids appears to be a requisite for the occurrence of hot flushes upon their withdrawal. Thus, hot flushes do not occur in women with gonadal dysgenesis[38] or Kleinfelter's syndrome[39], presumably because these women have never been exposed to elevated gonadal steroid levels. Yen[25] has reported that gonadal dysgenic women who are treated with estrogens and then withdrawn from the estrogen therapy develop hot flushes. It would appear then that the hot flush is one manifestation of a gonadal steroid withdrawal syndrome.

In this regard we have noted that the symptoms of gonadal steroid withdrawal are remarkably similar to the symptoms observed during opiate withdrawal[40]. Among the symptoms of opiate withdrawal are hot and cold flushes, perspiration, increased pulse rate, insomnia, depression, nervousness, irritability, anxiety, and aches in muscles and joints[41]. As indicated above, these same symptoms are reported for menopausal women, albeit, to a milder degree[3, 4]. Thus, we have proposed that the extragenital symptoms of gonadal steroid withdrawal may be a manifestation of withdrawal from endogenously released opioid peptides[40].

In this regard, evidence has accumulated which indicates that gonadal steroids influence the activity of endogenous opioid peptide (EOP) neurons. Using the LH secretory response to the narcotic antagonist, naloxone, as an index of EOP activity, several investigators have now observed that EOP activity is low during the early follicle phase, increased during the late follicular phase and is highest during the mid-luteal phase of the human menstrual cycle[41-44]. Similar observations have been made in the rhesus monkey[45]. More direct evidence for the stimulation of EOP neurons by gonadal steroid have been made in studies using the monkey. Ferin and colleagues[46] reported that ovariectomy reduced to undetectable levels of β-endorphin in the hypophyseal drainage of the medial basal hypothalamus. Additionally, as anticipated from the LH secretory response to naloxone[45], β-endorphin secretion increased progressively from menses (when both estradiol and progesterone levels are low) through follicular and luteal phase of the menstrual cycle of the monkey[46]. Interestingly, in ovariectomized monkeys, while estradiol treatment alone increased β-endorphin secretion, estradiol plus progesterone therapy was more effective in enhancing the secretion rate of this EOP[47]. Finally, in postmenopausal women, naloxone is unable to elicit LH secretion[48], suggesting the activity of EOPs are either absent or diminished. Hence, reduced gonadal steroid levels in menopausal women are associated with reduced activity in the β-endorphin neurons which impinge upon LHRH neurons in the medial basal hypothalamus. The aforementioned similarity in the symptoms of the menopause and opiate withdrawal support the contention that gonadal steroid decline at the menopause may precipitate a generalized decline in the activity of EOP neurons and the resulting withdrawal symptoms.

3. USE OF MORPHINE-DEPENDENT RATS AS A MODEL FOR THE MENOPAUSAL HOT FLUSH

In view of the aforementioned evidence for similarities between the symptoms of opiate withdrawal and the menopausal syndrome, we attempted to develop an animal model for the menopausal hot flush using the morphine-dependent rat. These studies were conducted to determine (a) if hot flushes accompany morphine withdrawal in the rat; and (b) if these flushes are associated temporally with other symptoms of the hot flush.

Morphine dependency was produced in female rats by subcutaneous (s.c.) implantation in one pellet containing 75 mg morphine (free base, Merck, St Louis, MO), 37.5 mg microcrystalline cellulose (avisil, FMC Corporation, Philadelphia, PA), 0.56 mg Cab-o-sil (Cabot Corp., Boston, MA) and 1.13 mg Mg Sterate (Fischer Chemical Co., Fair Lawn, NJ). Two days later an additional two morphine pellets were implanted. The pellets were compounded in our laboratory and this treatment regimen produced morphine dependency as measured by several tests of analgesia and withdrawal[49, 50]. Control animals were similarly treated, but received placebo pellets formulated with an additional 75 mg of microcrystalline cellulose that replaced the morphine base. Experiments were conducted 2 days after the last morphine pellets were implanted in a room with an ambient temperature of 26 ± 1 °C.

In an initial experiment, animals were lightly restrained in wire mesh tunnel cages with a wooden floor. Rectal temperature (Tr) and tail skin temperatures (TST) were measured at 5 min intervals. After being placed in the restraining cages, an acclimation period of 30 min was allowed before temperatures were monitored at 10 min intervals for an additional 30 min. At this time, animals were administered either naloxone HCl (1 mg/kg bodyweight (b.w.) s.c.) or saline, and temperatures were recorded at 5 min intervals for the next 90 min.

In morphine-dependent rats there was no difference in resting TST; however, naloxone treatment in these rats resulted in a rapid increase in TST and a subsequent decline in Tr. TST was significantly elevated by 5 min, peaked at 7.2 ± 0.2 °C above baseline by 10–15 min and returned to half of the maximal increase in temperature by 50 min post-naloxone (Fig. 21.1). In animals treated with placebo pellets, naloxone was ineffective

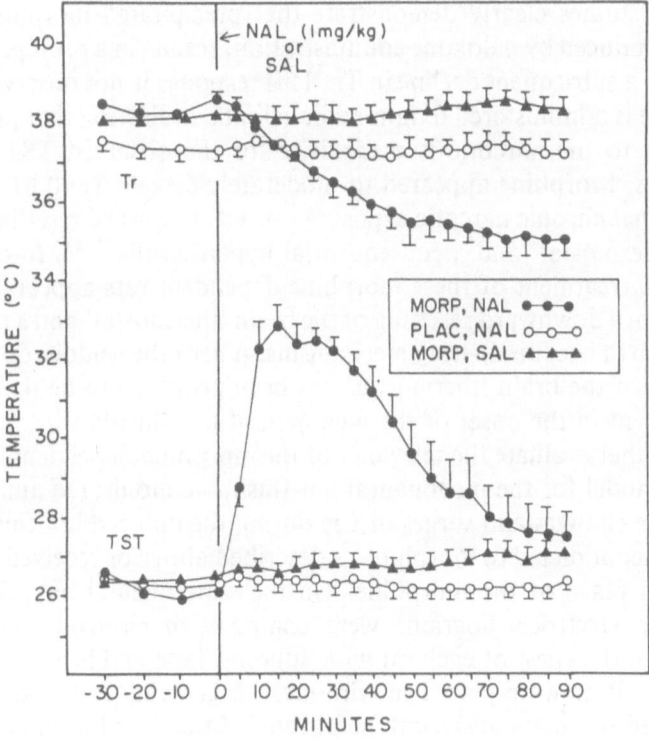

Figure 21.1 Effects of naloxone on tail skin temperature (TST) and rectal temperature (Tr) in morphine-dependent rats. Each point represents the mean and the vertical bar represents 1 standard error of the mean (SEM). The SEM bar is not presented when it is smaller than the symbol used to represent the mean or when it interferes with the expression of the mean value. MORP = morphine-dependent animals, PLAC = placebo-implanted animals, NAL = naloxone administration (1 mg/kg b.w., s.c.) and SAL = saline administration in place of naloxone. $N = 6$ rats per group

in altering TST or Tr (Fig. 21.1). Further, in morphine-dependent rats, saline treatment did not significantly affect TST or Tr (Fig. 21.1). Ovariectomy 2 weeks prior to morphine treatment did not alter naloxone-induced TST or Tr responses. In these ovariectomized rats, peak TST was $6.2 \pm 0.2\,°C$ above baseline and the maximum suppression of Tr was $4.3 \pm 0.3\,°C$. Thus, morphine-induced alterations in gonadal steroid secretion may not be a prerequisite for the observed TST or Tr reponses to naloxone.

Tr in morphine-addicted animals was $0.81\,°C$ higher than in placebo treated rats ($p < 0.05$). A significant decline in Tr was observed by 15 min after naloxone treatment and a maximum decline in Tr of $3.4\,°C$ was observed by 90 min. In placebo-treated rats given naloxone, and in morphine-dependent rats treated with saline, Tr did not change significantly over the 90 min period.

These studies clearly demonstrate that precipitated morphine withdrawal, induced by naloxone administration, results in a prompt surge in TST and a subsequent decline in Tr. This response is not observed when naloxone is administered to non-addicted rats, indicating that preceding exposure to the narcotic is a requisite for the observed TST and Tr responses. Morphine appeared to moderately elevate Tr (0.81 °C) suggesting that chronic narcotic exposure caused an upward resetting of the brain 'thermostat' and a consequential hyperthermia[51-53]. In contrast, naloxone treatment of these morphine-dependent rats appears to have resulted in a downward resetting of the brain 'thermostat' and a resultant activation of heat dissipatory mechanisms. A periodic, sudden downward resetting of the brain 'thermostat' has been proposed to be the precipitating event in the onset of the menopausal hot flush[12, 13].

To further evaluate the relevance of the morphine-dependent rat as an animal model for the menopausal hot flush, we monitored animals for heart rate changes and surges of LH during the induced hot flush. Rats were either addicted to morphine as described above or received placebo pellets in place of the morphine. On the experimental day, discs for recording electrocardiograms were coated with electrode paste and secured to the chest of each rat with adhesive tape and heart rates were recorded. Rats were placed in wire mesh cages and TST and Tr were monitored simultaneously with heart rates. After 1 h of acclimation, an initial resting (0 time) heart rate, TST and Tr were measured. Naloxone (1 mg/kg b.w., s.c.) was then administered and heart rate, TST and Tr were recorded every 3 min for the first 30 min and every 5 min for the remaining 50 min of the experiment.

To define the temporal association between TST and LH secretion, in a subsequent experiment, rats were addicted to morphine as described above. One day following the last morphine (or placebo) implants, an atrial catheter was inserted through the right jugular vein to allow for repeated blood sampling from unanesthetized animals. One day later, animals were lightly restrained and allowed a 1 h acclimation period after which TSTs were recorded at 10 min intervals. Prior to the administration of naloxone (1 mg/kg b.w., s.c.), a single 500 µl blood sample was withdrawn (0 time). Additional 500 µl blood samples were obtained at 5, 10, 15, 30 and 60 min after naloxone administration. TSTs were recorded at 5 min intervals throughout the 90 min experimental period. Each blood sample was immediately centrifuged, plasma was collected and frozen (− 20 °C) and red blood cells were resuspended in 500 µl of heparinized saline (5 IU/ml). To maintain a constant hematocrit, cells were returned to the animals after the subsequent blood sample was obtained. Plasma LH levels were determined by the RIA methods described in the NIAMDD Kits, generously provided by the Hormone Distribution Program. Plasma LH concentrations are expressed in terms of the reference preparation provided (LH-RP-1).

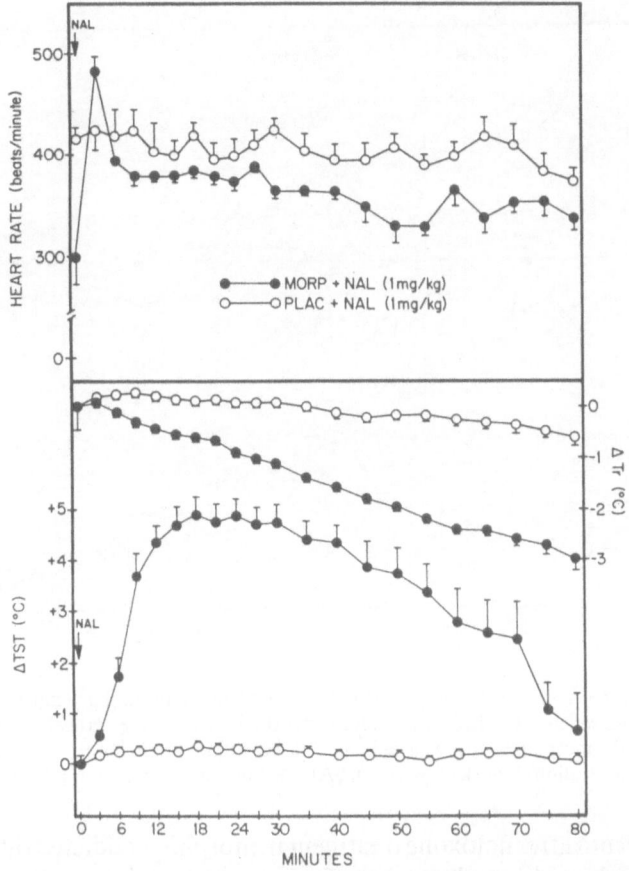

Figure 21.2 Effects of naloxone (NAL) on heart rate, tail skin temperature (TST) and rectal temperature (Tr) in morphine-dependent rats. Each point represents the mean and the vertical bar represents 1 SEM. MORP = morphine-dependent animals. PLAC = placebo-implanted animals, NAL = naloxone administration (1 mg/kg b.w., s.c.). $N = 6$ rats per group

Resting heart rate was 27% lower in MORP-dependent versus placebo implanted rats prior to naloxone treatment (Fig. 21.2). Although naloxone treatment had no significant effect on heart rate in placebo animals, naloxone treatment increased heart rate by 59% within 3 min in morphine-dependent rats (Fig. 21.2). Heart rates remained elevated above baseline by 20–30% through 40 min after naloxone treatment. In these animals TSTs were elevated significantly by 6 min, peaked at 4.9 ± 0.3 °C above baseline at 18 min and remained elevated through 70 min after naloxone treatment. Thus, the positive chronotropic effect of naloxone in the morphine-dependent rat precedes the peak TST response by 15 min. Tr showed a significant decline by 12 min, and decreased progressively

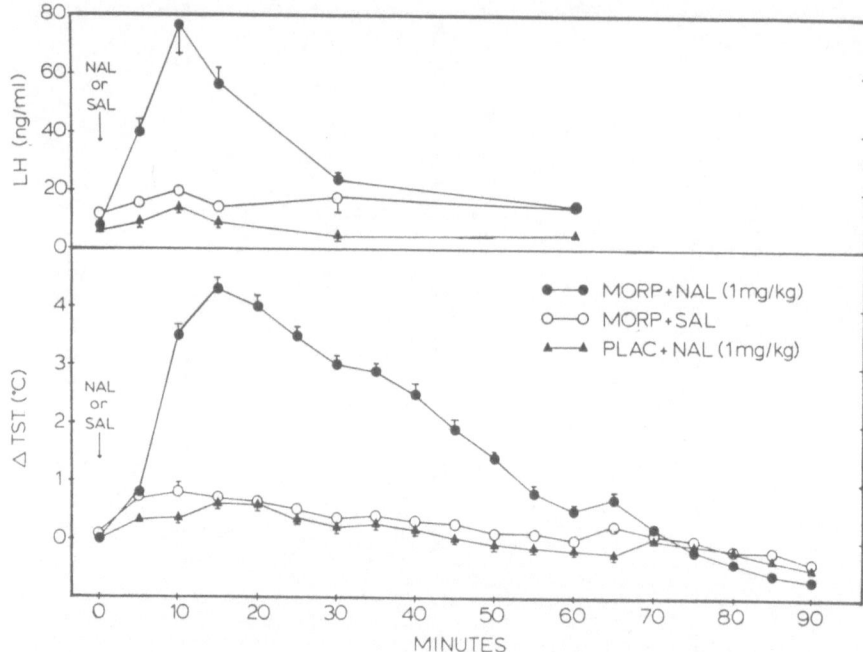

Figure 21.3 Effects of naloxone on plasma LH concentrations and tail skin temperature (TST) in morphine-dependent rats. Each point represents the mean and the vertical bar represents 1 SEM. MORP = morphine-dependent animals, PLAC = placebo-implanted animals, NAL = naloxone administration (1 mg/kg b.w., s.c.), SAL = saline administration. $N = 6$ rats per group

through 80 min after naloxone treatment in morphine-addicted rats, while placebo-implanted rats showed no Tr response to naloxone (Fig. 21.2).

Naloxone treatment in morphine-dependent rats caused a rapid increase in serum LH (Fig. 21.3). LH levels increased significantly by 5 min, peaked at 9 times basal levels by 10 min and remained elevated through 30 min after naloxone treatment. This marked hypersecretion of LH was not observed in placebo-implanted rats following naloxone treatment or in morphine-dependent rats treated with saline. In morphine-dependent rats, TST was moderately elevated by 5 min, peaked at 15 min and remained elevated through 65 min after naloxone treatment. In four of six morphine-dependent rats, the peak LH response preceded by 5 min the peak TST response, while in the remaining two animals LH and TST responses were coincident.

LH secretion appears to be tonically inhibited by opioid neurons in the rat since acute naloxone treatment enhances LH secretion by 2–3-fold in both male and female rats under a variety of experimental conditions[54–56]. In the morphine-addicted rat, naloxone resulted in a 9-fold increase in LH secretion which preceded or was coincident with the TST surge. This temporal association between LH secretion and the TST surge is of interest since hot flushes in women are consistently associated with an LH surge[12-14]. While in women it has been demonstrated that the LH surge itself is not necessary for generation of the hot flush[57-59], the involvement of neurons which secrete LHRH has been suggested. In the rat, LHRH perikarya has been observed in the preoptic area–anterior hypothalamus (POA-AH)[60]. This region is also a site of morphine-responsive, temperature-sensitive neurons[61, 62]. Additionally, injection of LHRH into the POA-AH results in a TST surge[63] which is similar in magnitude and duration to the alterations in TST induced by morphine withdrawal. Thus the present observation, that in morphine-addicted rats the naloxone-induced LH surge precedes or is coincident with the TST surge, is consistent with the involvement of LHRH neurons in the regulation of skin temperature.

While the mechanism by which withdrawal causes an acceleration in heart rate cannot be determined from the present study, the rapidity of the response implicates the adrenergic innervation of the heart. In view of our previous observation that naloxone-induced LH secretion is mediated by an adrenergic mechanism[56], and several reports of hyper-activity of noradrenergic neurons during withdrawal[64-66], some of the manifestations of withdrawal may be the consequence of a generalized sympathetic activation. In this regard it is of interest that an adrenergic involvement in the hot flush has been suggested[12-14], based upon the synchronized alteration in skin temperature, LH secretion and heart rate, all of which are under adrenergic regulation.

In a final experiment, six OVX rats were addicted to morphine while the remaining six OVX rats received placebo pellets as described above. Two days following placement of the last implants, the morphine (or placebo) pellets were surgically removed under light ether anesthesia. At 3, 24 and 53 h following removal of the pellets, TST and Tr were monitored for 2 h periods. Between these observation times animals were returned to their home cages.

Mean TSTs were not different among treatment groups or at any observation time (Table 21.1). However, the coefficient of variation (CV) of TST (an estimate of TST instability) was increased 5-fold, maximum amplitude of TST pulses were increased 7-fold and the number of TST pulses with amplitudes greater than 0.5 °C was increased 4-fold at 24–26 h of morphine withdrawal when compared to placebo controls (Table 21.1). In Fig. 21.4, six individual TST profiles for MORP and placebo-withdrawn rats are shown for the time interval at which maximum TST variability was observed. In the morphine-withdrawal group, one animal showed maximum TST instability at 3–5 h, four showed maximum TST instability at 24–26 h and one animal failed to exhibit significant TST instability at any of the observation times. By 26 h into morphine-abstention, a mild hypothermia was observed (Tr = 37.7 ± 0.2 °C for the

Table 21.1 Parameters of tail skin temperature of rats surgically withdrawn from morphine or placebo pellets

		Time interval after withdrawal		
Treatment	Parameter	3–5 h	24–26 h	53–55 h
Placebo	Average TST (°C)	27.0	27.0	27.1
	CV (%)[a]	0.64 ± 0.13	0.56 ± 0.09	0.57 ± 0.18
Morphine	Average TST (°C)	27.0	27.1	26.6
	CV (%)	1.44 ± 0.41	2.97 ± 1.07*	0.98 ± 0.41
Placebo	Maximum pulse amplitude (°C)[b]	0.43 ± 0.11	0.33 ± 0.07	0.27 ± 0.06
Morphine	Maximum pulse amplitude (°C)	1.08 ± 0.32	2.23 ± 0.84*	0.50 ± 0.06
Placebo	No. of pulses > 0.5 °C[c]	5	6	2
Morphine	No. of pulses > 0.5 °C	24	24	6

[a] CV = coefficient of variation = mean of all temperatures of 2 h ÷ standard deviation about the mean × 100%

[b] The single largest temperature pulse for each animal were grouped and are expressed as mean ± SEM

[c] The total number of skin temperature pulses of > 0.5 °C for all animals over the 2 h interval were grouped

* $p < 0.05$ vs appropriate placebo group. Six morphine- and six placebo-treated animals were employed for the determination of each parameter

placebo-withdrawn group versus 36.6 ± 0.2 °C for the morphine-withdrawn group).

Numerous studies have implicated brain opioids in the regulation of body temperature[51–53]. The above observations indicate that brain opioid neurons may participate in the genesis of the menopausal hot flush. Three consistently observed alterations associated with the hot flush are the rapid, regional skin temperature elevations, closely timed LH surges and a transient phase of tachycardia[12–14]. Each of these alterations is observed during naloxone-precipitated withdrawal. In rats the temporal organization of the peaks of these responses are tachycardia (3 min), LH surge (10 min) and TST surge (15–20 min). In women, tachycardia clearly precedes the hot flush[10], but the LH and skin temperature responses have not been dissociated temporally[12–14].

The role of the coincident LH surge and, presumably, the preceding increase in LHRH release from the basal hypothalamus, has been addressed in several studies. While it is clear that the enhanced LH release itself is not causative in the hot flush in women, the role of the presumed hypersecretion of LHRH has not been adequately addressed. Potent analogs of LHRH administered chronically cause a desensitization of the pituitary LH secretory mechanism and hence block the LH secretory response to endogenous LHRH[67]. Thus LHRH, while blocking the LH pulses associated with the hot flush, do not alter the magnitude or frequency of hot flushes[57, 58]. These results have been taken as evidence against the involvement of LHRH in the neuronal mechanism leading to the hot flush

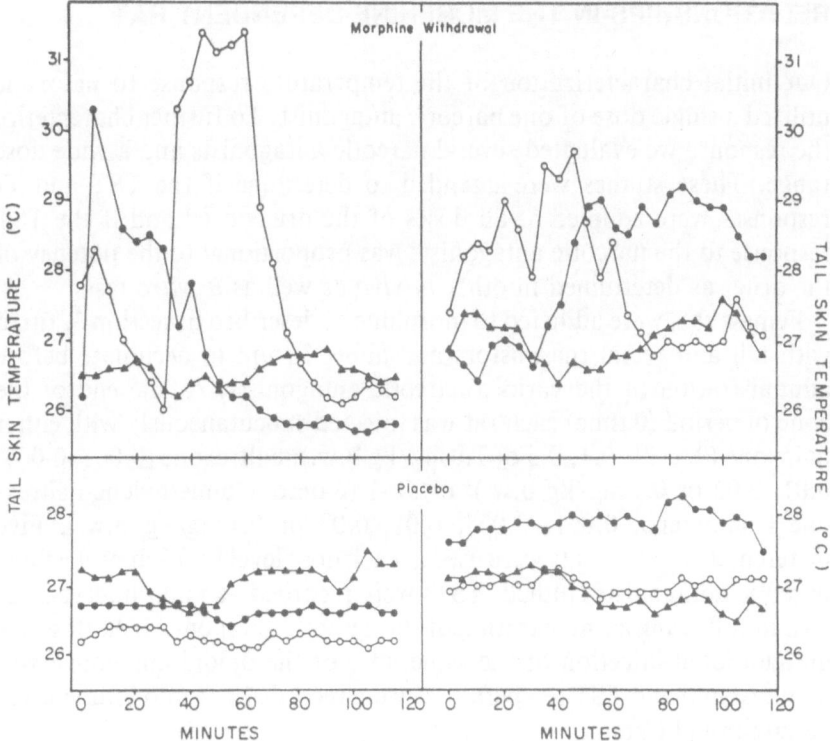

Figure 21.4 Tail skin temperature (TST) profiles of six individual morphine-dependent (upper two panels) or six individual placebo-implanted (lower two panels) rats after removal of morphine-containing or placebo pellets. The panels are separated for each treatment for convenience of expression of data. The three sets of symbols employed in each panel represent TST profiles of different animals

in women. However, it should be noted that systemically administered peptides do not readily cross the blood–brain barrier and, as such, it is unlikely that the LHRH analog could cause a desensitization of LHRH receptors in the POA-AH of the diencephalon. Thus, despite the blockade of LH secretion, the neuronal element in the brain which responds to LHRH likely remains functional. A resolution of the role of LHRH in the series of neuronal events which mediate the hot flush will await the development of LHRH analogs with sufficient lipid solubility to penetrate the blood–brain barrier, or the identification of an animal model (such as that which we have proposed[40]) which would allow the direct application of LHRH to the brain. In this regard, a single report[63], which has not yet be replicated, showed a TST response to LHRH after local administration to the POA-AH. The evaluation, using an appropriate animal model, of the role of LHRH and other neuropeptides is clearly a fruitful area for further evaluation of the hot flush.

4. NARCOTIC ANTAGONIST DOSE–TEMPERATURE RESPONSE RELATIONSHIPS IN THE MORPHINE-DEPENDENT RAT

Our initial characterization of the temperature response to naloxone utilized a single dose of one narcotic antagonist. To further characterize the response we evaluated several narcotic antagonists and a wide dose range. These studies were intended to determine if the TST and Tr responses were coupled at all doses of the drugs used and if the TST response to the narcotic antagonists was proportional to the potency of the drug, as determined in other *in vivo* as well as *in vitro* tests.

Female rats were addicted to morphine as described in section 3, fitted with tail and rectal thermistors and allow 30 min to acclimate before administration of the various narcotic antagonists. At the end of the control period (0 time) each rat was injected subcutaneously with either naloxone (0, 0.01, 0.1, 0.5 or 1.0 mg/kg b.w.); naltrexone (0.001, 0.005, 0.01, 0.02 or 0.1 mg/kg b.w.); or JF-1 (6-desoxy-6-methylene-naltrexone = nalmefene: 0.001, 0.005, 0.01, 0.02 or 0.1 mg/kg b.w.). Five different drug-naive rats were used at each dose level for each of the three narcotic antagonists studied. TSTs were recorded at 5 min intervals for 90 min following administration of the narcotic antagonists. At this time an additional injection of the same dose of the opioid antagonist was administered and TST temperatures were recorded at 5 min intervals for an additional 60 min.

There was no significant difference in resting TST among the groups evaluated. Resting TST for animals administered naloxone was $27.20 \pm 0.14\,°C$; for naltrexone, $27.05 \pm 0.15\,°C$; and for JF-1, $26.99 \pm 0.14\,°C$. Administration of naloxone resulted in a dose-dependent increase in the magnitude and duration of the TST response (Fig. 21.5). At the three highest doses of naloxone the TST was significantly elevated by 5 min and maximum responses were observed at 15–20 min after naloxone treatment (Fig. 21.5). The rectal temperature was significantly reduced at the two highest doses of naloxone. A similar dose-dependent increase in TST was observed following administration of the two other narcotic antagonists (Fig. 21.6).

Regression analysis between the maximal TST response observed and the drug dosage revealed that the dose–response curves for each antagonist were significantly different from each other. A similar relationship was observed when drug dosages and area under the 60 min TST response curve were evaluated. Additionally, when the area under the 60 min TST response curve was compared to the maximum TST response for each drug a linear relationship was observed. The correlation coefficients (r) between these variables were 0.839, 0.956 and 0.885 for naloxone, naltrexone and JF-1, respectively. Although not quantified in this this study, the characteristic wet dog shakes, diarrhea, and teeth chattering were

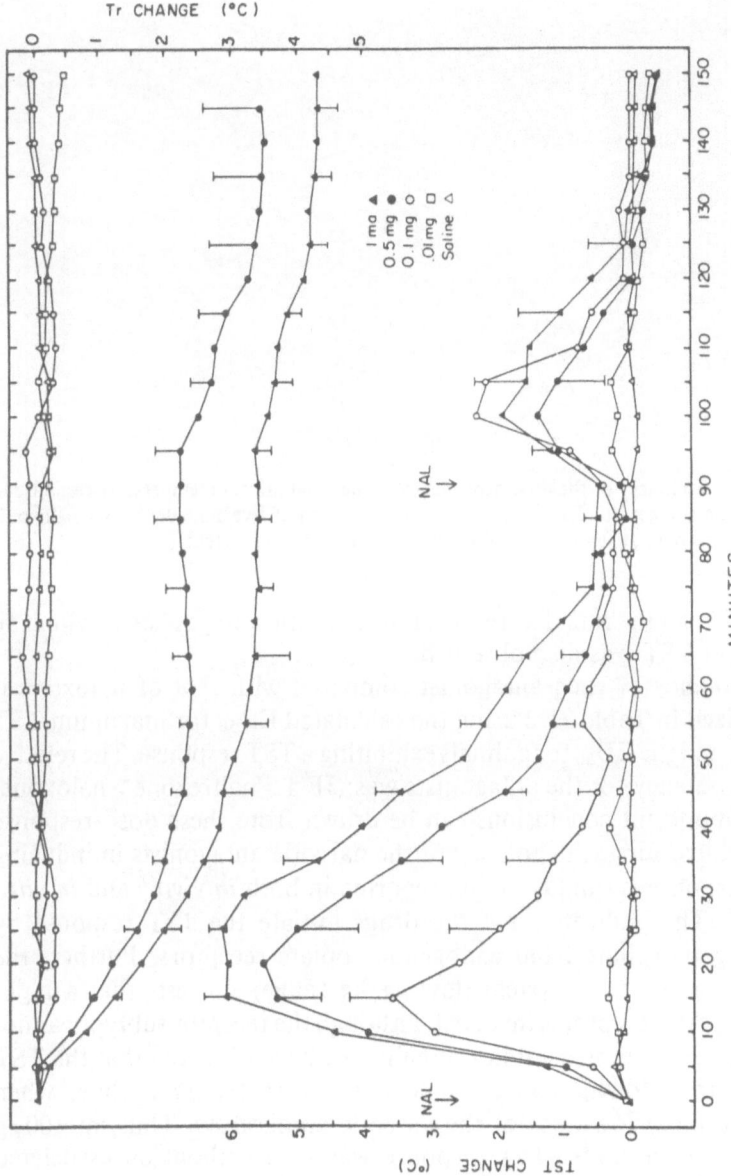

Figure 21.5 Dose dependency of the rectal (Tr) and tail skin temperature (TST) response to naloxone (NAL). Each point represents the mean and the vertical bar represents 1 SEM. Animals were addicted to morphine as described in the text and NAL was administered subcutaneously at the doses indicated

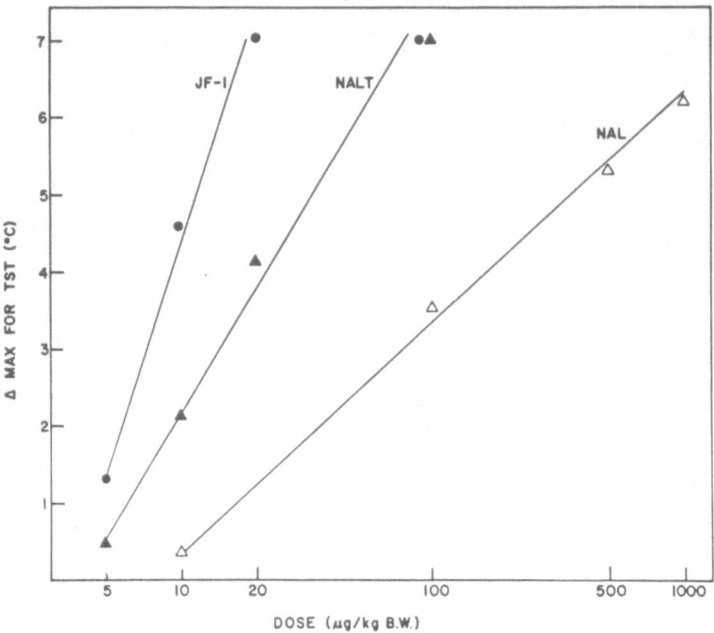

Figure 21.6 Summary of the dose-dependency of maximal tail skin temperature response to three narcotic antagonists. Each point represents the mean of five animals. NAL = naloxone, NALT = naltrexone, JF-1 = 6-desoxy-6-methylenenaltrexone (nalmefene)

observed in all the rats that received the narcotic antagonists in which an increase in TST was also observed.

The potency of each antagonist compared with that of naloxone is summarized in Table 21.2 using the calculated ED_{50} for maximum TST response and the ED_{50} for animals exhibiting a TST response. The relative order of potency for the antagonists was: JF-1 > naltrexone > naloxone.

Two important conclusions can be drawn from these dose–response relationships. First, the potency of the narcotic antagonists in inducing a TST response is similar to that reported in both *in vivo*[68] and *in vitro* studies[69]. This indicates that the drugs initiate the TST response by displacing morphine from endogenous opiate receptors. Further, the responsiveness of the system (low μg/kg range) suggests that a high-affinity opiate receptor is involved, although the receptor subtype cannot be determined by these studies. Finally, we have observed that the TST response to naloxone can be dissociated from the Tr decline, when administering a low dose of the narcotic antagonists. Thus, at 100 μg naloxone/kg, a 3.5 °C TST response was seen without an associated decline in Tr. The decline in Tr may not be a necessary result of a TST increase, and the two components of body temperature may be regulated independently.

Table 21.2 Comparison of potency of narcotic antagonists using tail skin temperature response in morphine-addicted rats

Potency	ED_{50} (μg/kg)[a]	ED_{50} (μg/kg)[b]	Relative	
			a	*b*
Naloxone	152.5	103.7	1	1
Naltrexone	11.5	8.8	13.1	11.8
DM-NALT	5.3	3.52	28.8	29.5

The method of Litchfield and Wilcoxon[100] was used to calculate the ED_{50} for each compound
[a] ED_{50} was calculated as the dose of drug at which 50% of the rats showed a 50% maximal response of TST. Maximal TST response was similar in the three groups, therefore the mean TST of all animals receiving the highest dose of opioid antagonists was the value used to calculate percentage maximal responses
[b] ED_{50} was calculated as the dose of drug at which 50% of the animals exhibited a TST response. A TST response was defined as the elevation in TST which was at least 50% greater than the mean TST response observed in saline-treated control rats

5. BRAIN MEDIATION OF THE TST RESPONSE TO NALOXONE IN MORPHINE-DEPENDENT RATS

The temporal association of the TST, heart rate and LH secretory response to naloxone administration (section 3), suggests that all three components of withdrawal are mediated by the activation of the CNS component of the sympathetic nervous system. As indicated above, a similar hypothesis has been proposed to explain the association of menopausal hot flushes with tachycardia and LH pulses. Direct testing of this hypothesis requires the application of methods to: (a) induce hot flush by activation of specific brain regions; (b) local application to specific brain regions of drugs which antagonized hot flushes; and (c) direct measurement of brain region neuronal activity during the hot flush. For obvious reasons these studies are not possible in human subjects, and appropriate animal models are needed. We have used the morphine-dependent rat to begin to resolve these issues of the brain locus and neurotransmitter systems which mediate the hot flush. The present study was undertaken to determine the brain locus of the naloxone-induced TST response in morphine-dependent rats.

To apply naloxone locally to various brain regions, guide cannulae were placed into the preoptic area–anterior hypothalamus (POA-AH), the medial basal hypothalamus (MBH), the locus coeruleus (LC) or the lateral ventricle (LV). Bilateral cannulas were placed in the POA-AH or MBH while a single cannula was placed in the LC or LV. The POA-AH was chosen for study because it is the major brain region which regulates body temperature[51–53, 62] and contains temperature-sensitive, morphine-responsive neurons[61, 62], as well as cell bodies for preopticotuberal LHRH neurons[60]. The MBH is the site of high concentrations of various

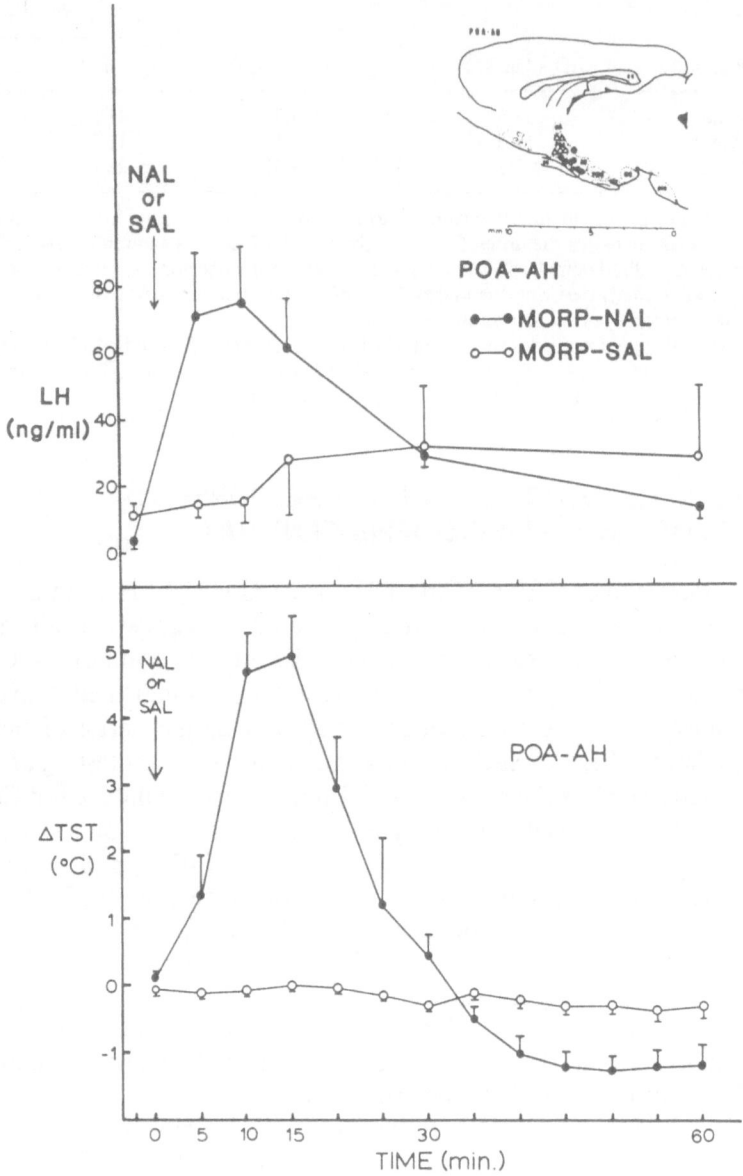

Figure 21.7 Effects of microinjection of naloxone into the preoptic area–anterior hypothalamus (POA-AH) on serum LH concentrations and tail skin temperature (TST) in morphine-dependent rats. Points represent the mean and vertical bars represent 1 SEM. MORP = morphine-dependent rats, NAL = naloxone injection ($40\,\mu g/4\,\mu l$), SAL = saline injection ($4\,\mu l$). The insert shows the loci of NAL (solid points) and saline (open triangles) injections

endogenous opioid peptides[70], opiate receptors[71] as well as nerve terminals of LHRH neurons[60]. The LC is a major site of origin of nor-adrenergic perikarya which project to the forebrain[72]. Finally, the LV was used as an injection site, since drugs administered here should be distributed to all of the aforementioned brain regions.

Following a 7-day recovery period, animals were subject to the morphine-addiction paradigm described in section 3. Naloxone (40 μg) was administered by microinjection (total volume of 4 μl) into the POA-AH, MBH, LC or LV. TST and LH levels were monitored as described in section 3 and after the experiment, brains were dissected to verify the injection site.

Microinjection of naloxone into the POA-AH resulted in a prompt hypersecretion of LH (MAX = 75 ± 17 ng/ml) which peaked at 10 min and a subsequent surge in TST (Fig. 21.7; MAX = 4.9 ± 0.5 °C) observed 5 min later. These peak responses in LH and TST were similar in onset, duration and magnitude to those observed following systemic administration of naloxone (Fig. 21.7).

Similar responses were observed following administration of naloxone into the LC. The peak surge in LH was 63 ± 16 ng/ml which was followed 5 min later by a maximal TST change of 4.9 ± 0.7 °C (Fig. 21.8).

Central microinjection of naloxone into the MBH (Fig. 21.9) also produced similar increases in serum LH (79 ± 11 ng/ml) and in the TST surge (2.6 ± 0.5 °C). The peak response times for both LH and TST were observed 10 min following administration of naloxone.

Administration of naloxone into the LV (Fig. 21.10) also resulted in a similar increase in serum LH (57 ± 17 ng/ml) and a 3.2 ± 0.7 °C surge in TST. However, the time courses for both the rise in LH and TST surge were extended by about 5 min to 15 and 20 min, respectively, when compared to that observed following microinjections into other brain sites.

In each of these four separate studies, administration of the vehicle, isotonic saline, in each brain area was ineffective in altering TST or serum LH. In each study the basal values for LH, TST and Tr were similar between all groups, as were the responses to microinjections of naloxone. Not shown were the maximal decreases of Tr observed following administration of naloxone in the POA-AH, MBH, LC and LV, which were similar in each study; -1.7 ± 0.5 °C, -1.6 ± 0.4 °C, -2.7 ± 0.6 °C, -2.8 ± 0.7 °C, respectively. Therefore, the overall responsiveness to central microinjection of naloxone was similar in all parameters to those previously described following systemic administration of naloxone. The only striking difference between the two routes of administration with the narcotic antagonist was a lack of a diarrhea response in the animals administered the naloxone centrally.

Since naloxone has a high lipophilicity and therefore may migrate rapidly away from the site of injection, we performed a subsequent experiment in which we administered [³H]naloxone into the cerebral

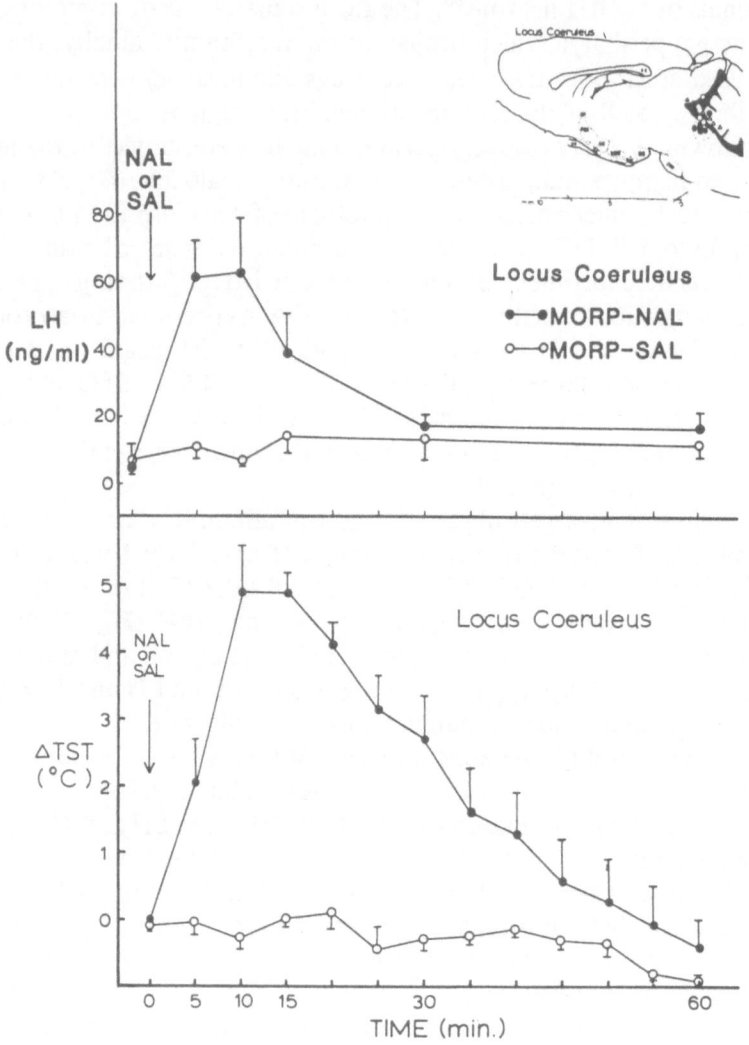

Figure 21.8 Effects of microinjection of naloxone into the locus coeruleus (LC) on serum LH concentrations and tail skin temperature (TST) in morphine-dependent rats. Points represent the mean and vertical bars represent 1 SEM. MORP = morphine-dependent rats, NAL = naloxone injection (40 μg/4 μl), SAL = saline injection (4 μl). The insert shows the loci of NAL (solid points) and saline (open triangles) injections

cortex and determined the concentration of naloxone recovered in the systemic blood and two other brain regions. The rats were fitted with a cannula into the frontal cortex and 2 days later they were addicted to morphine as previously described. Naloxone (40 μg/4 μl) was equally mixed with [³H]naloxone (1 μCi/μl, New England Nuclear). A total concentration of 40 μg of naloxone was administered into the frontal cortex

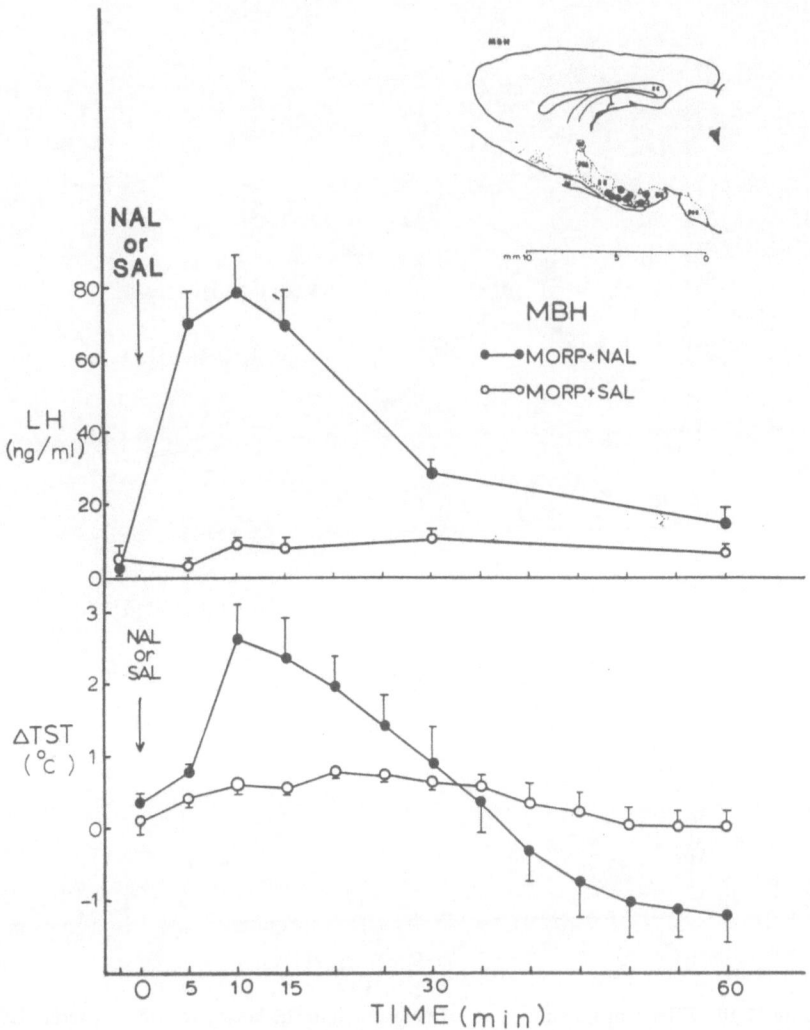

Figure 21.9 Effects of microinjections of naloxone into the medial basal hypothalamus (MBH) on serum LH concentrations and tail skin temperature in morphine-dependent rats. Points represent the mean and vertical bars represent 1 SEM. MORP = morphine-dependent rats, NAL = naloxone injection (40 μg/4 μl), SAL = saline injection (4 μl). The insert shows the loci of NAL (solid points) and saline (open triangles) injections

at the same 4 μl volume used in the previous studies. Animals were de-capitated 15 min following administration of naloxone, a time at which peak response of LH and TST had previously been shown to occur. At the time of sacrifice, trunk blood was collected and the brains were removed. The hypothalamus and its adjacent preoptic area were dissected using the caudal aspects of the olfactory tubercle as the rostral border, the

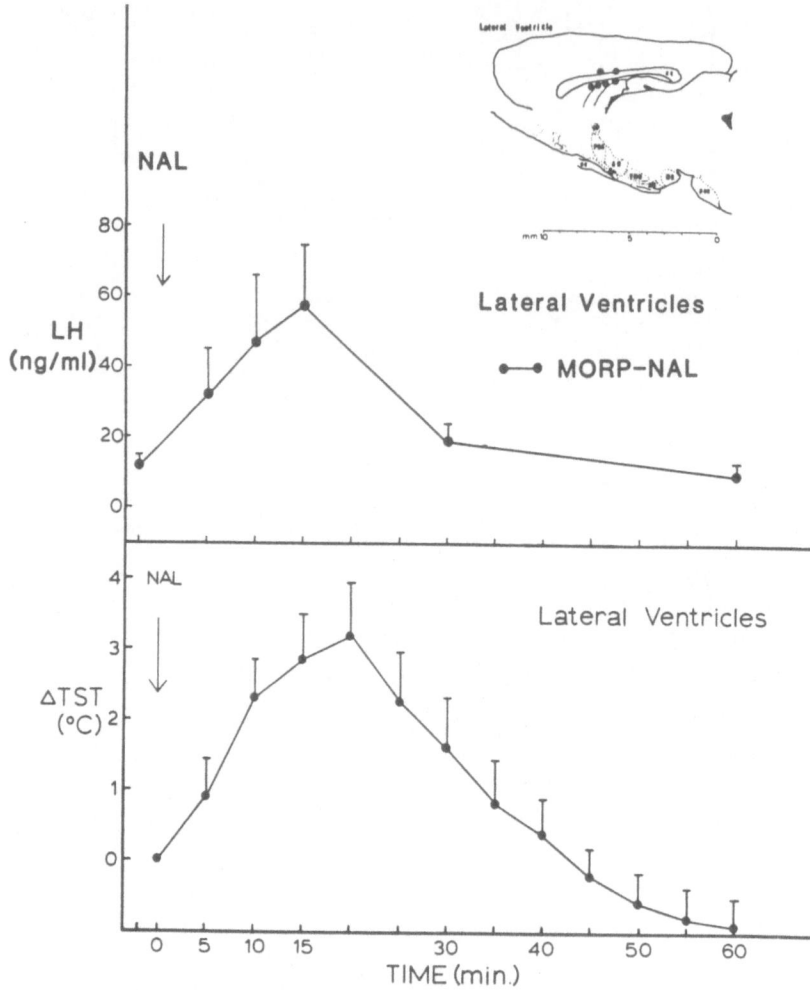

Figure 21.10 Effects of microinjection of naloxone into the lateral ventricle on serum LH concentrations and tail skin temperature (TST) in morphine-dependent rats. Points represent means and vertical bars represent 1 SEM. MORP = morphine-dependent rats, NAL = naloxone injection (40 μg/4 μl). The insert shows the loci of NAL injections (solid points)

hypothalamic sulci as the lateral border, and the rostral aspects of the mammillary bodies as the caudal borders. The midbrain–brainstem was also dissected out by removing the cerebellum and retaining the tissue between the superiormost aspects of the spinal cord and the cerebral peduncle. The [³H]naloxone was then extracted by a slight modification of procedures described by Sprague and Takemoi[73] and Owen and Cicero[74].

The results, as summarized in Table 21.3, suggest that less than 1% of the administered naloxone migrates to brain sites distant from the site of

Table 21.3 Estimate of movement of naloxone following administration of [³H]naloxone in the frontal cortex of the morphine-dependent female rat

Time after naloxone administration	Percentage of total counts (and calculated content of naloxone) recovered from		
	Hypothalamus	Brain stem	Systemic blood
15 min	0.029 ± 0.004^a (11.52 ± 1.80 ng)	0.062 ± 0.014 (24.68 ± 5.72 ng)	0.057.0.012 (22.80 ± 4.92 ng)

[a] Mean ± 1 SEM

injection or appears in the systemic circulation. The calculated concentration recovered in each area is also significantly lower than any minimal dosage of naloxone required to elicit a significant elevation in TST or serum LH. These results suggest that the diffusion of naloxone occurs rather slowly, and thus the major physiological effects of the administered naloxone should be restricted to the site of injection. Support for this suggestion is the 4.2 ± 0.6 °C surge in TST and the peak LH response of 93 ± 12 ng/ml that occurred 10–15 min following microinjection of naloxone ($40 \mu g/4 \mu l$) into the frontal cortex of morphine-addicted rats.

We had initially suspected that the POA-AH was the central anatomical site responsible for the increase in TST and LH response following administration of naloxone to morphine-addicted rats. The rationale for this hypothesis is that the POA-AH is the site of morphine-responsive, temperature sensitive neurons[61, 62] and is also a major CNS site for the regulation of body temperature. Therefore it was reasonable to anticipate the POA-AH would be a central site that mediated the TST surge observed in the morphine-addicted rats. The LC has also been shown to be integrally involved in enhanced noradrenergic activity associated with morphine withdrawal[75]. However, at this time there does not appear to be a 'specific brain site' that is responsible for the surge in TST and LH response associated with administration of naloxone in morphine-dependent rats. It appears that in all five brain regions evaluated, microinjection of naloxone results in similar behavioral manifestations of withdrawal; i.e. hyperactivity, licking behavior, and stereotypic gnawing and writhing. Additionally, regardless of the brain sites, the TST was significantly increased 3–5 °C and serum LH was elevated by 60–90 ng/ml over the control values. The peak LH surge preceded that of the TST by 5 min with both parameters reaching peak response within 20 min after administration of naloxone. The response observed following microinjection of naloxone into the LV was more prolonged than any other site, indicating that the drug first must be distributed out of the ventricle and into the neural tissue to mediate the appropriate responses. Collectively, these data indicate that, in morphine-dependent rats, TST and LH surges can be induced by local administration of naloxone to several brain regions at concentrations much lower than those that could elicit the responses when naloxone is administered systemically. Therefore, the effect of naloxone appears to be mediated subsequent to a locally initiating spreading activation of central neurons, similar to seizure-type responses associated with epilepsy.

6. EFFECTS OF MORPHINE WITHDRAWAL ON NOREPINEPHRINE AND DOPAMINE METABOLISM IN THE POA-AH AND THE MBH

The evidence for the involvement of brain sympathetic nerves in the series of events which mediates the menopausal hot flush, is largely derived from inference and certain pharmacological observations. The association of the hot flush with other symptoms of acute sympathetic outflow from the brain has led to the suggestion of an instability of the sympathetic component of the brain mechanism which regulates body temperature[12-14]. Clonidine, a specific α_2-adrenergic receptor agonist[76, 77], reduces the symptoms of hot flush in menopausal women[78, 79]. This effect is observed at doses of clonidine which exert antihypertensive effects, and presumably the two actions of the drugs are mediated by the same mechanism. The preponderance of evidence indicates that the antihypertension action of clonidine results from the stimulation of α_2-adrenoceptors on presynaptic noradrenergic neurons[76, 77]. Stimulation of these auto-receptors reduces activity in noradrenergic neurons[80, 81]. Thus in the menopausal women it is presumed that clonidine reduces the incidence of hot flushes by preventing (or reducing) the acute discharge of brain norepinephrine associated with the flush.

Like the menopausal hot flush, opiate withdrawal results in the symptoms associated with brain sympathetic outflow[40, 41], and these symptoms are ameliorated by clonidine treatment[82, 83]. In animals, morphine treatment reduces noradrenergic neuronal activity[75, 83] and in morphine-dependent rodents withdrawal is associated with enhanced norepinephrine turnover[75, 85-87]. Collectively, these studies suggest that opiate withdrawal symptoms, including the hot flush which we have described[40], is mediated by brain noradrenergic neurons. Additionally, activity in other neuronal systems is altered during opiate withdrawal although the role in its symptomatology is less certain. To further document the role of brain catecholaminergic neurons in the etiology of the rat hot flush, we evaluated NE and DA turnover during the time of the naloxone-induced TST surge.

Morphine-dependency was produced in female rats as described in section 3. After 4 days of exposure to the narcotic, withdrawal was precipitated by naloxone (1 mg/kg b.w., s.c.) and rats were killed by decapitation 5, 15, 30 or 60 min later. A control group of morphine-dependent rats was treated with the saline vehicle rather than naloxone and was killed 5 min later. The POA-AH and the MBH were immediately dissected, homogenized in PCA and frozen for later assay of catecholamines and their metabolites by HPLC and amperometric methods.

During the course of naloxone-induced withdrawal in morphine-dependent rats, concentrations of NE in the MBH were reduced by 26% and 28% by 30 and 60 min respectively (Fig. 21.11). Similarly, in the POA-AH, a 29% and 40% decrease in NE concentrations occurred over the same time period (Fig. 21.11). In both tissues the decline in NE concentrations was preceded by a 2–3-fold increase in the concentration of normetanephrine (NME). Elevated NME levels persisted through 60 min in the MBH and 30 min in the POA-AH. In contrast, DA

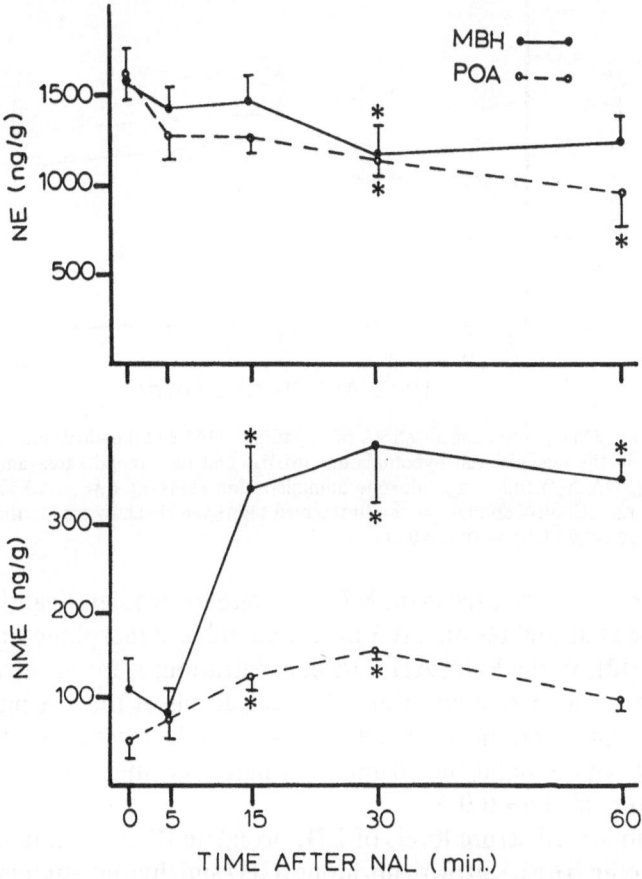

Figure 21.11 Changes in concentrations of norepinephrine (NE) and normetanephrine (NME) in the medial basal hypothalamus (MBH) and the preoptic area–anterior hypothalamus (POA-AH) following naloxone administration (1 mg/kg b.w., s.c.) to morphine-dependent rats. Control animals (time = 0) received saline vehicle and were sacrificed at 5 min after injection. $*p < 0.05$ vs time = 0 group

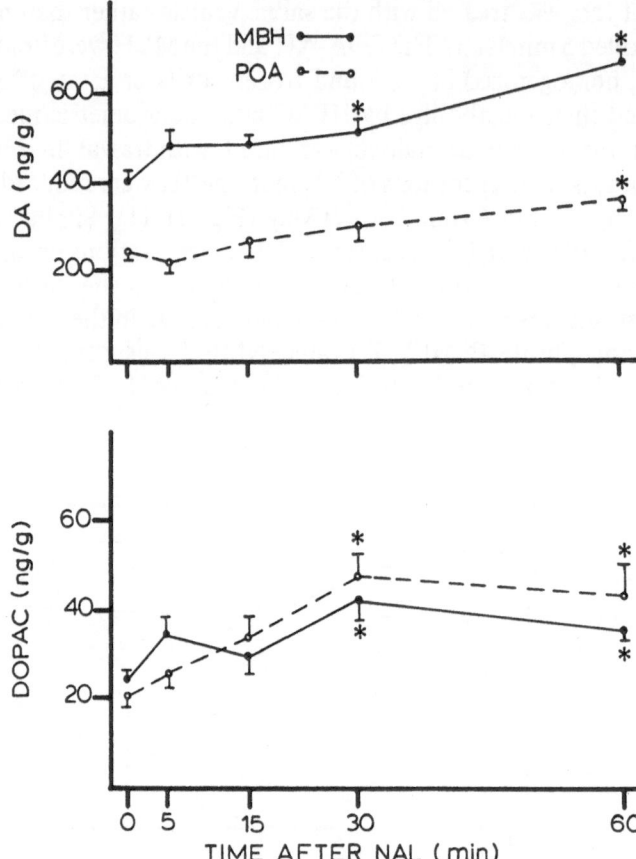

Figure 21.12 Changes in concentrations of dopamine (DA) and dihydroxyphenylacetic acid (DOPAC) in the medial basal hypothalamus (MBH) and the preoptic area–anterior hypothalamus (POA-AH) following naloxone administration (1 mg/kg b.w., s.c.) to morphine-dependent rats. Control animals (time = 0) received saline vehicle and were sacrificed at 5 min after injection. $*p < 0.05$ vs time = 0 group

concentrations increased in the MBH, being elevated significantly by 21% and 40% at 30 and 60 min after naloxone-induced morphine withdrawal (Fig. 21.12). In the POA-AH, DA concentrations were elevated 34% at 60 min after naloxone injection. Concentrations of the DA metabolite, dihydroxyphenylacetic acid (DOPAC), were increased in both hypothalamic regions at 30 and 60 min after naloxone injection to morphine-dependent rats ($p = 0.05$).

We monitored serum levels of LH, prolactin (PRL), immunoreactive β-endorphin (IRβE), growth hormone (GH) and thyroid-stimulating hormone (TSH) during the course of naloxone-induced morphine withdrawal. As expected, naloxone caused a prompt, large increase in serum LH concentrations (see sections 3 and 5) with peak levels occurring at 5 min into withdrawal (Fig. 21.13). Interestingly, IRβE levels increased coincident

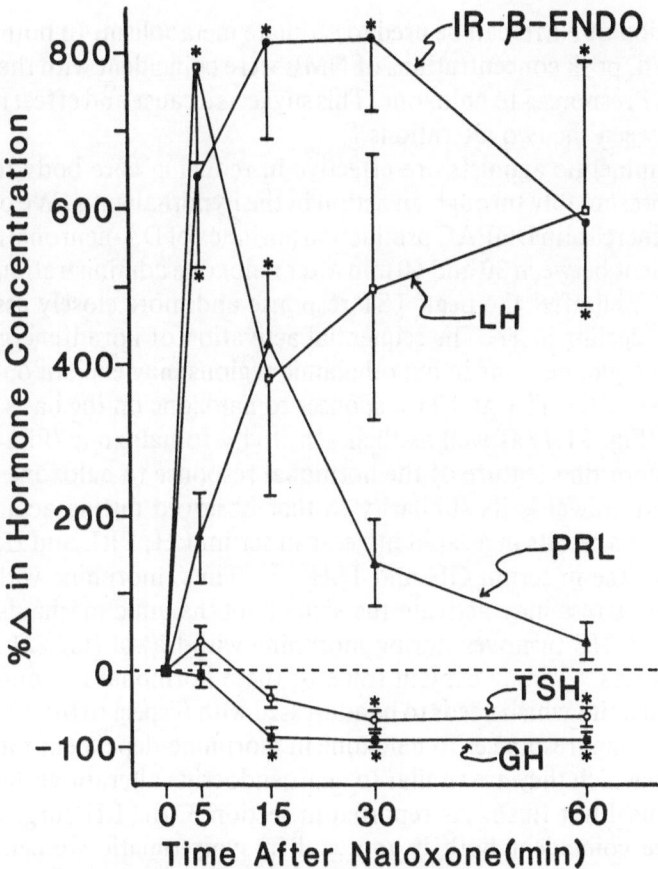

Figure 21.13 Percentage changes in serum immunoreactive β-endorphin (IR-β-ENDO), luteinizing hormone (LH), prolactin (PRL), thyroid stimulating hormone (TSH) and growth hormone (GH) concentrations in morphine-dependent rats following injection of naloxone (1 mg/kg b.w., s.c.). Control animals (time = 0) received saline vehicle and were sacrificed 5 min after injection. *$p < 0.05$ vs. time = 0 group

with the LH surge at 5 min but peaked at 15–30 min and remained elevated through 60 min after naloxone administration (Fig. 21.13). Serum PRL levels were increased at 30 min only. In marked contrast to the hypersecretory responses of LH, IRβE and PRL, serum levels of GH and TSH were reduced from 15 to 60 min into naloxone precipitated withdrawal (Fig. 21.13).

The present results indicate that associated with naloxone-induced morphine withdrawal is a prompt activation of hypothalamic noradrenergic and dopaminergic neurons. For noradrenergic neurons in both the POA-AH and the MBH, this activation was expressed as an increase in concentrations of NME, the 3-O-methylated metabolite of NE. NME is formed by the action of catecholamine-O-methyl transferase (COMT) on NE[88]. Since COMT is located postsynaptically, among other sites, the production of NME can be used to estimate metabolism. In both regions examined, peak concentrations of NME were coincident with the time of peak TST responses to naloxone. This suggests a cause and effect relationship between the two alterations.

Dopaminergic agonists are effective in reducing core body temperature[89], presumably through an action in the hypothalamus. We observed that the increase in DOPAC production (an index of DA-neuronal activity) was evident between 30 and 60 min after naloxone administration, a time which is well after the peak TST response and more closely associated with the decline in Tr. The sequential activation of noradrenergic, then dopaminergic, neurons in hypothalamic regions may explain our ability to dissociate the TST and Tr responses to naloxone on the basis of their latency (Fig. 21.1) as well as their sensitivity to naloxone (Fig. 21.5).

An interesting feature of the hormonal response to naloxone precipitated withdrawal is its similarity to that observed during acute stress. Acute stress results in a rapid increase in serum LH, PRL and IRβE[90–92] and a decline in serum GH and TSH[93, 94]. Thus, morphine withdrawal and acute stress may activate the same hypothalamic mechanism. The increase in NE turnover during morphine withdrawal (Fig. 21.11) and during stress[95, 96] may explain some of these hormonal responses.

A final point which needs to be addressed with respect to these neuronal and hormonal responses to naloxone in morphine-dependent rats, is the extent to which they are similar to neuroendocrine alterations during the menopausal hot flush. As reported in section 3, the LH surge and hot flush are coincident both in rats and in symptomatic women. Initial reports have failed to observe a consistent secretory response of PRL associated with the hot flush[12, 13]. However, β-endorphin, which is released in concert with adrenocorticotropin (ACTH), is released during the hot flush[18]. This release of β-endorphin/ACTH likely explains the coincident release of adrenal steroids during hot flushes[14]. In light of recent evidence for the release of adrenal epinephrine during the hot flush in women[17], it can be concluded that in women, central sympathetic activation is associated with, and likely causative in, the hot flush.

7. ROLE OF α-ADRENERGIC NEURONS IN THE SKIN TEMPERATURE RESPONSE TO NALOXONE IN MORPHINE-DEPENDENT RATS

The aforementioned evidence for the coincident hyperactivity of noradrenergic neurons in the POA-AH and the MBH and the TST surge during the induced hot flush provides supportive, albeit circumstantial, evidence for the involvement of a brain adrenergic mechanism in the series of neuronal events leading to the hot flush. If acute hyperactivity of brain noradrenergic neurons is involved in the induced hot flush, the TST alteration during withdrawal should be responsive to pharmacological interruption of noradrenergic neurotransmission. In the present study we used our animal model for the hot flush to determine the effects of clonidine on the naloxone-induced flush. Additionally, we evaluated the effects of blockade of postsynaptic α-adrenergic receptors on the flush.

Female rats were fitted with a stainless steel cannula into the lateral ventricle and addicted to morphine as described in sections 3 and 5. Again, control animals received placebo implants formulated without morphine.

To specifically evaluate the role of brain noradrenergic neurons in the TST response to naloxone in morphine-dependent rats, the adrenergic agonist and antagonist were administered intracerebroventricularly (i.c.v.). Clonidine HCl was administered to both placebo-implanted and morphine-dependent rats at doses of 0.53, 10 or 50 μg/rat. Phentolamine was given to morphine-dependent rats only at doses of 11.9, 30 or 60 μg/rat. A volume of 4 μl was used for all i.c.v. administration of drugs and vehicle (saline, SAL). In some studies the adrenergic drugs were administered 10 min prior to naloxone HCl (1 mg/kg b.w., s.c.). This dose and route of administration was chosen for naloxone because it causes a maximal TST response in morphine-dependent rats (section 4). The dose ranges for clonidine[97] and phentolamine[97, 98] were chosen on the basis of their ability to alter core body temperature.

As we observed previously, naloxone treatment in morphine-dependent rats caused a prompt significant rise in TST (Δmax TST $= 5.0 \pm 0.3$ °C) (Fig. 21.14). This naloxone-induced elevation in TST was associated with a 1.3 ± 0.1 °C decline in Tr by 60 min after injection. Saline injection, in place of naloxone, failed to alter either TST or Tr. Injection (i.c.v.) of a low dose of clonidine (0.53 μg) also failed to modify TST or Tr when compared to saline-injected controls. Clonidine at doses of 10 or 50 μg elevated TST by about 1.5 °C. This response was significantly greater than that caused by saline and the low dose of clonidine but significantly less than the naloxone response. Despite the modest TST response to clonidine, the Δmax for Tr was reduced in a time- and dose-dependent manner.

In view of the TST and Tr responses to clonidine in morphine-dependent rats, we determined temperature responses to this adrenergic agonist in control rats. In placebo-treated rats the TST response to clonidine was evident only at the highest dose of clonidine, and it was not different from that observed in morphine-dependent rats (Fig. 21.15). As in morphine-dependent rats, clonidine causes a dose-dependent decline in Tr (Fig. 21.15). Thus morphine treatment appeared to modify only the TST response to the intermediate dose (10 μg) of clonidine.

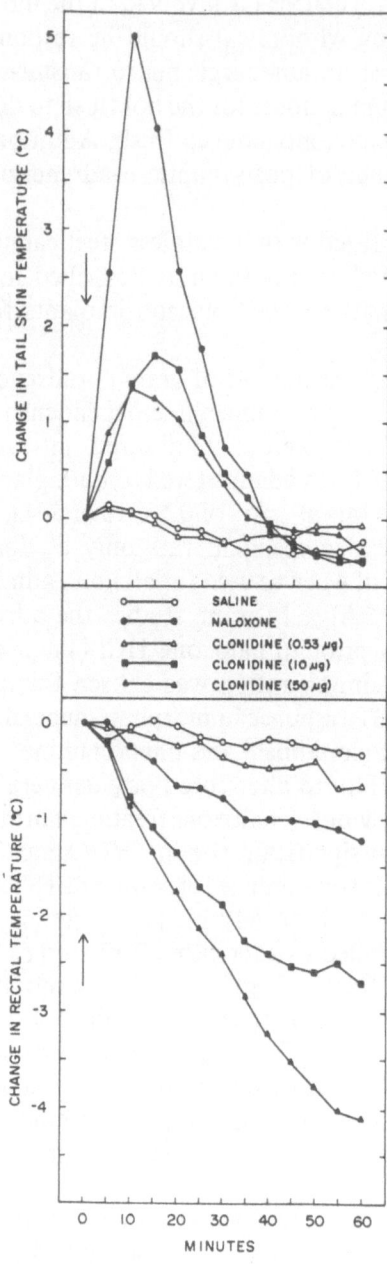

Figure 21.14 Effects of naloxone and clonidine on tail skin temperature (TST) and rectal temperature (Tr) in morphine-dependent rats. Rats were administered saline or clonidine i.c.v. at time 0 (arrow). For comparison, naloxone was administered s.c. at a dose (1 mg/kg b.w.) which causes a maximal TST response. Represented here are mean changes in TST and Tr for each group at specific times after drug administration

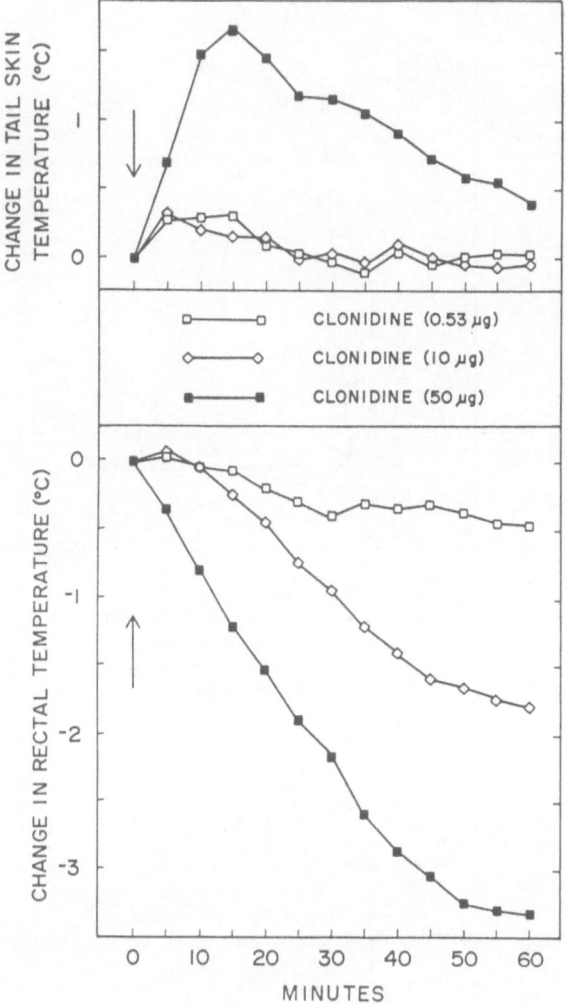

Figure 21.15 Effects of clonidine on TST and Tr in placebo-implanted rats. Rats were administered clonidine i.c.v. at time 0 (arrow). Represented here are mean changes in TST and Tr for each group at specific times after drug administration

In view of the evidence that clonidine can reduce NE release by an action on presynaptic α_2-adrenergic receptor activity[76, 77, 80, 81], we evaluated the effect of central administration of clonidine on the capacity of systemically administered naloxone to precipitate a TST surge in the morphine-dependent rat. In animals treated i.c.v. with the saline vehicle, naloxone caused a prompt TST surge (Δmax TST = 4.5 ± 0.9 °C) (Fig. 21.16). The low dose of clonidine (0.53 μg), which in placebo- or morphine-treated animals failed to modify TST or Tr, also failed to block the TST

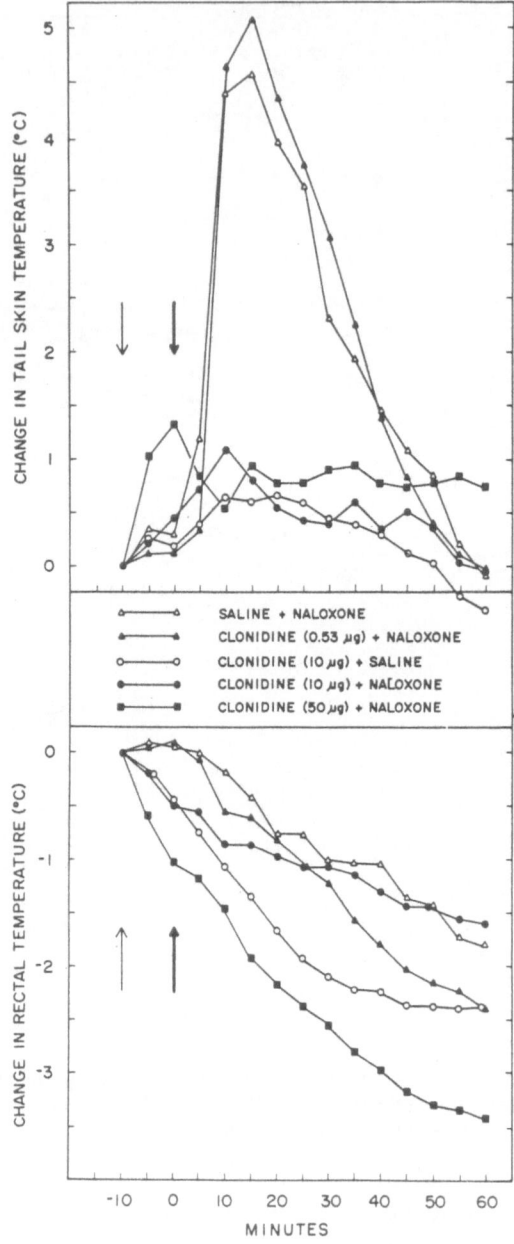

Figure 21.16 Effects of clonidine pretreatment on the response of tail skin temperature (TST) and rectal temperature to naloxone in morphine-dependent rats. Rats were administered clonidine or saline, i.c.v. (small arrow, − 10 min) and 10 min later received naloxone (1 mg/kg b.w.) or saline s.c. (bold arrow, time 0). Represented here are the mean changes in TST and Tr for each group at specific times after drug administration

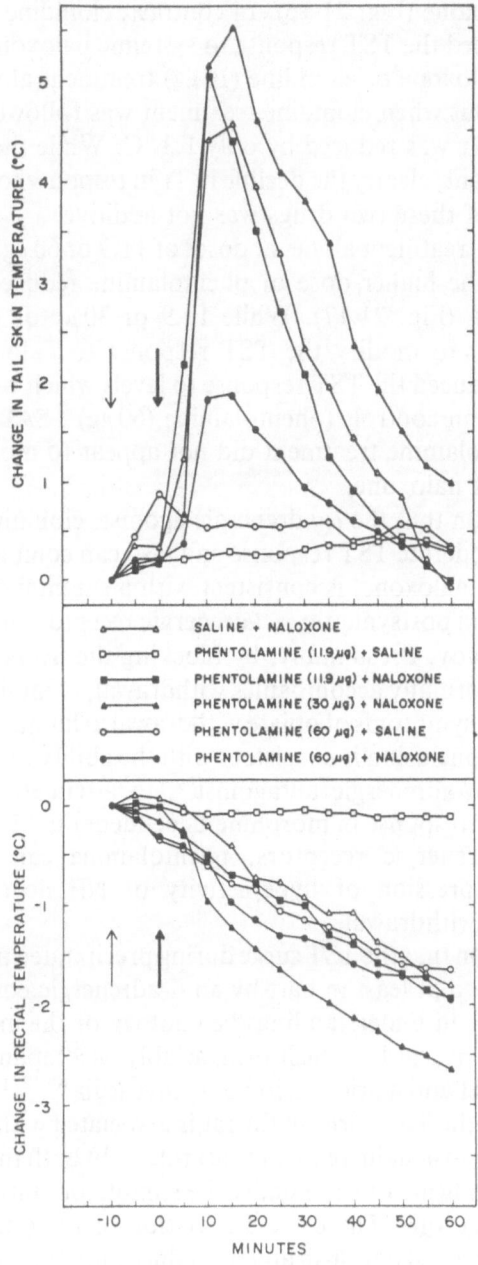

Figure 21.17 Effects of phentolamine pretreatment on the response of tail skin temperature (TST) and rectal temperature (Tr) to naloxone in morphine-dependent rats. Rats were administered phentolamine or saline, i.c.v. (small arrow, −10 min) and 10 min later received naloxone (1 mg/kg b.w.) or saline s.c. (bold arrow, time 0). Represented here are the mean changes in TST and Tr for each group at specific times after drug administration

response to naloxone (Fig. 21.16). In contrast, clonidine at doses of 10 or 50 μg suppressed the TST response to systemic naloxone (Fig. 21.16). Interestingly, naloxone or clonidine (10 μg) treatment alone reduced Tr by about 2 °C, but when clonidine treatment was followed 10 min later with naloxone, Tr was reduced by only 1.3 °C. While these differences were not significant, clearly the decline in Tr in response to the sequential administration of these two drugs was not additive.

Phentolamine treatment alone, at doses of 11.9 or 60 μg, failed to alter TST, although the higher dose of phentolamine reduced Tr by 1.5 ± 0.3 °C by 60 min (Fig. 21.17). While 11.9 or 30 μg of the α-receptor antagonist failed to modify the TST response to naloxone, 60 μg of phentolamine reduced the TST response to levels which were not significantly greater than controls (phentolamine (60 μg) + SAL) (Fig. 21.17). However, phentolamine treatment did not appear to modify the hypothermic effect of naloxone.

Our observation that the α-adrenergic agonist, clonidine[76, 77] can, by itself, cause a moderate TST response and also can completely block the TST response to naloxone, is consistent with a simultaneous activation of presynaptic and postsynaptic α_2-adrenergic receptors at the doses used in the present study. Presumably, by blocking the hyperactivity of NE neurons which normally accompanies withdrawal, clonidine can prevent the expression of symptoms of opiate withdrawal in human addicts as well as the rat. This conclusion is consistent with the ability of phentolamine, a non-selective α-adrenergic antagonist[99], to attenuate the naloxone-precipitated TST response in morphine-dependent rats. By antagonizing postsynaptic adrenergic receptors, phentolamine can attenuate the physiological expression of hyperactivity of NE neurons occurring during morpine withdrawal.

Our observation that the TST surge during precipitated morphine withdrawal is mediated at least in part by an α-adrenergic component, may be of importance in understanding the etiology of the menopausal hot flush. The menopausal hot flush is invariably accompanied by a surge in secretion of LH and a brief period of tachycardia[10, 12–14]. Similarly we have shown that the TST surge in the rat is associated with a surge in LH secretion and a transient increase in heart rate[40]. In both the rat and man, LH secretion and heart rate are under the stimulatory influence of brain noradrenergic neurons. The close association of these three responses during the menopausal hot flush and the induced hot flush in rats suggests that a common mechanism is involved. It is not surprising then that clonidine treatment reduces the incidence of hot flushes in menopausal women[78, 79], and as we presently report, blocks the naloxone-induced TST surge in morphine-dependent rats. In both cases clonidine may be acting to block the hyperactivity of brain noradrenergic neurons associated with rapid skin temperature fluctuations.

8. SUMMARY AND CONCLUSIONS

We have demonstrated that naloxone-precipitated morphine withdrawal in the rat causes a hot flush which is similar to the menopausal hot flush in its amplitude and duration, and like the menopausal hot flush is associated temporally with a transient tachycardia and a surge in LH, and β-endorphin secretion. Additionally, abstention-induced withdrawal is associated with tail skin temperature instability characterized by transient pulses in surface temperature. This response to morphine withdrawal is mediated by the central nervous system, and shows an amplitude and duration which are related to the dose of the narcotic antagonist adminis-tered. Using this animal model we have been able to demonstrate that a rapid increase in NE activity is associated with the TST response and a delayed increase in DA neuronal activity. Consistent with this observation, stimulation of NE autoreceptors with clonidine, which reduces NE release, blocks the naloxone-induced TST response. Additionally, phen-tolamine, an α-adrenergic antagonist, can attenuate the amplitude of the TST response to naloxone.

Collectively, these data indicate that the proposed animal model is useful in determining the neurochemical substrates for the hot flush and in evaluating new and existing drugs for their usefulness in treating this menopausal vasomotor syndrome.

Acknowledgements

Part of the research described herein was supported by Grants AG02021 and HD18133 and a Grant from Key Pharmaceuticals, Inc.

REFERENCES

1. Lauritzen, C. (1973). In van Keep, P. A. and Lauritzen, C. (eds.) *Aging and Estrogens*. Vol. 2, pp. 2–21. (Basel: Karger)

2. Neugarten, B. L. and Kraines, R. J. (1965). *Psychosom. Med.*, **27**, 266–73

3. Jaszmann, J. (1973). In van Keep, P. A. and Lauritzen, C. (eds.) *Aging and Estrogens*. Vol. 2, pp. 22–34. (Basel: Karger)

4. Jaszmann, J., van Lith, N. D. and Zaat, J. C. A. (1969). *Med. Gynaecol. Sociol.*, **4**, 268–77

5. McKinlay, S. M. and Jeffreys, M. (1974). *Br. J. Prev. Soc. Med.*, **28**, 108–15

6. Korenmann, S. G. (1982). *Arch. Intern. Med.*, **142**, 1131–6

7. Mulley, G. and Mitchell, J. R. A. (1976). *Lancet*, **1**, 1397–8

8. Sturdee, D. W., Wilson, K. A., Pipili, E. and Crocker, A. D. (1978). *Br. Med. J.*, **2**, 79–80

9. Voda, A. M. (1980). *Maturitas*, **3**, 73-90

10. Molnar, G. W. (1981). *Obstet. Gynecol.*, **57**, 525-55

11. Hannan, J. H. (1927). In *The Flushings of the Menopause*. pp. 1-22. (London: Baillière, Tindall and Cox)

12. Casper, R. F., Yen, S. S. C. and Wilkes, M. M. (1979). *Science*, **205**, 823-5

13. Casper, R. F. and Yen, S. S. C. (1981). *J. Clin. Endocrinol. Metab.*, **53**, 1056-8

14. Meldrum, D. R., Shamonki, I. M., Frumar, A. M., Tataryn, I. V., Chang, R. J. and Judd, H. L. (1979). *Am. J. Obstet. Gynecol.*, **135**, 713-17

15. Molnar, G. W. (1975). *J. Appl. Physiol.*, **38**, 499-503

16. Molnar, G. W. (1979). *Am. J. Physiol.*, **237**, R306-R310

17. Kronenberg, F., Cote, L. J., Linkie, D. M., Dyrenfurth, I. and Downey, J. A. (1984). *Maturitas*, **6**, 31-43

18. Genazzani, A. R., Facchinetti, F., Ricci-Danero, M. G., Parrini, D., Petraglia, F., LaRosa, R. and D'Antona, N. (1981). *J. Endocrinol. Invest.*, **4**, 375-8

19. Rivier, C., Brownstein, M., Spiess, J., Rivier, J. and Vale, W. (1982). *Endocrinology*, **110**, 272-8

20. Collett, M. E. (1949). *J. Appl. Physiol.*, **1**, 629-39

21. Kalra, S. P., Kalra, P. S. and Simpkins, J. W. (1981). In McKerns, K. W. (ed.) *Reproductive Processes and Contraception*. pp. 27-45. (New York: Plenum)

22. Tilders, F. J. H., Berkenbosch, F. and Smelik, P. G. (1982). *Endocrinology*, **110**, 114-20

23. Fox, R. H., Wilkins, D. C., Bell, J. A., Bradley, R. D., Browse, N. L., Cranston, W. I., Foley, T. H., Gilby, E. D., Hebden, A., Jenkins, B. S. and Rawline, M. D. (1973). *Br. Med. J.*, **2**, 693-5

24. Penfield, W. (1929). *Arch. Neurol. Psychiatry*, **22**, 358-74

25. Yen, S. S. C. (1977). *J. Reprod. Med.*; **18**, 287-96

26. Erlik, Y., Meldrum, D. R. and Judd, H. L. (1982). *Obstet. Gynecol.*, **59**, 403-7

27. Judd, H. L. (1983): In Meites, J. (ed.) *Neuroendocrinology of Aging*. pp. 173-202. (New York: Plenum)

28. Sherman, B. M., West, J. H. and Korenman, S. G. (1976). *J. Clin. Endocrinol. Metab.*, **42**, 629-36

29. Askel, S., Schomberg, D. W., Tyrey, L. and Hammond, C. B. (1976). *Am. J. Obstet. Gynecol.*, **126**, 165-9

30. Stone, S. C., Mickal, A. and Rye, P. H. (1975). *Obstet. Gynecol.*, **45**, 625-7

31. Hutton, J. D., Murray, M. A. F., Jacobs, H. S. D. and James, V. H. T. (1979). *Lancet*, **1**, 678-81

32. Abe, T., Furuhashi, N., Yamaya, Y., Wada, Y., Hoshiai, A. and Suzuki, M. (1977). *Am. J. Obstet. Gynecol.*, **129**, 65–7

33. Sherman, B. M. and Korenman, S. G. (1975) *J. Clin. Invest.*, **55**, 699–706

34. Meldrum, D. R., Davidson, B. J., Tataryn, I. V. and Judd, H. J. (1981). *Obstet. Gynecol.*, **57**, 624–8

35. Sherman, B. M., West, J. H. and Korenman, S. G. (1976). *J. Clin. Endocrinol. Metab.*, **42**, 629–36

36. Vermeulen, A. (1976). *J. Clin. Endocrinol. Metab.*, **42**, 247–53

37. Judd, H. L., Shamonki, I. M., Frumar, A. M. and Lagasse, L. D. (1982). *Obstet. Gynecol.*, **59**, 680–6

38. Yen, S. S. C., Tasai, C. C., Vandenberg, G. and Rebar, R. (1972). *J. Clin. Endocrinol. Metab.*, **35**, 897–904

39. Bullock, J. L., Massey, F. M. and Gambrell, D., Jr. (1975). *Obstet. Gynecol.*, **46**, 165–8

40. Simpkins, J. W., Katovich, M. J. and Song, I.-C. (1983). *Life Sci.*, **32**, 1957–66

41. Gold, M. S., Redmond, D. E., Jr. and Kieber, H. D. (1978). *Lancet*, **2**, 599–602

42. Quigley, M. E. and Yen, S. S. C. (1980). *J. Clin. Endocrinol. Metab.*, **51**, 179–81

43. Blankstein, J., Reyes, F. I., Winter, J. S. D. and Faiman, C. (1981). *Clin. Endocrinol. (Oxf.)*, **14**, 287–94

44. Ropert, J. F., Quigley, M. E. and Yen, S. S. C. (1981). *J. Clin. Endocrinol. Metab.*, **52**, 583–5

45. Van Vugt, D. A., Lam, N. Y. and Ferin, M. (1984). *Endocrinology*, **115**, 1095–101

46. Wehrenberg, W. B., Wardlaw, S. L., Frantz, A. G. and Ferin, M. (1982). *Endocrinology*, **111**, 879–81

47. Wardlaw, S. L. Wehrenberg, W. B., Ferin, M., Antunes, J. L. and Frantz, A. G. (1982). *J. Clin. Endocrinol. Metab.*, **55**, 877–81

48. Reid, R. L., Quigley, M. E. and Yen, S. S. C. (1983). *J. Clin. Endocrinol. Metab.*, **57**, 1107–10

49. Wei, E. and Way, E. L. (1975). In Ehrenpress, S. (ed.) *Methods in Narcotic Research*. pp. 243–59. (New York: Dekker)

50. Way, E. E., Loh, H. H. and Shen, F. H. (1969). *J. Pharmacol. Exp. Ther.*, **167**, 1–8

51. Lotti, V. J., Lomax, P. and George, R. (1966). *Int. J. Neuropharmacol.*, **5**, 35–42

52. Cox, B., Ary, M. and Lomax, P. (1976). *Pharmacol. Biochem. Behav.*, **4**, 259–62

53. Cox, B., Ary, M., Chesarak, W. and Lomax, P. (1976). *Eur. J. Pharmacol.*, **36**, 33–9

54. Cicero, T. J., Owens, D. P., Schmoeker, P. F. and Meyer, E. R. (1983). *J. Pharmacol. Exp. Ther.*, **225**, 35–41

55. Gabriel, S. M., Simpkins, J. W. and Kalra, S. P. (1983). *Endocrinology*, **113**, 1806-11

56. Kalra, S. P. and Simpkins, J. W. (1981). *Endocrinology*, **109**, 776-82

57. Casper, R. F. and Yen, S. S. C. (1981). *J. Clin. Endocrinol. Metab.*, **53**, 1056-8

58. Lightman, S. L., Jacobs, H. S. and Maguire, A. K. (1982). *Br. J. Obstet. Gynaecol.*, **89**, 977-80

59. Mulley, G., Mitchell, J. R. A. and Tattersall, R. B. (1977). *Br. Med. J.*, **1**, 1062

60. Setalo, G., Vigh, S., Schally, A. V., Arimura, A. and Flerko, B. (1976). *Brain Res*, **103**, 597-602

61. Lotti, V. J., Lomax, P. and George, R. (1965). *J. Pharmacol. Exp. Ther.*, **150**, 135-9

62. Baldino, F., Jr., Beckman, A. L. and Adler, M. W. (1980). In Cox, B. *et al.* (eds.) *Thermoregulatory Mechanisms and Their Therapeutic Implications.* pp. 157-8. (Basel: Karger)

63. Lomax, P., Bajorek, J. G., Chesarek, W. and Tataryn, I. V. (1980). In Cox, B. *et al.* (eds.) *Thermoregulatory Mechanisms and Their Therapeutic Implications.* pp. 208-11. (Basel: Karger)

64. Paalzow, L. (1974). *J. Pharm. Pharmacol.*, **26**, 361-3

65. Paalzow, G. and Paalzow, L. (1976). *Naunyn-Schmiedeberg's Arch. Pharmacol.*, **292**, 119-26

66. Paalzow, G. (1978). *Naunyn-Schmiedeberg's Arch. Pharmacol.*, **304**, 1-4

67. Rabin, D. and McNeil, L. W. (1980). *J. Clin. Endocrinol. Metab.*, **51**, 873-6

68. Hahn, E., Fishman, J. and Heilman, R. D. (1975). *J. Med. Chem.*, **18**, 259-62

69. Creese, I. and Snyder, S. H. (1975). *J. Pharmacol. Exp. Ther.*, **194**, 205-19

70. Chan, J. S. D., Lu, C. L., Seidah, N. G. and Chretien, M. (1982). *Endocrinology*, **111**, 1388-90

71. Drouva, S. V., Epelbaum, J., Taia-Arancibia, L., Laplante, E. and Kordon, C. (1981). *Neuroendocrinology*, **32**, 163-7

72. Moore, R. Y. and Bloom, F. E. (1979). *Ann. Rev. Neurosci.*, **2**, 113-68

73. Sprague, G. L. and Takemoi, A. E. (1979). *J. Pharm. Sci.*, **68**, 660-2

74. Owens, D. P. and Cicero, T. J. (1981). *J. Pharmacol. Exp. Ther.*, **216**, 135-41

75. Aghajanian, G. K. (1978). *Nature*, **276**, 186-8

76. Kobinger, W. and Welland, A. (1967). *Eur. J. Pharmacol.*, **2**, 155-62

77. Kobinger, W. (1973). In Onesti, O. *et al.* (eds.) *Hypertension Mechanisms and Management.* pp. 369-82. (New York: Grune & Stratton)

78. Clayden, J. R., Bell, J. W. and Pollard, P. (1974). *Br. Med. J.*, **1**, 409-12

79. Metz, S. A., Halter, J. B., Porte, D. and Robenson, R. P. (1978). *J. Clin. Endocrinol. Metab.*, **46**, 83-90

80. Starke, K. and Montel, H. (1973). *Neuropharmacology*, **12**, 1073-80

81. Starke, K., Montel, H., Gayk, W. and Merker, R. (1974). *Naunyn-Schmiedeberg's Arch. Pharmacol.*, **285**, 133-50

82. Tseng, L. F., Loh, H. H. and Wei, E. T. (1975). *Eur. J. Pharmacol.*, **30**, 93-9

83. Vetulani, J. and Bednarczyk, K. (1977). *J. Pharm. Pharmacol.*, **29**, 567-8

84. Guaza, C., Torrellas, A., Borrell, S. and Borrell, J. (1980). *Psychopharmacology*, **68**, 43-9

85. Brodie, M. E., Laverty, R. and McQueen, E. G. (1983). *Naunyn-Schmiedeberg's Arch. Pharmacol.*, **313**, 135-8

86. Distefano, P. S. and Brown, O. M. (1982). *Fed. Proc.*, **41**, 1055

87. Reis, D. J., Hess, P. and Armitia, E. C., Jr. (1970). *Brain Res.*, **20**, 309-12

88. De Met, E. and Halaris, A. E. (1979). *Biochem. Pharmacol.*, **28**, 3043-50

89. Clark, W. G. (1980). *Neurosci. Biobehav. Rev.*, **3**, 179-231

90. Euker, J., Meites, J. and Riegle, G. D. (1975). *Endocrinology*, **96**, 85-92

91. Rossier, J., French, E. D., Rivier, C., Ling, N., Guillemin, R. and Bloom, F. E. (1977). *Nature*, **270**, 618-20

92. Ajika, K., Kalra, S. P., Fawcett, C. P., Krulich, L. and McCann, S. M. (1972). *Endocrinology*, **90**, 707-15

93. Du Ruseau, P., Tache, Y., Brazeau, P. and Collu, R. (1979). *Neuroendocrinology*, **29**, 90-9

94. Krulich, L., Hefco, E., Illner, P. and Read, C. B. (1974). *Neuroendocrinology*, **16**, 293-311

95. Nakagawa, R., Tanaka, M., Kohno, Y., Noda, Y. and Nagasaki, N. (1981). *Pharmacol. Biochem. Behav.*, **14**, 729-32

96. Roth, K. A., Mefford, I. M. and Barchas, J. D. (1982). *Brain Res.*, **239**, 417-24

97. Clark, W. G. and Clark, Y. L. (1980). *Neurosci. Biobehav. Rev.*, **4**, 281-375

98. Lin, M. T., Chandra, A. and Fung, T. C. (1979). *Can. J. Physiol. Pharmacol.*, **57**, 1401-6

99. Weiner, N. (1980). In Gilman, A. G. *et al.* (eds.) *The Pharmacological Basis of Therapeutics*. p. 176. (New York: Macmillan)

100. Litchfield, J. T., Jr. and Wilcoxon, F. (1949). *J. Pharmacol. Ther.*, **96**, 99-113

Chapter 22

Vascular responses in menopausal flushers

J. Ginsburg and B. O'Reilly

The menopausal hot flush is an evanescent, short-lived circulatory phenomenon. In order to assess what is actually happening during the flush itself, it is essential to use a technique which is capable of detecting changes in the circulation occurring not only every few minutes or minute but over 30 or even 15 s. For this purpose, therefore, when studying what happens during the menopausal flush in the limbs, we used a time-honoured, well-validated technique – venous occlusion plethysmography – which measures the arterial inflow into a segment of the limb by occluding the venous return from that part. The method is simple, atraumatic and gives reproducible results[1, 2], and while we can swim with the electronic computerized tide and add a fancy recording device, the basis of the instrument remains macrotechnology. Besides the choice of an appropriate technique for recording what is happening during the flush, there is the problem that women who state in the clinic that they flush frequently – as much as six times an hour or more – may not flush at all when they are in the laboratory for 3 h, even when we attempt to provoke a flush by a standardized stressful spell of mental arithmetic. Additionally, there is the problem that when women flush they are frequently agitated and move; this affects the recording device and it may be impossible to obtain valid measurements of limb blood flow. Thus we had to study several women in order to get one reliable recording session of what happens during the flush. After over 50 women had been studied in the laboratory, we ended up with 18 recording sessions from which meaningful data could be obtained[3].

Nevertheless, a consistent pattern of vascular response was observed during the flush. A marked rapid rise in hand flow occurred with the onset of sensations of the flush. Hand flow remained elevated for 3–4 min and fell to control values over a further 3 min. Forearm blood flow also rose simultaneously but to a lesser extent, falling to basal levels at a time when hand blood flow was still elevated. Pulse rate rose concurrently but less than either hand or forearm flow, and fell to control levels when the limb flow was still elevated. There was no change in blood pressure during this period. Vasodilatation in other regional vascular beds did not therefore occur, or there would have been a marked fall in blood pressure. Indeed, there may have been a slight reduction in flow in certain regional vascular beds in order to maintain systemic pressure constant. The fact that there was no fall in blood pressure during this period suggests further that the flush is unlikely to be due to a circulating vasodilator with a generalized effect, rather that the alteration in forearm and hand flow reflects changes in local vasomotor activity.

Circulation through the hand – which is largely composed of skin – is essentially controlled by release of vasoconstrictor tone. This is the classic mechanism for dissipating heat as when the ambient temperature rises, or in fever. Vasodilator nerves have not been demonstrated to supply the skin of the hand. On the other hand, dilator mechanisms are known to be active in forearm skin. Thus the rise in forearm flow could reflect active vasodilatation in skin vessels but could also relate to an increase in flow in the underlying skeletal muscle. However, as already discussed, this is probably not generalized in skeletal muscle vessels or a significant reduction in blood pressure would have been observed.

The menopausal hot flush is generally considered an exclusively female response. However, there are reports in the literature[4–6] suggesting that, in the appropriate circumstances, men may also experience such symptoms, although expression of the phenomenon in the male generally requires a dramatic event such as orchidectomy. We have recently studied a man of 60 who experienced frequent disabling hot flushes after bilateral orchidectomy for disseminated carcinomatosis of the prostate.

Our patient's response during a hot flush showed the same pattern as in the menopausal female with a marked rapid rise in hand flow and an associated lesser rise in forearm flow and pulse rate[7]. The fact that in the male, as in the female, a reduction in sex steroids after gonadectomy may herald the onset of intermittent episodes of altered vasomotor activity characterized by the climacteric hot flush, has obvious implications for the etiology of the phenomenon in women. It has hitherto been accepted that the trigger *par excellence* for the onset of menopausal flushing is the acute reduction in estrogen levels which occurs at the menopause, after ovariectomy, or if estrogen therapy is suddenly withdrawn in menopausal women. Our observations that an apparently identical phenomenon can occur in the male after orchidectomy suggest that the signal for the initiation of hot flushes need not necessarily be a fall in estrogen or even testosterone levels but perhaps the lack of an as yet unidentified compound, common to both ovary and testis and in whose absence activity of the hypothalamic centres controlling vasomotor activity and temperature regulation is disturbed.

It is well known that emotional or other stress may provoke a hot flush in susceptible individuals. However, comparison of the relative changes in limb flow and pulse rate during stressful mental arithmetic and the menopausal hot flush, whether spontaneous or induced by arithmetical stress, shows that both the degree of change and the hemodynamic response as a whole differ in the two phenomena. Thus a significant rise in blood pressure may occur during emotional stress and stressful mental arithmetic[8] and a variable change in hand flow (with a fall in some subjects and a rise in others) and a lesser increase in forearm flow than in the menopausal hot flush. The increase in peripheral blood flow observed during the menopausal flush is therefore a specific part of the response and not a consequence of the 'stress' induced by the symptoms associated with the hot flush.

Treatment of menopausal flushing is currently empirical and frequently unsatisfactory. Estrogens may alleviate the symptoms but this is not invariable and estrogen therapy, particularly when given in sufficient dosage to control the symptoms, may have unacceptable side-effects or be contraindicated. An alpha-adrenergic agonist, clonidine, used in the treatment and prophylaxis of migraine, has been found to exert a beneficial effect on menopausal flushes[9], in particular by decreasing their intensity. In the light of our observations of the peripheral vasodilatation associated with the hot flush, we wondered whether the alleviating effect of clonidine on sensations of the flush might be mediated through an influence on vascular activity.

We therefore investigated vascular responsiveness to the administration of naturally occurring vasoactive agents in menopausal women suffering from severe hot flushes and undergoing treatment with clonidine. The result of our study demonstrated an influence of the drug on peripheral vascular responsiveness and provides a possible explanation of the beneficial effects of clonidine in patients with either migraine or menopausal flushing.

In this study we observed the effects of physiological doses of noradrenaline, adrenaline and angiotensin – three vasoactive amines normally released in the course of exercise, etc., in the human and whose action on the circulation is well documented. The response to noradrenaline in the forearm is normally a slight dilator response. This was reduced in women after clonidine treatment for at least 6 weeks, the difference in flow being statistically significant. With adrenaline, which causes a classical biphasic pattern of vasodilatation in the human forearm – the adrenaline 'yawn' and the second sustained dilator phase 2 are likewise reduced in women after treatment with clonidine and these differences in forearm flow are all statistically highly significant. There is a similar pattern of response with angiotensin, in fact even more dramatic in that the vasodilator response in the forearm to angiotensin is converted to vasoconstriction. Similar changes occurred in respect of the pulse rate responses during the various infusions with a lesser increase in rate with adrenaline when this was infused after patients had received clonidine. With both noradrenaline and angiotensin, there was a greater fall in pulse rate than in the control infusions performed before administration of clonidine.

Since the menopausal hot flush is characterized by peripheral vasodilatation, one would expect a drug which reduced peripheral dilator responsiveness as we have demonstrated to be the case with clonidine, might also alleviate the sensations associated with the menopausal flush. Similarly, with migraine, in which the cerebral vessels are thought to be dilated, the effect that we have demonstrated could explain the therapeutic benefit of clonidine in the prophylaxis of migrainous attacks. It is also of interest that the action of clonidine is not apparently confined to an influence on adrenergic mechanisms as exemplified by the reduction in dilator responses to adrenaline and to noradrenaline, but also modifies the vascular response to angiotensin. This may have implications for the etiology and mechanism of the vascular changes occurring during the menopausal hot flush and likewise in migraine.

Although the hot flush is the commonest symptom of the menopause, estimated to occur in around 70% of women[9-11], some women never flush or do so for only a very short while whilst others may have severe and disabling episodes of flushing persisting for several years. The factors which determine the duration and severity of the symptoms in different women are not known but from clinical observation we know that women who flush are also conscious of increased body heat. They are frequently intolerant of a warm ambient temperature which is acceptable to younger women and to men, and wear lighter clothes when undertaking physical work than was the case before the menopause. This led us to consider the possibility of a different vascular responsiveness between women who flushed and those who did not.

We are currently studying peripheral blood flow and various vascular responses in menopausal women who complain of frequent hot flushes, and comparing this with those who have never flushed or did so for only a very short while. The preliminary results are based on data obtained in 33 women complaining of severe menopausal flushing – 'flushers' – and 15 women who had either never flushed at all or who had experienced flushes for a short while, the last episode being at least 1 year ago.

Resting forearm flow in the flushers was significantly ($p < 0.05$) higher than that recorded in non-flushers – 4.0 ($\pm$0.5) and 2.6 ($\pm$0.2) ml/100 ml tissue per minute respectively. During stressful mental arithmetic, forearm flow increased significantly more ($p<0.05$) in flushers than in non-flushers, the respective means being 7.0 ($\pm$1.1) and 3.9 ($\pm$0.4) ml. After cessation of mental arithmetic, forearm flow remained significantly higher in the flushers at 4.6 ($\pm$0.6) ml than in the non-flushers – 2.8 ($\pm$0.2) ml ($p<0.05$), and whilst forearm flow in the non-flushers rapidly approached that recorded in the initial control period, mean forearm flow after the stress of mental arithmetic did not fall to control level in flushers but remained significantly elevated ($p<0.02$) above that recorded in the initial control period.

Resting pulse rate was slightly but not significantly higher in flushers compared with non-flushers – 71.1 ($\pm$3.0) and 68.3 ($\pm$2.0) beats per minute respectively and remained elevated in flushers compared with non-flushers when pulse rate increased with mental arithmetic. During the recovery period, pulse rate remained significantly elevated at 74.1 ($\pm$2.0) compared with 71.1 ($\pm$3.0) beats per minute above that recorded in the control period in these women, whereas pulse rate in the non-flushers fell rapidly to control values.

There was no significant difference in hand flow as between flushers and non-flushers, whether in the control period, during the application of mental arithmetic or in the recovery period therefrom.

A similar difference in responsiveness to vasoactive amines in the forearm was demonstrated between the flushers and non-flushers with higher levels during noradrenaline infusion in the flushers compared with non-flushers and similarly in response to adrenaline.

Thus the subjective distinction between menopausal women who flush and those who do not, has an objective physiological parallel with a higher level of forearm flow at rest in those who flush compared with those who do not flush. Resting tone in forearm vessels is under adrenergic vasomotor control and it would seem therefore that adrenergic vasomotor tone in menopausal flushers may be altered. The altered responses in menopausal women to the administration of adrenaline and noradrenaline are consonant with this view.

The precise mechanism of these differences and the extent to which influences at hypothalamic level are different in the two groups, or whether there may be even a specific difference in the peripheral vasculature, is a matter for speculation and investigation. We may, however, conclude that menopausal women who have frequent hot flushes are a distinct population with an apparent physiological difference from those of the same age and who do not flush. The mechanisms underlying these differences are obviously crucial to the elucidation of the etiology of the flush and for the instigation of rational treatment for these disabling symptoms.

Acknowledgement

Barbara O'Reilly's work was supported by the British Heart Foundation.

REFERENCES

1. Ginsburg, J. (1958). Observations of the peripheral circulation in hypertrophic pulmonary osteoarthropathy. *Q. J. Med.*, **27**, 335–52
2. Ginsburg, J. and Cobbold, A. F. (1960). Effects of adrenaline, noradrenaline and iso-propylnoradrenaline in man. In Wolstenholme, G. E. W. and O'Connor, M. (eds.) *The Ciba Foundation Symposium on Adrenergic Mechanisms.* pp. 173–89. (London: Churchill)
3. Ginsburg, J., Swinhoe, J. and O'Reilly, B. (1981). Cardiovascular responses during the menopausal hot flush. *Br. J. Obstet. Gynaecol.*, **88**, 925–30
4. Feldman, J. M., Postlethwaite, R. W. and Glenn, J. F. (1976). Hot flushes and sweats in men with testicular insufficiency. *Arch. Intern. Med.*, **136**, 606–8
5. Steinfeld, A. D. and Reinhardt, C. (1980). Male climacteric after orchidectomy in a patient with prostatic cancer. *Urology*, **16**, 620–2
6. Linde, R., Doelle, G. C., Alexander, N. *et al.* (1981). Reversible inhibition of testicular steroidogenesis and spermatogenesis by a potent gonadotrophin-releasing hormone agonist in normal men: an approach toward the development of a male contraceptive. *N. Engl. J. Med.*, **305**, 663–7
7. Ginsburg, J. and O'Reilly, B. (1983). Climacteric flushing in a man. *Br. Med. J.*, **287**, 262–3
8. Fencl, V., Hejl, Z., Jirka, J., Madlafousek, J. and Brod, J. (1959). Changes of blood flow in forearm muscle and skin during an acute emotional stress (mental arithmetic). *Clin. Sci.*, **18**, 491–8
9. Clayden, J. R., Bell, J. W. and Pollard, P. (1974). Menopausal flushing: double-blind trial of a non-hormonal medication. *Br. Med. J.*, **1**, 409–12
10. Thompson, B., Hart, S. A. and Dunro, D. (1973). Age and symptomatology in general practice. *J. Biosoc. Sci.*, **5**, 71–5
11. McKinley, S. M. and Jeffreys, M. (1974). The menopausal syndrome. *Br. J. Prev. Soc. Med.*, **28**, 108–14

Chapter 23

Description of the hot flash: sensations, meaning and change in frequency across time

A. M. Voda, B. M. Feldman and E. Gronseth

The purpose of this chapter is to present a reality-based clinical description of the menopausal or climacteric hot flash. Two questions of importance to menopausal women will be addressed: 'What is the hot flash?' and 'How long will it last?'

INTRODUCTION

Menarche and menopause are definitive developmental landmarks and universal events for all women; both events are associated with physiological, hormonal and biochemical adjustments in women's bodies. During the reproductive years the manifestations of these adjustments in the form of fluctuating physical and behavioral activity are signals that all is well, that woman is prepared and able to insure the survival of the species through reproductive capacity. Yet throughout recorded time these very same messages of life have become the object of horrific and mythical superstitions, superstitions that have been interpreted in such a way that woman by-and-large has been reduced to her reproductive capacity. Even in today's enlightened society we remain ignorant of what being a woman means from a woman's perspective. The menopause is no exception; it is but a point in time in the total process of change from reproductive life to vital years ahead. Yet despite scientific advances and sophistication in research methods, stereotypes about menopausal women persist. The most consistent stereotype is that menopause is a crisis, is catastrophic, that menopausal women are inferior and incapable of functioning, that menopausal women are estrogen-deficient, and that the changes associated with the transition, such as hot flash, are symptoms of disease.

MENOPAUSE AS A DEFICIENCY STATE?

The overriding assumption that menopause is an estrogen-deficiency disease with hot flash as a symptom of disease has led to a proliferation of research on hormone replacement: how much hormone, 'what kind, how long?' . . . these are the research questions that emanate from the stereotype of menopausal woman being conceptualized as estrogen-deficient. According to MacPherson[1, 2] we are witness to the social construction of a metaphor, the medicalization of the natural ending of woman's reproductive life. Until recently, most biomedical research on menopause unquestionably assumed that women were estrogen-deficient. Studies based on this assumption were designed with control and objectivity uppermost in mind, and women were viewed as data-producing objects. In this context the experience of menopause was interpreted and described by others, and little information was found in the literature describing menopause from the perception or perspective of the women experiencing the event.

HOT FLASH AS A SYMPTOM OF DISEASE?

Until the 1970s, hot flashes in women were either ignored or treated as a symptom of disease. Research on hot flash, *per se*, was not a serious line of scientific investigation. Subjective information on hot flash reported in the literature prior to 1970 and in the 1970s, with few exceptions, was that incorporated into the findings of survey or epidemiological research[3-14]. Most biomedical research on hot flash prior to and since the classic physiological descriptive work of Molnar[15] in 1975 has followed either a biological, vasomotor or neurohormonal line of investigation[16-52]. These studies are important in that they validate the objective reality of the hot flash experience for women and provide unequivocal support that hormone replacement alleviates and/or eliminates hot flash. These descriptions of hot flash have broken new ground in that they identify that all subjective hot flashes are associated with a measurable increase in peripheral skin temperature; that a subjective experience precedes the objective physiological measurement; that changes in physiological correlates may occur in the absence of a perceived hot flash; that hormonally there is disagreement about the role of and/or changes in gonadotropin level associated with hot flash.

These studies do not prove, however, that hot flash is either a symptom of or a disease. Work by Voda[53] and others[54-56] suggests that the hot flash is more than an objective measurable phenomenon. It is an event that is associated with a variety of sensations and feelings, it is perceived as a normal event by women, and it has been found to be highly prevalent among menopausal women. Recent work by Feldman et al.[57], employing the random-digit dialing survey method, estimates hot flash prevalence at 89%. The high prevalence estimate strongly suggests not only that hot flash is a normal and expected somatic event but that it may be as universal as menopause itself.

Removing the metaphor of disease allows one to ask research questions related to meaning and value of the event for women. Different perspectives lead to different theoretical underpinnings of research which necessitate different research designs and methods. Based on the assumption that menopause is a normal event and the hot flash is a normal body change, it was my choice to consider the women experiencing hot flash as the experts on the subjective aspects of the event. In order to answer a question of importance to women, I combined objective and subjective methods of data collection and analysis in order to generate data on hot flash frequency, the hope being that such data will both add to and complement the large body of objective knowledge which has been generated.

STUDY DESIGN AND METHODS OF PROCEDURE

The design was descriptive/exploratory; the intent was to combine qualitative and quantitative methods of data collection and to collect data on hot flash frequency over a 3-year period. Underpinning the research are the following assumptions: Hot flash is a valid and reliable concept. It is a real vasomotor/physiological event; it is not in women's heads. Women are capable of cognitively processing perceived bodily sensations associated with the hot flash and are able to report these experiences accurately. Menopause and the hot flash are normal physiological and growth and developmental events in women.

The research questions

(1) What is the hot flash?
(2) How long does it last? Does it change over time?

Methods

To answer the research questions, data were obtained as follows.

(1) open-ended interview to obtain self-report descriptions of the hot flash using subjects' own words;

(2) body diagrams filled out by subjects to capture the perceived somatic aspects of the origin and spread of the hot flash;

(3) a self-report record card/diary for subjects to record origin and spread of hot flash and hot flash frequency;

(4) thermal measurement of peripheral skin temperature before, during and after hot flash in a controlled laboratory setting.

A detailed description of methods 2 and 3 has been described previously[53]. Subjects of the study were 70 perimenopausal women randomly selected from a pool of 300 women experiencing hot flash. (Perimenopausal, by definition, is the date of onset of the first hot flash. The term is defined differently than that proposed by the Menopause Congress[59].) Subjects' ages ranged from 38 to 73 years.

Analyses of interviews, body diagrams, 2 weeks of daily entries into the self-report card/diary and interviews conducted following hot flashes in the laboratory evolved the subjective characteristics associated with a hot flash and thus the description of the hot flash.

Data on hot flash frequency were collected over a 3-year period using subject self-report of hot flash frequency and objective measurement of hot flash in the laboratory. Specifically, using the self-report diary method[53], a subset sample of 25 of the 70 subjects recorded hot flash frequency on a daily basis for a 2-week period during the months of January and February from 1980 to 1983. Of these 25 subjects, 14 were experiencing a natural menopause; 11 had had menopause induced surgically through removal of uterus and both ovaries.

To obtain an objective estimate of hot flash frequency, the same subset sample of 25 subjects underwent thermal monitoring once each year for an average of 2.5 hours per year. Peripheral skin temperatures were measured using Yellow Springs No. 427 thermistors. Placement of the thermistors on the body was based on self-report of each subjects's origin and spread of the hot flash. All measurements were made in an environmentally controlled room. During the measurements, subjects were asked to indicate verbally the onset and end of a hot flash, and this information was entered into a computerized system of data acquisition, storage and retrieval. Frequency of hot flashes that occurred in the laboratory during thermal monitoring was calculated from temperature change data accessed by the thermistors. A temperature change from baseline was accepted as data that indeed a hot flash had occurred when the change was associated with a subject's subjective report, 'I'm having a hot flash'. In this way an objective method of observing, measuring and thus validating subjects' hot flash origin, spread, and frequency was obtained.

The mean age of the subset sample on entry into the study in 1980 was 51.92 years for the naturally menopausal subjects ($n = 14$) and 52.00 years for the induced menopausal group ($n = 11$). Age at which subjects experienced the first hot flash was 46 years for the natural group and 47.31 for the induced group. Age of first menstrual period for the natural group was 13.39 years and 12.36 for the induced group. Age when menstrual periods became irregular, that is, changes in the quantity and quality of bleeding, was 44.67 years for the natural group and 45.90 years for the induced group. These demographic and menstrual-life characteristics are summarized in Table 23.1.

Table 23.1 Subject profile on self-report of hot flash frequency, 1980–83[a]

	Natural menopause group (n = 14) (years)	Induced menopause group (n = 11) (years)
Age at entry into study	51.92	52.00
Age of first hot flash	46.50	46.81
Age, last menstrual period	48.54	47.31
Age, first menstrual period	13.39	12.36
Age when periods (bleeding) change in quantity and quality of menstrual flow	44.67	45.90

[a] Subject profile of 25 subjects who kept self-reports of hot flash frequency for 3 years, 1980–83, and who had hot flash measured in the laboratory for the same time period

RESULTS

Research question 1: What is the hot flash?

Analysis of self-report data from 69 of 70 women ages 38–73 who comprised the original convenience sample suggests that the hot flash is not perceived as a symptom of disease. Instead, subjects viewed it as a sign that the end of one stage of life was at hand with another beginning. Consistent with the findings previously reported[58], the subjects described a variety of sensations associated with hot flashes as well as different intensities. Specifically, a hot flash was described as the increase and perception of heat located within and/or on the body, having both an origin and a spread which may last from ½ min to 12 min or more. It is sometimes accompanied by a variety of bodily sensations, sometimes by a skin color change, which is a 'hot flush', ranging from pink to bright red, and of differing intensities which may range from mild to severe.

A *mild* hot flash was described as a warm feeling all over the body, lasting less than 1 min to 2 min, sometimes barely noticeable, sometimes accompanied by dampness, sweat, slight flushing, and at times including sensations of tingling and rushing blood.

A *moderate* hot flash was described as a warm to extremely warm feeling, lasting from less than 1 min to 5 min or more, having a precise origin and spread, often accompanied by sweat and sometimes by flushing. It may include tingling, throbbing, rushing blood, light-headed-ness, chills, swelling of extremities, a need to urinate yet with little inter-ruption of normal activity.

In contrast a *severe* hot flash was described as an intense or extremely hot feeling which could last less than 1 min or longer than 12 min, almost always accompanied by profuse sweat or flushing, which had a precise origin and spread, was extremely unbearable and discomforting and requiring disruption of normal activity to seek relief. It may also include a feeling of waves of heat, dizziness, chills, suffocation, inability to con-centrate, not wanting to be touched or communicate in any way, and chest pains.

Research question 2: How long does the hot flash last? Does it change over time?

Analysis of hot flash frequency data showed that the occurrence of hot flash decreased over the 3-year period. For the total group of 25 subjects a decrease from year 01 of 1802 hot flashes to 1127 in year 03 was recorded via the self-report method. In the laboratory calculation of the hot flash frequency via objective methods of thermal monitoring showed a decrease in hot flash frequency from year 01 of 73 to 39 hot flashes in year 03. These data are summarized in Table 23.2.

Table 23.2 Hot flash frequency based on two methods of data collection[a] $(n = 25)$

| | Hot flash frequency | | | |
Method	Year 01	Year 02	Year 03	Total
Self-report daily record over a 2-week period times 3 years	1802	1494	1127	4423
Laboratory measurement average 2.30 hours per year times 3 years	73	43	39	155

[a] Hot flash frequency calculated over a 3 year (1980–83) period based on two methods of data collection: self-report and laboratory measurement

The percent change ($\%\Delta$) in hot flash frequency based on the two methods of data collection is displayed in Table 23.3. A greater $\%\Delta$ was reflected from year 01 to 03 in self-report and laboratory calculation. A more gradual decrease across time is reflected in the self-report data from year 01 to 03. A $\%\Delta$ of 17.00 occurred from year 01 to 02; a $\%\Delta$ of 24.60 from year 02 to 03; and from year 01 to 03 a $\%\Delta$ of 37.50. Hot flash frequency decreased from year 01 to 02 in data collected using objective methods in the laboratory, specifically a $\%\Delta$ of 41.10 with a lesser increment of change from year 02 to 03, $\%\Delta$ 9.30, than that recorded via self-report method from year 02 to 03.

Table 23.3 Percentage change in hot flash frequency[a]

Year	%Δ Laboratory	%Δ Self-report
01 to 02	41.10	17.10
02 to 03	9.3	24.56
01 to 03	46.58	37.46

[a] Percentage change in menopausal hot flash frequency for 25 subjects who kept self-report records over same 2 week period and who were measured in the laboratory over 3 years

The decrease in hot flash frequency from year 01 to 03 was reflected in the records and peripheral temperature changes of both natural and induced menopausal subjects. As shown in Table 23.4, a consistent and similar decrease in frequency from 985 in year 01, 719 in year 02, to 617 for year 03 was recorded by the natural group using self-report. For the induced group, hot flash frequency in year 01 was 817, 775 in year 02 and 510 for year 03. In the laboratory, hot flash frequency in the induced group decreased from 37 to 17 to 12 from year 01 to 03. For the natural menopausal subjects, however, no decrease in hot flash number was observed in year 03. Instead, hot flash frequency increased in year 03 to 27, up from 26 in year 02.

Table 23.4 Hot flash frequency and percentage change in frequency for natural and induced ($n = 14$) menopausal subjects[a]

Method	Natural menopause status (n = 14)		Induced menopause status (n = 11)	
	Hot flash frequency	%Δ	Hot flash frequency	%Δ
Self-report				
Year 01	985		817	
Year 02	719	27.00	775	5.15
Year 03	617	14.20	510	34.20
Totals	2321	37.40	2102	37.37
Laboratory				
Year 01	36		37	
Year 02	26	27.78	17	54.05
Year 03	27	3.84	12	29.41
Totals	89	25.00	66	67.57

[a] Hot flash frequency calculated over a 3-year period (1980–83) based on two methods of data collection: self-report and laboratory measurement

DISCUSSION

The findings of this study on a small sample of menopausal women support information found in gynecological texts and self-care manuals for women that indeed the hot flash does decrease in frequency with time.

While this study may appear to be reporting the obvious, and thus appear to be simplistic and of little import, it does address a question of interest to women and does invalidate the information that is provided to women regarding the duration of hot flashes. Data summarized in Table 23.1 show that the subjects were at different points in the climacterium. The average number of years of onset of the first hot flash for subjects was 5–6 years prior to entry into the study with some subjects reporting a hot flash experience for 12–13 years. All 25 subjects continued to experience hot flashes at the termination of the study, 3 years later, which meant that in 1983 the average duration of hot flash experience was 8–9 years. This finding contradicts information found in texts and journals that the duration of the hot flash is about 2 years.

Women, researchers and care-providers need to know that the exact parameters for hot flash duration are unknown. Women need to use this information when making decisions regarding whether to be a hormone user as a way of managing the hot flash. In other words, for women who choose hormone replacement, they need to know that the time frame for replacement will, in all probability, be more than a 2-year period. It is speculated that the intensity of the hot flash decreases as hot flash frequency subsides. Intensity data on this sample of subjects are in the process of analysis.

For menopause researchers, to avoid methodological flaws, it is critical to realize that when women are recruited into studies they are not a homogeneous group with respect to stages within the climacteric. Women in this study were experiencing hot flashes for an average of 5–6 years. Some of the subjects were premenopausal, some postmenopausal. What is needed in menopause research is an noninvasive indirect indicator of changing internal milieu with respect to fluctuating hormones. More attention to recording the onset of the first hot flash in relation to menopause may be one way of selecting more homogeneous samples of subjects in the climacteric to determine whether the variability in the totality of the menopause experience from woman to woman is the norm or the exception. Obviously, more work is needed and more precise criteria need to be evolved in order to select and then compare menopausal subjects and studies one with the other. Variability in the frequency and intensity and sensation of the hot flash may be an indirect indicator of placement within the climacterium.

The use of estrogen by subjects in this study was not a variable that affected change in hot flash frequency. Only one natural menopausal subject had to resort to estrogen use in the third year of the study. Those subjects who had had menopause induced surgically and who were estrogen users in year 01 continued on the same dosage through year 03. For the induced subjects, for the most part, estrogen use was contra-indicated.

Information generated by subject self-report on the variability of the hot flash experience as an event that has both somatic and affective characteristics expands the description of the hot flash as reported in literature from one of a purely objective detached definition of a scientific interest to one that can be operationalized and meaningful for women and care-providers. It appears that hot flash frequency does indeed decrease with time; unfortunately, the precise parameters in terms of duration in numbers of years women will experience it are unknown.

In conclusion, it appears that women can expect to experience hot flashes as a normal sequela of transit through the climacteric. They can also expect that the event will present with variability from woman to woman and across time in the same woman. What is unknown and needs to be the focus of future research is not only how long women can expect to be blessed with such warmth, but what effect age of first hot flash, estrogen use, pregnancies, family history of menstrual and reproductive illness, date of first menstrual period, mother's menstrual history, date of menopause, body composition and other unknown variables have on the hot flash experience.

Acknowledgements

The authors wish to thank Stacey Levine, Suresh Dholakia, Wendy Visscher, and Diane Lemke for technical assistance, and Joyce Rathbun for the secretarial expertise. This study was funded by Grant No. RU01 NU 00961, H and HS, Nursing Research and Analysis Branch, Bureau of Health Professions, HRSA, Division of Nursing.

REFERENCES

1. MacPherson, K. I. (1981). Menopause as disease: the social construction of a metaphor. *Adv. Nurs. Sci.*, 3(2), 95-113
2. MacPherson, K. I. (1985). Osteoporosis and menopause: a feminist analysis of the social construction of a syndrome. *Adv. Nurs. Sci.*, 7(4), 11-22
3. Neugarten, B. L. and Kraines, R. J. (1965). Menopausal symptoms in women of various ages. *Psychosom. Med.*, 27, 266-73
4. Jaszmann, L., van Lith, N. D. and Zatt, J. C. A. (1969). The perimenopausal-symptoms: the statistical analysis of a survey. Part (a). *Med. Gynaecol. Sociol.*, 4, 268-77
5. Thompson, B., Hart, S. A. and Durno, D. (1973). Menopausal age and symptomatology in a general practice. *J. Biosoc. Sci.*, 5, 71-82
6. Aitken, J. M., Davidson, A., England, P., Govan, A. D. T., Hart, D. M., Kelly, A., Lindsay, R. and Moffatt, A. (1974). The relationship between menopausal vasomotor symptoms and gonadotropin excretion in urine after oophorectomy. *J. Obstet. Gynaecol Br. Commonw.*, 80, 150-4
7. McKinlay, S. and Jefferys, M. (1974). The menopausal syndrome. *Br. J. Prev. Soc. Med.*, 28, 108-15
8. Ballinger, C. B. (1975). Psychiatric morbidity and the menopause: screening of general population sample. *Br. Med. J.*, 3, 344-6
9. Stadel, B. V. and Weiss, N. (1975). Characteristics of menopausal women: a survey of King and Pierce counties in Washington, 1973-1974. *Am. J. Epidemiol.*, 102, 209-16

10. Dennerstein, L. and Burrows, G. D. (1978). A review of studies of the psychological symptoms found at the menopause. *Maturitas*, 1, 55-64
11. Batrinos, M. L., Panitsa-Faflia, C., Pitoulis, S., Piaditis, G., Alexandridis, T. and Liappi, C. (1979). The clinical features of the menopause and its relation to the length of pregnancies and lactation. *Maturitas*, 1, 261-8
12. Flint, M. P. and Garcia, M. (1979). Culture and the climacteric. *J. Biosoc. Sci.*, 6 (Suppl.), 197-215
13. Severne, L. (1979). Psycho-social aspects of the menopause. In Haspels, A. A. and Musaph, H. (eds.) *Psychosomatics in Peri-menopause.* pp. 101-20. (Baltimore: University Park Press)
14. Moore, B. (1981). Climacteric symptoms in an African community. *Maturitas*, 3, 25-29
15. Molnar, G. W. (1975). Body temperature during menopausal hot flashes. *J. Appl. Physiol.*, 38, 499-503
16. Munsick, R. A. (1959). Serotonin and the menopausal flush. *Am. J. Obstet. Gynecol.*, 78, 147-51
17. Ferriman, D. and Purdie, A. W. (1965). Mechanism of menopausal hot flushes indicated by the effect of a dithiocarbamylhydrazine. *J. Endocrinol.*, 31, 173-4
18. Clayden, J. R. (1972). Effect of clonidine on menopausal flushing. *Lancet*, 2, 1361
19. Clayden, J. R., Bell, J. W. and Pollard, P. (1974). Menopausal flushing: double-blind trial of a non-hormonal medication. *Br. Med. J.*, 1, 409-12
20. Lauritzen, C. (1975). The hypothalamic anterior pituitary system in the climacteric age period. *Front. Horm. Res.*, 3, 20-31
21. Aksel, S., Schomberg, D. W., Tyrey, L. and Hammond, C. B. (1976). Vasomotor symptoms, serum estrogens, and gonadotropin levels in surgical menopause. *Am. J. Obstet. Gynecol.*, 126, 165-9
22. Campbell, S. (1976). Intensive steroid and protein hormone profiles on post-menopausal women experiencing hot flashes, and a group of controls. In Campbell, S. (ed.) *Management of the Menopause and Postmenopausal Years.* pp. 63-77. (Baltimore: University Park Press)
23. Thompson, J. and Oswald, I. (1977). Effect of oestrogen on the sleep, mood, and anxiety of menopausal women. *Br. Med. J.*, 2, 1317-19
24. Coope, J., Williams, S. and Patterson, J. S. (1978). A study of the effectiveness of propranolol in menopausal hot flushes. *Br. J. Obstet. Gynaecol.*, 85, 472-5
25. Dennerstein, L., Burrows, G. D., Hyman, G. and Wood, C. (1978). Menopausal hot flushes: a double blind comparison of placebo, ethinyl oestradiol and norgestrel. *Br. J. Obstet. Gynaecol.*, 85, 852-6
26. Sturdee, D. W., Wilson, K. A., Pipili, E. and Crocker, A. D. (1978). Physiological aspects of menopausal hot flush. *Br. Med. J.*, 2, 79-80
27. Casper, R. F., Yen, S. S. C. and Wilkes, M. M. (1979). Menopausal flushes: a neuroendocrine link with pulsatile luteinizing hormone secretion. *Science*, 205, 823-5
28. Lightman, S. L. and Jacobs, H. S. (1979). Naloxone: non-steroidal treatment for postmenopausal flushing? *Lancet*, 2, 1071
29. Meldrum, D. R., Shamonki, I. M., Frumar, A. M., Tataryn, I. V., Chang, R. J. and Judd, H. L. (1979). Elevations in skin temperature of the finger as an objective index of postmenopausal hot flashes: standardization of the technique. *Am. J. Obstet. Gynecol.*, 135, 713-17
30. Molnar, G. W. (1979). Investigation of hot flashes by ambulatory monitoring. *Am. J. Physiol.*, 237, 306-10
31. Schiff, I., Regestein, Q., Tulchinsky, D. and Ryan, K. J. (1979). Effects of estrogens on sleep and psychological state of hypogonadal women. *J. Am. Med. Assoc.*, 242, 2405-7
32. Sturdee, D. W. and Reece, B. L. (1979). Thermography of menopausal hot flushes. *Maturitas*, 1, 201-5
33. Tataryn, I. V., Meldrum, D. R., Lu, K. H., Frumar, A. M. and Judd, H. L. (1979). LH, FSH and skin temperature during the menopausal hot flash. *J. Clin. Endocrinol. Metab.*, 49, 152-4
34. Edington, R. F., Chagnon, J. P. and Steinberg, W. M. (1980). Clonidine (Dixarit) for menopausal flushing. *Can. Med. Assoc. J.*, 123, 23-6
35. Meldrum, D. R., Tataryn, I. V., Frumar, A. M., Erlik, Y., Lu, K. H. and Judd, H. L. (1980). Gonadotropins, estrogens and adrenal steroids during the menopausal hot flash. *J. Clin. Endocrinol. Metab.*, 50, 685-9

36. Morrison, J. C., Martin, D. C., Blair, R. A., Anderson, G. D., Kincheloe, D. W., Bates, G. W., Hendrix, J. W., Rivlin, M. E., Forman, E. K., Propst, M. G. and Needham, R. (1980). The use of medroxyprogesterone acetate for relief of climacteric symptoms. *Am. J. Obstet. Gynecol.*, **138**, 99-104

37. Tataryn, I. V., Lomax, P., Bajorek, J. G., Chesarek, W., Meldrum, D. R. and Judd, H. L. (1980). Postmenopausal hot flushes: a disorder of thermoregulation. *Maturitas*, **2**, 101-7

38. Albecht, B. H., Schiff, I., Tulchinsky, D. and Ryan, K. J. (1981). Objective evidence that placebo and oral medroxyprogesterone acetate therapy diminish menopausal vasomotor flushes. *Am. J. Obstet. Gynecol.*, **139**, 631-5

39. Casper, R. F. and Yen, S. S. C. (1981). Menopausal flushes: effect of pituitary gonadotropin desensitization by a potent luteinizing hormone-releasing factor agonist. *J. Clin. Endocrinol. Metab.*, **53**, 1056-8

40. Erlik, Y., Meldrum, D. R., Lagasse, L. D. and Judd, H. L. (1981). Effect of megestrol acetate on flushing and bone metabolism in post-menopausal women. *Maturitas*, **3**, 167-72

41. Erlik, Y., Tataryn, I. V., Meldrum, D. R., Lomax, P., Bajorek, J. and Judd, H. L. (1981). Association of waking episodes with menopausal hot flushes. *J. Am. Med. Assoc.*, **245**, 1741-4

42. Lightman, S. L., Jacobs, H. S., Maguire, A. K., McGarrick, G. and Jeffcoate, S. L. (1981). Climacteric flushing: clinical and endocrine response to infusion of naloxone. *Br. J. Obstet. Gynaecol.*, **88**, 919-24

43. Molnar, G. W. (1981). Thyrotropin-releasing hormone and the menopausal hot flash. *Maturitas*, **3**, 115-23

44. Nesheim, B. I. and Saetre, T. (1981). Reduction of menopausal hot flushes by methyldopa: a double blind crossover trial. *Eur. J. Clin. Pharmacol.*, **20**, 413-16

45. Tataryn, I. V., Lomax, P., Meldrum, D. R., Bajorek, J. G., Chesarek, W. and Judd, H. L. (1981). Objective techniques for the assessment of postmenopausal hot flashes. *Obstet. Gynecol.*, **57**, 340-4

46. Erlik, Y., Meldrum, D. R. and Judd, H. L. (1982). Estrogen levels in postmenopausal women with hot flashes. *Obstet. Gynecol.*, **59**, 403-7

47. Harrison, R. F. (1981). Ethamsylate in the treatment of climacteric flushing. *Maturitas*, **3**, 31-7

48. Jones, M. M., Pearlman, B., Marshall, D. H., Crilly, R. G. and Nordin, B. E. C. (1982). Dose-dependent response of FSH, flushes and urinary calcium to estrogen. *Maturitas*, **4**, 285-90

49. Laufer, L. R., Erlik, Y., Meldrum, D. R. and Judd, H. L. (1982). Effect of clonidine on hot flashes in postmenopausal women. *Obstet. Gynecol.*, **60**, 583-6

50. Lightman, S. L., Jacobs, H. S. and Maguire, A. K. (1982). Down-regulation of gonadotropin secretion in postmenopausal women by a superactive LHRH analogue: lack of effect on menopausal flushing. *Br. J. Obstet. Gynaecol.*, **89**, 977-80

51. Nesheim, B. I. and Saetre, T. (1982). Changes in skin blood flow and body temperatures during climacteric hot flushes. *Maturitas*, **4**, 49-55

52. Paterson, M. E. L. (1982). A randomized, double-blind, cross-over study into the effect of sequential mestranol and norethisterone on climacteric symptoms and biochemical parameters. *Maturitas*, **4**, 83-94

53. Voda, A. (1981). 'Climacteric hot flash.' *Maturitas*, **3**, 73-90

54. Moore, B. (1981). Climacteric symptoms in an African community. *Maturitas*, **3**, 25-9

55. Sharma, V. K. and Saxena, M. S. L. (1981). Climacteric symptoms: a study in the Indian context. *Maturitas*, **3**, 11-20

56. Kay, M., Voda, A., Olivas, G., Rios, F. and Imle, M. (1982). Ethnography of the menopause-related hot flash. *Maturitas*, **4**, 217-27

57. Feldman, B. F., Voda, A. M. and Gronseth, E. (1985). Prevalence of menopausal hot flash. *Res. Nurs. Health*, **8**, 261-8

58. Voda, A. M. (1982). Coping with the menopausal hot flash. *Patient Counsel. Health Educ.*, **2**, 80-3

59. Van Keep, P. A., Greenblatt, R. and Albeaux-Fernet, M. (eds.) (1976). *Proceedings of the International Congress on the Menopause*. (Lancaster: MTP Press)

Chapter 24

Therapy for hot flushes

D. W. Sturdee

HISTORY

Treatment of the hot flush, the most characteristic feature of the climacteric syndrome, has provoked controversy throughout the ages, though it is not until relatively recently that the medical profession, and gynecologists in particular, have accepted that such therapy does merit general consideration rather than being left to the preserve of fringe medical practitioners. Much of this attitude was a result of the lack of an explanation for what Tyler Smith[1] described as 'this curious malady', so that for centuries women were reassured that they were only suffering from 'the change of life' and at best were offered sedation. Until the mechanics of the ovarian cycle and menstruation were first appreciated many believed that the 'heats and chills of the body were due to vascular plethora resulting from non-secretion of the catamenia increasing nervous excitability'[1]. Tilt[2] considered that flushes were cases of pathological blushing and he supported Tyler Smith's view of the 'toxaemic effect of retention of the menstrual fluid', which provided his rationale for treatment by phlebotomy and the application of leeches. Other remedies proposed at this time included the sedatives bromide and valerian, and tepid bathing of the skin to diminish the excess sensibility. The writings of these times do not record the effectiveness of such therapies and there was certainly no appreciation of the importance of the double-blind controlled trial.

As the 19th century progressed medical opinion inclined to the view that a glandular disturbance was responsible and thyroid deficiency in particular, so that thyroid extract was a popular prescription[3]. Gradually more and more attention was focused on the ovary and treatment with ovarian extracts was initiated by Brown-Séquard, who is reported to have prescribed two sheep's ovaries a day sandwiched between slices of un-leavened bread. However, injections of extracts proved more acceptable and were given initially at the Landau Clinic in Berlin from 1896 and also in Paris[4]. It was not until 1923 when Allen and Doisy first demonstrated the estrogenic activity of follicular fluid from hog's ovaries and subse-quently isolated estrone from the urine of pregnant women[5], that any real progress was possible. Subsequently estradiol and estriol were also isolated but they were all comparatively inactive when given by mouth and frequent injections were necessary so that this form of therapy was unsuitable on a large scale. The development of the synthetic non-steroid stilboestrol[6] provided an effective oral therapy and later the semi-synthetic estrogens ethinyl estradiol and mestranol were produced, which were much more potent[7]. Today conjugated natural estrogen preparations form the basis of oral therapy.

Although the effectiveness of estrogen therapy for the relief of hot flushes has been accepted by most doctors with an interest in the climac-teric, there has been a persistent fear that estrogens might be carci-nogenic, and this has been a major factor in limiting the wider usage of hormone replacement therapy (HRT). In addition the lack of informa-tion on the etiology of the flush has fuelled the controversies concerning the rationale and safety of exogenous hormone replacement[8, 9]. The lack of knowledge of the underlying mechanisms of flushing has resulted in a multitude of alternative therapies.

NON-ESTROGENIC REMEDIES

Because of the belief that excess production of pituitary gonadotrophins had a role in the etiology of flushing, irradiation of the pituitary gland was advocated by Geist and Mintz[10]. They treated 75 postmenopausal women and 25 controls, and apparently produced considerable relief for up to 6 weeks, but this approach has not proved popular. More recently danazol, a specific anti-gonadotrophin agent, has been shown to suppress the elevated gonadotrophin levels of the climacteric but without any significant effect on flushing[11].

Vitamin E has been proposed for the treatment or prevention of many sex-related problems but although the rationale for its use to treat flushes is not explained, McLaren[12] found that it was successful in 30 out of 47 patients compared with only one of 18 who were receiving a placebo. Once again such enthusiasm has not been persuasive.

Sedatives and tranquilizers have been widely prescribed for over a century, ranging from bromide and valerian, nux vomica to barbituates, diazepam and similar drugs, but often such therapy has only added to the lethargy of which so many flushing women also complain. A combination of phenobarbitone, belladonna and ergotamine marketed as Bellergal retard (Sandoz) had some popularity for many years[13], but as it is no longer available even the pharmaceutical company must have accepted that it was not a satisfactory alternative to estrogen.

Agents which alter the responsiveness of the peripheral vasculature have wide therapeutic potential. Clonidine, an alpha-adrenergic agonist, is an effective prophylaxis for migraine and in high doses as an antihypertensive agent. Clayden et al.[14] supervised a multicentre double-blind placebo-controlled crossover study on 100 women and reported a significant effect in controlling the duration and severity of flushes with minimal side-effects (Fig. 24.1). It is of note, though, that as with so many similar studies until the crossover of therapy there was no difference in the response between the two groups. These findings have been supported by some workers[15] but others have failed to confirm any difference from placebo treatement[16].

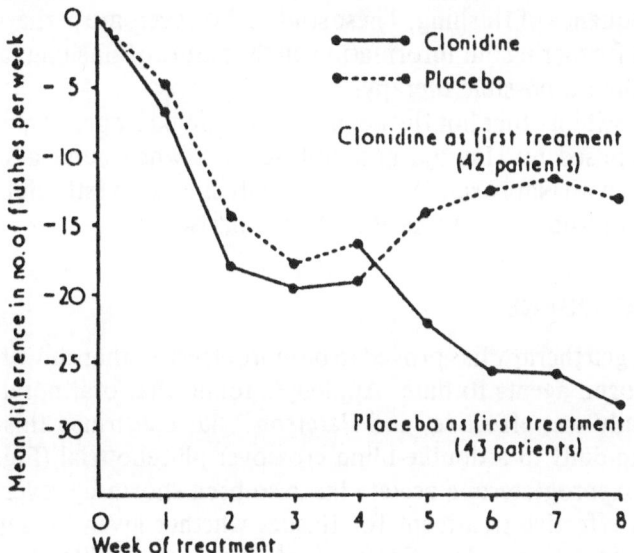

Figure 24.1 Double-blind crossover trial of clonidine in women with severe flushes[14] – mean change in number of flushes from initial values

Ethamsylate is a non-hormonal agent used principally for the treatment of menorrhagia and is considered to act by increasing capillary strength. Harrison[17] reported on a double-blind trial of 12 weeks duration in 20 flushing women in which the ethamsylate group showed a significant reduction in the frequency of flushes with no side-effects.

The effect of propranolol, which causes peripheral and central beta-blockade, has been studied with conflicting results. Coope et al.[18], in a prospective double-blind randomized trial in 25 flushing women, found no difference with placebo or any effect on other symptoms, whereas Alcoff et al.[19] found a statistically significant reduction in the frequency and severity of vasomotor symptoms in 37 women who received propranolol 40 mg twice daily.

Methyldopa, which depletes noradrenaline stores by preventing the conversion of dopa to dopamine and also interferes with the formation of 5-hydroxytryptamine (serotonin), seems to be yet another possible alternative therapy[20].

The drug opipramol, which has some antidepressant properties similar to imipramine and may inhibit the uptake of noradrenaline and serotonin in the hypothalamus, has also been shown to cause significant suppression of hot flushes[21].

The possibility that flushing is related to the activation of opiate receptors prompted assessments of naloxone by intravenous infusion. Lightman et al.[22] noted a significant reduction in the frequency of flushes but De Fazio and colleagues[23], using identical dosage, found no change in the frequency of flushing. These studies, however, are perhaps of more value for furthering our information on the nature of flushing rather than in providing a possible therapy.

The possibility that hot flushes may be mediated by prostaglandins has been proposed by Haataja and colleagues[24], who found a significant reduction with Naproxen 250 mg twice daily similar to estradiol 1 mg b.d. but they did not have a placebo for comparison.

PROGESTOGENS

Progestogen therapy has proved to be more effective than any of the other non-estrogen agents to date. Appleby[25] found that oral norethisterone 10 mg daily was effective, and Paterson[26] has confirmed this response with 5 mg daily in a double-blind crossover placebo trial (Fig. 24.2).

Medroxyprogesterone acetate has also been shown by several studies to be an effective treatment for flushes whether given by depot intramuscular injections – depo Provera[27, 28]; in doses from 50 to 150 mg every few months or 20 mg orally per day[29, 30]. There are also several further studies being reported in this book.

Megestrol acetate is also effective in suppressing flushes, and Erlik et al.[31] suggest that this form of therapy may also reduce postmenopausal bone resorption.

The mode of action of progestogens in this context is not clear. Serum gonadotrophin levels are lowered but there is no improvement in other symptoms or changes that indicate metabolism to estrogenic products; rather it is most likely that they have a direct effect in their own right[26].

A synthetic steroid – Org OD14 – which has weak estrogenic, progestogenic and androgenic properties, is being evaluated as a safe alternative

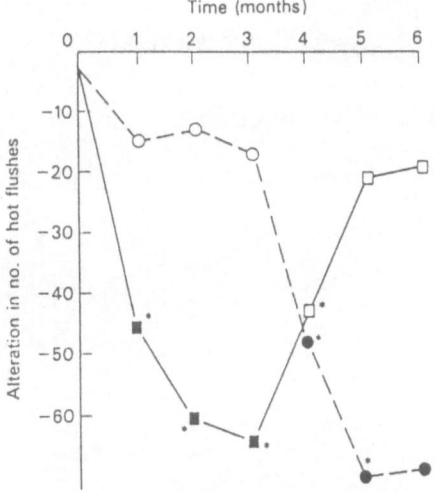

Figure 24.2 Double-blind crossover trial of norethisterone 5 mg daily[26]. Alteration in number of flushes per week after each month of therapy. O---● Placebo/active; ■—□ active/placebo. Significance of differences: * $p < 0.01$

to estrogen therapy[32]. It has a greater effect on relieving hot flushes than placebo, but without a stimulatory effect on the endometrium. There are further reports on this preparation in this book.

ESTROGEN

Although estrogen deficiency is not a fundamental cause of hot flushes, the superiority of estrogen therapy over all other medications is now surely beyond dispute. Earlier reports of the relative merits of estrogen preparations over placebo[33-35] have been criticized for their failure to counter the considerable placebo contribution. This placebo response is so strong in menopausal women that only double-blind randomized crossover placebo-controlled trials can establish the true value of therapy. These criteria are satisfied by two studies.

Coope et al.[36] studied 30 menopausal women in a 6-month crossover trial with Premarin 1.25 mg. After 3 months both groups of women had noticed a significant reduction in hot flushes, though this was much greater in those receiving estrogen first. After the crossover those who changed to placebo had a rapid return of flushes whereas the others had a further significant reduction in flushing with the addition of Premarin (Fig. 24.3). Campbell and Whitehead[37] conducted a 4- and 12-month crossover study also with Premarin 1.25 mg, and produced a statistically significant reduction in hot flushes during estrogen therapy compared to placebo (Fig. 24.4). Both these studies confirmed the powerful therapeutic

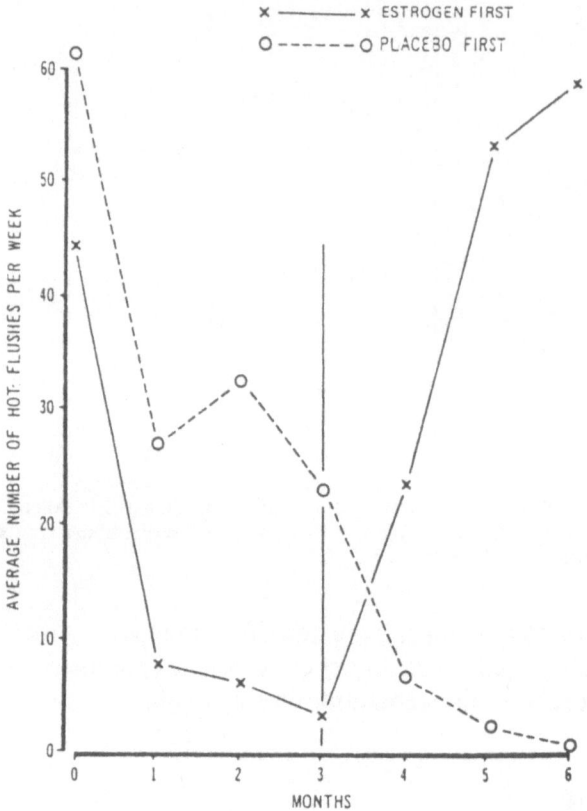

Figure 24.3 Hot flush count during a 6-month crossover trial with Premarin 1.25 mg[36]

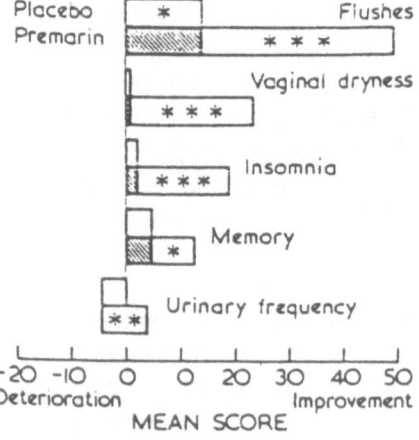

Figure 24.4 Differences in graphic rating scale scores for Premarin 1.25 mg and placebo therapy in a 12-month study[37]. ***$p < 0.001$; **$p < 0.01$; *$p < 0.05$

response in those who received placebo first, but invariably the switch from estrogen first to placebo caused a rapid return of flushing.

There are now many types of HRT containing estrogen, most of which have a similar effect on flushes. In addition subcutaneous implants of estradiol with or without testosterone may be a preferred route of administration and the effect on hot flushes is equally satisfactory[38, 39].

Estrogen may also be administered in a cream to be absorbed either per vaginam or transcutaneously[40, 41], but although this route may cause fewer biochemical changes the effect on flushing may be less satisfactory[42].

CLINICAL APPLICATION

For women with hot flushes of the climacteric estrogen therapy is the treatment of choice. Continuous daily estrogen seems preferable to the traditional cyclical regimen as many women complain of a return of flushes during the tablet-free week. For women who have not had a hysterectomy the addition of progestogen to the regimen of therapy that is continued beyond a few months' initial trial is obligatory in order to protect the endometrium from over-stimulation[43, 44], but the role of additional progestogen in protecting the breast in a similar manner is less clear[44].

The initial response to treatment is usually dramatic with an effect noticed within a few days and elimination of flushing achieved well before the end of the first cycle of therapy (Fig. 24.5). An adjustment of the dosage may be required but most will have symptomatic relief at the lowest doses of the currently available preparations.

With such dramatic relief from flushing, as well as the other benefits of hormone therapy, many women are reluctant to consider stopping treatment. If untreated, flushes may continue for only a few weeks or for many years and their duration cannot be predicted. When cessation of therapy is desired, however, it is less likely to be followed by a return of flushes if the dose of estrogen is gradually reduced over several weeks rather than by a precipitous and sudden withdrawal.

OTHER TREATMENTS

For those who are unable to take or tolerate estrogen therapy, progestogen alone seems to be the best alternative. However, although many non-estrogen treatments may reduce or eliminate flushing they do not influence other climacteric symptoms such as vaginal atrophy which can be a cause of even greater distress.

PLEASE RECORD FOR EACH DAY AS FOLLOWS:

Bleeding = Write B for bleeding. Write S for spotting.
Flushes = Write number of flushes per 24 hours. Write O for no flushes.
Tablets = Write T for tablet taken. Leave blank for tablet omitted.

Day of Month (Each vertical column represents one day).

		1	2	3	4	5	6	7	8	9	10	11	12	13	14	15	16	17	18	19	20	21	22	23	24	25	26	27	28	29	30	31
APRIL	Bleeding																															
	Flushes			8	8	8	15	8	5	7	6	8	11	11	12	9	11	10	10	7	5	5	4	4	2	4	3	1	1	0	0	B
	Tablets	T	T	T	T	T	T	T	T	T	T	T	T	T	T	T	T	T	T	T	T	T	T	T	T	T	T	T	T	T	T	T
MAY	Bleeding					B	B																								B	B
	Flushes	O	O	O	O	O	O	O	O	O	1	O	O	O	O	O	O	O	O	O	O	O	O	O	O	O	O	1	O	O	O	O
	Tablets	T	T	T	T	T	T	T	T	T	T	T	T	T	T	T	T	T	T	T	T	T	T	T	T	T	T	T	T	T	T	T
JUNE	Bleeding						B	B																								
	Flushes	O	O	O		O	O																									
	Tablets	T	T	T																												
	Bleeding																															
	Flushes																															
	Tablets																															

WRITE IN MONTHS

Figure 24.5 A patient calender card record indicating the change in frequency and severity of hot flushes at the start of an estrogen and progestogen regimen of therapy

FLUSHES IN MEN

The existence of a male climacteric is questionable, but men who suffer loss of testicular function through atrophy, surgery or disease can experience the same distressing vasomotor symptoms as menopausal women[45, 46]. Testosterone replacement by intramuscular injections every 2-4 weeks eliminates the flushes and restores libido and potency[45, 47, 48]. Alternatively cyproterone acetate can also be helpful, though the mode of action is not understood[49].

SUMMARY

The multitude of apparently effective treatments for the hot flush is a reflection of our lack of knowledge of the underlying mechanism. It is the easiest climacteric symptom to quantify and treat but the development and assessment of new treatments is complicated by the high placebo response and wide inter-patient variation. With greater recognition of the safety of hormone therapy, estrogen for women and testosterone for men will continue to be the most effective remedy, and even when the cause is identified and a specific treatment found, they will remain popular because of the additional benefits they bring to those who are also experiencing other symptoms of sex hormone deficiency.

The successful treatment of what is often a distressing complaint that can so alter the quality of life of menopausal women is easily achieved. Therapy has progressed dramatically from the leeches of the last century but after so many years of the availability of estrogen therapy it is disappointing that so many women are still denied this benefit.

REFERENCES

1. Tyler Smith, W. (1849). The climacteric disease in women. *Lond. J. Med.*, **7**, 601-9
2. Tilt, E. J. (1857). *The Change of Life in Health and Disease*, 2nd edn. (London: Churchill)
3. Leith Napier, A. D. (1897). *The Menopause and its Disorders*. (London: Scientific Press)
4. Novak, E. (1940). The management of the menopause. *Am. J. Obstet. Gynecol.*, **40**, 589-95
5. Doisy, E. A., Veler, C. D. and Thayer, S. (1930). The preparation of the crystalline ovarian hormone from the urine of pregnant women. *J. Biol. Chem.*, **86**, 499-509
6. Dodds, E. C., Goldberg, L., Lawson, W. and Robinson, R. (1938). Oestrogenic activity of certain synthetic compounds. *Nature*, **141**, 247-8
7. Swyer, G. I. (1959). The oestrogens. *Br. Med. J.*, **1**, 1029-31
8. Mulley, G. and Mitchell, J. R. (1976). Menopausal flushing: does oestrogen therapy make sense? *Lancet*, **1**, 1397-9
9. Strickler, R. C., Borth, R. and Woolever, C. A. (1977). The climacteric syndrome: an estrogen replacement dilemma. *Can. Med. Assoc. J.*, **19**, 586-7
10. Geist, S. H. and Mintz, M. (1937). Pituitary radiation for the relief of menopausal symptoms. *Am. J. Obstet. Gynecol.*, **33**, 643-5
11. Bohler, C. S. and Greenblatt, R. B. (1974). The pathophysiology of the hot flush. In Greenblatt, R. B. *et al.* (eds.) *Menopausal Syndrome*. pp. 29-37. (New York: Medcom Press)
12. McLaren, H. C. (1949). Vitamin E in the menopause. *Br. Med. J.*, **2**, 1378-82

13. Kelly, M. J., Power, R. M. and Arromet, G. H. (1961). Management of the perimenopausal syndrome. *Obstet. Gynecol.*, **17**, 328-32
14. Clayden, J. R., Bell, J. W. and Pollard, P. (1974). Menopausal flushing: double-blind trial of a non-hormonal preparation. *Br. Med. J.*, **1**, 409-12
15. Edington, P. T., Chagnon, J.-P. and Steinberg, W. M. (1980). Clonidine (dixarit) for menopausal flushing. *Can. Med. Assoc. J.*, **123**, 23-6
16. Lindsay, R. and Hart, D. M. (1978). Failure of response of menopausal vasomotor symptoms to clonidine. *Maturitas*, **1**, 21-5
17. Harrison, R. F. (1981). Ethamsylate in the treatment of climacteric flushing. *Maturitas*, **3**, 31-7
18. Coope, J., Williams, S. and Patterson, J. S. (1978). A study of the effectiveness of propranolol in menopausal hot flushes. *Br. J. Obstet. Gynaecol.*, **85**, 472-5
19. Alcoff, J. M., Campbell, D., Tribble, D., Oldfield, B. and Cruess, D. (1981). Double-blind, placebo-controlled, cross-over trial of propranolol as treatment for menopausal vasomotor symptoms. *Clin. Ther.*, **3**, 356-64
20. Nesheim, B.-I. and Saetre, T. (1981). Reduction of menopausal hot flushes by methyldopa. A double-blind cross-over trial. *Eur. J. Clin. Pharmacol.*, **20**, 413-16
21. van Lith, N. D. and Motké, J. C. (1983). Opipramol in the climacteric syndrome. A double-blind, placebo-controlled trial. *Maturitas*, **5**, 17-23
22. Lightman, S. L., Jacobs, H. S., Maguire, A. K., McGarrick, G. and Jeffcoate, S. L. (1981). Climacteric flushing: clinical and endocrine response to infusion of naloxone. *Br. J. Obstet. Gynaecol.*, **88**, 919-24
23. De Fazio, J., Verheugen, C., Chetkowski, R., Nass, T., Judd, H. L. and Meldrum, D. R. (1984). The effects of naloxone on hot flashes and gonadotrophin secretion in postmenopausal women. *J. Clin. Endocrinol. Metab.*, **58**(3), 578-81
24. Haataja, M., Paul, R., Grönroos, M., Erkkola, R., Punnonen, R., Rauramo, L. and Nieminen, A.-L. (1984). Effect of prostaglandin inhibitor and oestrogen on climacteric symptoms and serum free fatty acids. *Maturitas*, **5**, 263-9
25. Appleby, B. (1962). Norethisterone in the control of menopausal symptoms. *Lancet*, **1**, 407-9
26. Paterson, M. E. (1982). A randomized double-blind cross-over trial into the effect of norethisterone on climacteric symptoms and biochemical profiles. *Br. J. Obstet. Gynaecol.*, **89**, 464-72
27. Bullock, J. L., Massey, F. M. and Gambrell, R. D. (1975). Use of medroxyprogesterone acetate to prevent menopausal symptoms. *Obstet. Gynecol.*, **46**, 165-8
28. Morrison, J. C., Martin, D. C., Blair, R. A., Anderson, G. D., Kincheloe, B. W., Bates, G. W., Hendrix, J. W., Rivlin, M. E., Forman, E. K., Propst, M. G. and Needham, R. (1980). Use of medroxyprogesterone acetate for relief of climacteric symptoms. *Am. J. Obstet. Gynecol.*, **138**, 99-104
29. Schiff, I., Tulchinsky, D., Cramer, D. and Ryan, K. J. (1980). Oral medroxyprogesterone in treatment of postmenopausal symptoms. *J. Am. Med. Assoc.*, **244**, 1443-5
30. Albrecht, B. H., Schiff, I., Tulchinsky, D. and Ryan, K. J. (1981). Objective evidence that placebo and oral medroxyprogesterone acetate therapy diminish menopausal vasomotor flushes. *Am. J. Obstet. Gynecol.*, **139**, 631-5
31. Erlik, Y., Meldrum, D. R., Lagasse, L. D. and Judd, H. L. (1981). Effect of megestrol acetate on flushing and bone metabolism in post-menopausal women. *Maturitas*, **3**, 167-72
32. Trevoux, R., Dieulangard, P. and Blum, A. (1983). Efficacy and safety of Org OD14 in the treatment of climacteric complaints. *Maturitas*, **5**, 89-96
33. Greenblatt, R. B., Barfield, W. E., Ganner, J. F., Calk, G. L. and Harrod, J. P. (1950). Evaluation of an estrogen, androgen, estrogen-androgen combination and a placebo in the treatment of the menopause. *J. Clin. Endocrinol.*, **10**, 1547-58
34. Kupperman, H. S., Blatt, M. H., Wiesbader, H. and Filler, W. (1953). Comparative clinical evaluation of estrogenic preparations by the menopausal and amenorrhoeal indices. *J. Clin. Endocrinol.*, **74**, 685-94
35. Martin, P. L., Burnier, A. M., Segre, E. J. and Huix, F. J. (1971). Graded sequential therapy in the menopause: a double-blind study. *Am. J. Obstet. Gynecol.*, **111**, 178-86
36. Coope, J., Thomson, J. M. and Poller, L. (1975). Effects of 'natural oestrogen' replacement therapy on menopausal symptoms and blood clotting. *Br. Med. J.*, **4**, 139-43-

37. Campbell, S. and Whitehead, M. I. (1977). Oestrogen therapy and the menopausal syndrome. In Greenblatt, R. and Studd, J. W. (eds.) *The Menopause; Clinics in Obstetrics and Gynaecology*, vol. 4, pp. 31-47. (London, Philadelphia and Toronto: Saunders)
38. Brincat, M., Magos, A., Studd, J. W., Cardozo, L. D., Wardle, P. J. and Cooper, D. (1984). Subcutaneous hormone implants for the control of climacteric symptoms. *Lancet*, 1, 16-18
39. Nagamani, M., Lin, T. J., McDonough, P. G., Watatani, H., McPherson, J. C. and Mahesh, V. B. (1978). Clincical and endocrine studies in menopausal women after estradiol pellet implantation. *Obstet. Gynecol.*, 50, 541-7
40. Campbell, S. and Whitehead, M. I. (1982). Potency and hepato-cellular effects of oestrogens after oral, percutaneous and subcutaneous administration. In van Keep, P. A. *et al.* (eds.) *The Controversial Climacteric.* pp. 103-25. (Lancaster: MTP Press)
41. Sitruk-Ware, R., de Lignieres, B., Basdevant, A. and Mauvais-Jarvis, P. (1980). Absorption of percutaneous oestradiol in postmenopausal women. *Maturitas*, 2, 207-11
42. Laufer, L. R., De Fazio, J. L., Lu, J. K., Meldrum, D. R., Eggena, P., Sambhi, M. P., Hershman, J. M. and Judd, H. L. (1983). Estrogen replacement therapy by transdermal estradiol administration. *Am. J. Obstet. Gynecol.*, 146, 533-40
43. Thom, M. H., White, P. J., Williams, R. M., Sturdee, D. W., Paterson, M. E., Wade-Evans, T. and Studd, J. W. (1979). Prevention and treatment of endometrial pathology in climacteric women receiving oestrogen therapy. *Lancet*, 2, 455-7
44. Gambrell, R. D. (1982). The menopause: benefits and risks of estrogen–progestogen replacement therapy. *Fertil. Steril.*, 37, 457-74
45. Feldman, J. M., Postlethwaite, R. W. and Glenn, J. F. (1976). Hot flashes and sweats in men with testicular insufficiency. *Arch. Intern. Med.*, 136, 606-8
46. Ginsburg, J. and O'Reilly, B. (1983). Climacteric flushing in a man. *Br. Med. J.*, 287, 262
47. Hendy, M. S. and Burge, P. S. (1938). Climacteric flushing in a man. *Br. Med. J.*, 287, 423
48. De Fazio, J., Meldrum, D. R., Winer, J. H. and Judd, H. L. (1984). Direct action of androgen on hot flushes in the human male. *Maturitas*, 6, 3-8
49. Eaton, A. C. and McGuire, N. (1983). Cyproterone acetate in treatment of post-orchidectomy hot flushes. *Lancet*, 2, 1336-7

Workshops

Workshops

Workshop 1

The breast

Chairman: R. D. Gambrell, Jr (USA)
Co-chairman: G. B. Melis (Italy)

R. J. B. King (UK)
H. Vorherr (USA)
N. Siddle (UK)
K. I. Bland (USA)
J. B. Buchanan (USA)
R. B. Greenblatt (USA)

Carcinoma of the breast strikes 1 in 11 women in the United States. Breast cancer is the most frequent malignancy in American females, accounting for 27% of all cancers. It is also the leading cause of death from cancer in women, causing 19% of all cancer deaths in women in the United States. The mortality from breast carcinoma varies from a high of 25.7:100000 women in England to a low of 0.2:100000 women in Honduras. The mortality from breast cancer of 22.1:100000 female population has not changed around the world during the past 45 years, while death from uterine corpus cancer declined from 27:100000 in 1930 to 7.7:100000 during 1975. The incidence rates of breast cancer have increased only slightly during the past 28 years, from 70:100000 of the female population in 1947 to 75:100000 during 1975. The American Cancer Society estimated that 115 900 new cases of breast carcinoma would be diagnosed in the United States in 1984 and that 37 300 women would die in that country from this tumor in 1984. This is 12 times the number of deaths each year from endometrial adenocarcinoma. The incidence of breast cancer increases throughout the female life span. In this respect the incidence of this malignancy differs from cervical, endometrial, and ovarian cancer, which peak in the 40s, 50s, and 60s, respectively, and then either decline or plateau. Since estrogens are the growth hormone of normal breast tissue and either endocrine ablative surgery or antiestrogen therapy such as tamoxifen may at least temporarily arrest the progression of some metastatic breast carcinomas, concern has been rightfully expressed over the role of the sex steroids, especially estrogen replacement therapy.

Melis presented data on fibrocystic mastopathy, where many hormonal alterations have been reported. In 271 women where fibrocystic mastopathy was diagnosed by history and physical examination, evaluations of plasma LH, FSH, prolactin, progesterone and 17β-estradiol were performed throughout their menstrual cycles. Normal ovulatory cycles were found in only 19.9% of patients, while the others were affected by short luteal phase or luteal insufficiency (35.7%), hyperprolactinemia (24.7%), polycystic ovaries (11.1%), and anovulatory cycles (8.5%). Imbalance in the ratio of progesterone to estradiol was observed in the luteal phase of the patients with fibrocystic disease, which was significantly lower ($p < 0.0005$) than the controls. In 106 patients, sulpiride (5 mg i.v. bolus) induced a prolactin release that was significantly higher ($p < 0.0005$) than in control subjects. These data suggest that an inapparent hyperprolactinemia is present in patients with fibrocystic mastopathy. Bromocriptine 5 mg daily was administered for 3 months to 78 patients. A significant decrease ($p < 0.0005$) of prolactin levels was associated with a significant improvement ($p < 0.0005$) of progesterone secretion. Consequently the ratio of progesterone to estradiol became similar to normal. Subjective and objective breast symptoms were relieved in more than 70% of the patients and remission continued for 3–6 months after cessation of bromocriptine therapy.

King stated that steroid receptor assays provide useful data that help determine treatment schedules for breast cancer. However, the current assays using [^{3}H]steroids have limitations: (1) the assay is not simple because of the lability of the [^{3}H]steroid binding; (2) no practical method exists for locating the receptors in tissue sections; (3) relatively large amounts of tissue are required. Most of the problems could be overcome if antibodies to the receptor protein were available. The Imperial Cancer Research Fund have generated monoclonal antibodies against an antigen qualitatively and quantitatively related to estradiol receptors (ER) that will react with ER from several human tissues but not with other human steroid binding proteins or with ER from other species. Both an immunoradiometric assay (IRMA) and a histochemical assay have been developed that correlate very highly with the [^{3}H]estradiol binding assays. The IRMA is much more robust than present methods and should enable more widespread use of such assays. The histochemical method offers several avenues of exploitation; analyses can be made on wax-embedded samples and needle biopsies. Furthermore the heterogeneous staining patterns seen in some sections may provide important clues as to why some ER positive tumors do not respond to endocrine therapy. Immunological probes for estradiol receptors in breast tumors have also been developed.

Vorherr reviewed the endocrinology of breast cancer, stating that although many hormones have been related to the pathobiology of mammary malignancy, prolactin and mainly estrogens have been more closely connected to fibrocystic breast disease and carcinoma of the breast. In the case of prolactin, however, most studies fail to show an association with breast cancer[1]. In hypophysectomized rats lacking prolactin it was observed that estrogens induce fibrocystic disease to the same or greater extent than in intact animals (Vorherr, H. and Vorherr, V., unpublished observations, 1983). Only premenopausal breast cancer is thought to be hormone-sensitive[2]. However, in postmenopausal patients breast cancer is more often ER-positive (60%) than during the premenopause (40%). In postmenopausal women progesterone levels are low and ductal epithelium can be stimulated for proliferation by small amounts of estrogens. Intraductal epithelial proliferation is observed in 40% of older women, despite estrogen deficiency. It is possible that local estrogen synthesis in ductal epithelium or, more so, conversion of androstenedione to estrone in periductal fat and diffusion of estrogen to adjacent ductal epithelium produce epithelial proliferation. The risk of breast cancer is up to fivefold increased in patients with epithelial proliferation. Hyperproliferation of ductal epithelium may favor development of epithelial atypia that may progress to carcinoma (Fig. W1.1). Understandably so, estrogen replacement therapy, unopposed by progestogen, has been related to an increased risk of breast cancer. Conversely, in postmenopausal women receiving estrogen therapy opposed by progestogen, breast cancer incidence was

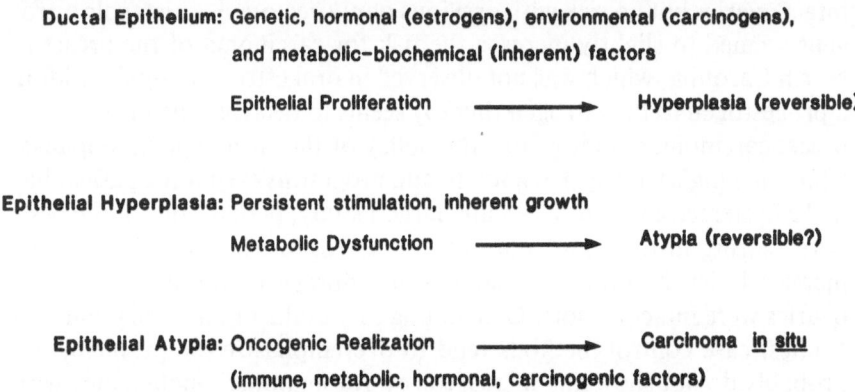

Ductal Epithelium: Genetic, hormonal (estrogens), environmental (carcinogens), and metabolic–biochemical (inherent) factors

Epithelial Proliferation   ⟶   Hyperplasia (reversible)

Epithelial Hyperplasia: Persistent stimulation, inherent growth

Metabolic Dysfunction   ⟶   Atypia (reversible?)

Epithelial Atypia: Oncogenic Realization   ⟶   Carcinoma *in situ* (immune, metabolic, hormonal, carcinogenic factors)

Figure W1.1 Pathophysiology of epithelial proliferation. Hormonal (estrogens) and other factors stimulate ductal epithelial proliferation leading to epithelial hyperplasia and possibly via epithelial atypia to carcinoma *in situ*.

only half that of patients taking estrogens alone[3]. The protective effect of progestogen from hyperstimulation of breast and endometrium is brought about by: (1) downregulation of estrogen receptor levels and increasing intracellular metabolism of estrogens; (2) inhibiting androstenedione conversion to estrone; and (3) lowering the rate of mitosis while inducing epithelial differentiation.

In estrogen-dependent breast carcinomas, growth may become accelerated by endogenous or exogenous estrogens. On the other hand, estrogens can inhibit cancer growth in patients with an ER-negative tumor that has grown in an estrogen-poor environment. Thus, estrogens can be carcinoma-promoting or carcinoma-inhibiting but this is often difficult to ascertain on an individual basis. The diagnosis of breast cancer is a collective one, including a patient population with probably more than 20 tumor subsets, i.e., patients that have an individually different tumor pathobiology, endocrinology, and prognosis. Hormone measurements in plasma and urine cannot define patients at high risk for breast cancer and cannot yield information as to the prognosis of mammary malignancy. Progess in the endocrinology of breast cancer can be achieved by prospective studies where hormones are determined in normal breast tissue, ductal fluid, cyst fluid, and breast cancer tissue, and are correlated to respective concentrations in plasma and urine.

Siddle reviewed the epidemiologic studies of breast cancer in postmenopausal estrogen users. In the 20 published studies, factors that must be considered include the type of menopause, age at menopause, age at parity, and age at first term birth. In one study of 1891 patients it was suggested that there may be an increased risk of breast cancer from long-term estrogen use of more than 12 years, especially in those women with fibrocystic disease of the breast[4]. Another study observed a slightly increased risk of carcinoma from long-term estrogen use in patients with intact ovaries but no risk with previous oophorectomy[5]. Injectable estrogens seemed to slightly increase the risk for carcinoma of the breast in North Carolina, which was not observed in oral estrogen users[6]. Adding a progestogen to the estrogen therapy seems to decrease the incidence of breast carcinoma[3], so it is now the policy of the Academic Menopausal Clinic at King's College Hospital to add progestins even if the patient has had a hysterectomy. The latest and largest study, perhaps one of the best, is reassuring in that non-contraceptive estrogen use did not show any increased risk of breast cancer for any dosage or duration, whether ovaries were intact or not[7]. Concluding the results of all these published studies, case control methods tend to overemphasize the problem, but probably do not show any increased risk for mammary malignancy with estrogen replacement therapy. However, there may be some subgroups of women who are at risk for breast carcinoma so patients should be screened for risk factors. Estrogen therapy should be kept to the minimal dosage that relieves symptoms and a progestogen should be added even if the patient has had a hysterectomy.

Gambrell presented an update of the data from Wilford Hall USAF Medical Center, with 5 years of prospective study plus 4 years of follow-up. The incidence of breast cancer continues to decline at this institution with the ever-increasing addition of progestogens to postmenopausal estrogen therapy. The lowest incidence of mammary malignancy was observed in the estrogen–progestogen users (66.8 : 100 000) and has remained remarkably consistent in the unopposed estrogen users (142.3 : 100 000) despite ever-increasing estrogen usage. The highest incidence was found in the non-hormone users (343.6 : 100 000), most likely because of the prevalence of risk factors such as family history and fibrocystic disease of the breast.

Bland discussed risk factors for carcinoma of the breast and presented guidelines for who should be screened. A family history of breast cancer is a major indicator in that 50% of individuals in the direct genetic lineage have the cancer phenotype[8–12]. The mainstay of management among non-affected asymptomatic high-risk relatives is surveillance. Precancerous fibrous mastopathy increases the risk 2.5 times over normal females.

Dupont and Page[10] recently evaluated women with benign proliferative breast lesions. Women having proliferative disease without atypical hyperplasia had a risk of cancer that was 1.9 times the risk in women with non-proliferative lesions. However, the risk for women with atypical hyperplasia (atypia) was 5.3 times that in women with non-proliferative lesions. The proportional hazards – relative risks shown in Table W1.1 – are useful to compare the relative risks for different subgroups within the same study. A family history of breast cancer had little effect on the risk for women with non-proliferative lesions. However, the risk for women with atypia and a family history of breast cancer was elevenfold that for women who had non-proliferative lesions without a family history (95% confidence interval, 5.5–24). The authors observed calcification to elevate the cancer risk if the biopsy confirmed proliferative disease. The presence of cysts and a family history of breast cancer enhanced the risk 2.7 times that for women without either of these risk factors (95% confidence interval, 1.5–4.6). These authors conclude that the majority of women (70%) having breast biopsy for benign disease are not at increased risk for cancer. These data do corroborate the above findings of an increased cancer risk on the basis of atypical hyperplasia and a family history of breast cancer. Figure W1.2 denotes the proportion of patients free of invasive cancer as a function of time since biopsy. A 2- or 3-fold increase may have little clinical importance if the risk in the reference population is small. The adverse effect of positive family history for the patient with atypical hyperplasia becomes appreciable at approximately 20 years post-biopsy.

The aforementioned clinicopathological studies reflect the opinion that proliferative lesions of epithelial duct origin provide circumstantial and

Table W1.1 The effect of hyperplasia, age, family history, and calcification on the risk of breast cancer[a]

Numerator of relative risk	Denominator of relative risk	Relative risk[b]	95% confidence interval	p value
PDWA, age 20–45	Non-PD, age 20–45	1.9	1.2–3.2	0.012
PDWA, age 46–55	Non-PD, age 46–55	1.4	0.57–3.3	0.49
PDWA, age >55	Non-PD, age >55	5.6	0.69–46	0.11
PDWA with CAL	Non-PD without CAL	2.3	1.2–4.3	0.008
AH with CAL	Non-PD with CAL	8.6	2.5–29	0.0006
AH with CAL	Non-PD without CAL	8.3	3.5–19	<0.0001
Cysts without FH	Neither cysts nor FH	1.3	0.88–2.0	0.19
Cysts with FH	No cysts but FH	2.1	0.78–5.5	0.14
Cysts with FH	Neither cysts nor FH	2.7	1.5–4.6	0.0004
PDWA	Non-PD	1.9	1.2–2.9	0.003
AH	Non-PD	5.3	3.1–8.8	<0.0001
CAL	No CAL	1.3	0.87–2.0	0.19
PDWA without FH	Non-PD without FH	1.9	1.2–3.0	0.007
PDWA with FH	Non-PD with FH	2.0	0.63–6.1	0.25
PDWA with FH	Non-PD without FH	2.7	1.4–5.3	0.004
AH without FH	Non-PD without FH	4.3	2.4–7.8	<0.0001
AH with FH	Non-PD with FH	8.4	2.6–27	0.0003
AH with FH	Non-PD without FH	11.0	5.5–24	<0.0001

[a] PDWA = proliferative disease without atypia; AH = atypical hyperplasia; CAL = calcification; FH = family history of breast cancer (mother, sister, or daughter); Age = age at time of entry biopsy
[b] As compared with the risk in women from Atlanta (Third National Cancer Survey)
From ref. 18

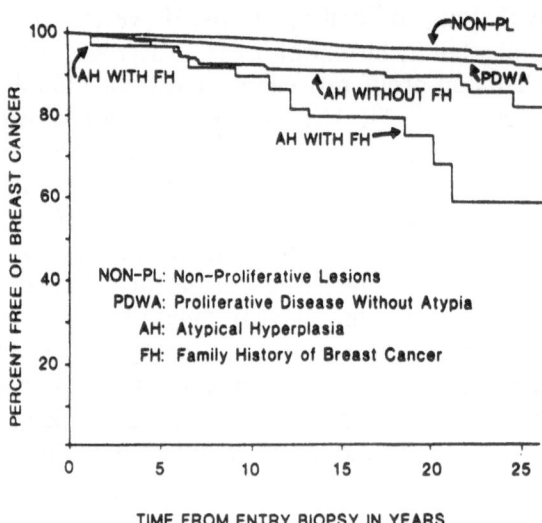

Figure W1.2 Proportion of patients free of invasive breast cancer as a function of the time since the entry biopsy (from ref. 18)

objective data as prognostic markers for increased cancer risk in certain age groups. A differentiation of proliferative pathological elements in tissue sampling appears important to maximize prognostic accuracy and to enhance end-result reporting. These data further support the utilization of the breast biopsy report for pathological indicators which may optimize identification of the high-risk patient with and without other commonly recognized clinical risk factors for breast carcinogenesis. Previous carcinoma in one breast has a 5-fold greater risk of carcinoma in the other breast at a rate of 0.7–1% per year. Equally important determinants for the multifactorial etiology of breast cancer include age, sex, and parity. Over 99% of breast cancers occur in women, and one-third of these tumors occur in postmenopausal patients. The importance of parity seems to be related to age of first birth, with a decrease in risk of 3–4-fold if the first birth was before age 18. Conversely, an increased risk is noted in infertile or unmarried women with fewer than three children, and those whose first child was born after age 34[9]. Less important risk factors include immuno-suppression, viruses, radiotherapy, high-fat diets, obesity, and excess methylxanthine ingestion. The following guidelines were given for screening asymptomatic individuals with *major* risk factors. With a family history of breast cancer in mother or sister, baseline xeromammography should be obtained before age 35 and clinical examination performed every 6 months. After age 35, xeromammogram should be obtained every 2 years. With precancerous fibrous mastopathy, clinical examination should be done every 4 months following diagnosis by biopsy or aspiration, and xeromammogram every 2 years following baseline study at age 35. In patients with carcinoma in one breast surveillance of the opposite breast every 3–6 months by a physician, breast self-examination education, and annual xeromammograms should be done. For patients under age 35 with *minor* risk factors, monthly self breast examination should be taught. After age 35, they should have baseline xeromammography, semi-annual examination, and interval xeromammogram as indicated between ages 35 and 45 years. Patients over 45 years should have monthly breast self-examination and annual xeromammogram with annual examination[11, 12].

Bland *et al.*[11] have successfully employed physical examination with high-quality serial xeromammography to enhance the detection of mammary carcinoma in a national screening clinic. Minimal cancers were more prevalent in this screened population (29%) than for the unscreened population (< 5%) and were detected almost exclusively via xeromammography.

Buchanan presented information on mammography, especially the xeroradiographic process, which produces superior results of breast soft tissue imaging[13]. In the routine xeromammography, two views are taken at right angles to each other, the craniocaudal and mediolateral, which yields less than 500 millirads of radiation. The value of xeromammography as a complement for a clinical breast examination in the symptomatic patient is well established. Evidence is currently available that annual mammographic screening in women over the age of 40 seems prudent[14]. Certainly a baseline examination utilizing mammography at age 40 seems indicated at this time. Radiation dosages in breast cancer screening have decreased 10-fold in the past few years. The absorbed dose to the breast midpoint is now so low that decision-making in regard to mammography need no longer include concern over radiation exposure. Using the techniques available to us today and linear extrapolation accepted by the most severe critics of mammography, the estimated risk becomes a hypothetical figure of one induced breast cancer per 10 million women screened[15]. Physicians can no longer address only the hypothetical estimate of a small number of radiation-induced cancers in women in the later years of life. What must be considered is the great number of breast cancer deaths in younger women – deaths that might be prevented with proper application of a proven diagnostic and screening technique.

Greenblatt pointed out that the breast is more than a target organ. While estrogens, androgens, progesterone, prolactin, insulin, thyroid and growth hormones influence breast growth and activity, the breast is also capable of producing hormones. The study of fluid obtained in gross cystic

Table W1.2 Polypeptide hormones in women with multiple cysts (performed at the same time)

Patient	Age	β-hCG	LH	FSH	PRL	TSH
N.N.	43	5.8	11.3	11.2	6.4	10.7
		6.4	13.5	11.2	5.1	8.9
M.P.	43	2.7	13.0	—	—	—
		54.1	28.5	0.4	—	—
B.C.	45	<5.0	—	—	—	—
		5.9	—	—	—	—
H.B.	59	72.5	—	—	—	—
		10.8	—	—	—	—
B.R.	41	22.4	—	—	—	—
		3.9	13.9	7.2	4.0	7.5
C.D.	51	10.8	11.4	5.8	≤1.0	9.4
		4.8	13.7	9.4	4.8	—
E.W.	55	2.5	12.3	—	8.1	10.0
		3.8	10.9	6.9	7.0	9.6
B.B.	61	2.4	8.3	—	—	—
		28.7	62.5	—	—	—
		2.1	12.4	—	—	—
K.L.	42	<1.0	24.7	—	—	—
		21.0	—	—	—	—
		<1.0	11.7	11.7	—	—
		4.0	9.6	7.0	3.0	10.1
D.M.L.	44	0.9	6.5	10.4	0	11.3
		4.5	15.8	8.2	0.5	—
		1.9	18.0	15.2	0	11.0
		1.5	17.0	4.6	0	—

From ref. 16

Table W1.3 Comparison of polypeptide hormone levels in blood and cyst fluid in three representative cases

Patient	Age		β-hCG	LH	FSH	PRL	TSH
A.H.	53	Serum	<5.0	5.7	10.2	7.9	2.0
		Cyst fluid	194.0	40.7	7.8	8.4	1.8
E.G.	53	Serum	<5.0	7.3	11.2	13.3	4.5
		Cyst fluid	11.0	11.0	5.6	5.2	11.5
D.McL.	44	Serum	<5.0	7.9	22.8	312.0[a]	4.9
		Cyst fluid	<5.0	6.5	10.4	<1.0	11.3

[a] Blood taken during anesthesia (stress raises prolactin levels). Serum β-hCG in all cases were <5. TSH level in cyst fluid was higher than in serum in almost every instance. FSH was usually higher in serum than cyst fluid
From ref. 16

disease of the breast frequently reveals greater than normal values for β-hCG and TSH, and more or less normal FSH, LH and prolactin levels[16] (Tables W1.2 and W1.3). Such hormonal values indicate that the adult breast either stores polypeptide hormones in cysts or produces such hormones *de novo*. Increased cellular activity in the epithelium lining the cyst wall may be reflected in a capacity to produce aberrant β-hCG and may prove a marker to warn the clinician. The relationship between temperature and disease has long occupied the interest of scientists and physicians. For several years liquid crystal thermal imaging has been available to determine changes in symmetry of heat produced by the breast. If a basic period of 10 min of breast cooling is employed, normal breast tissue cools while lesions with increased cellular proliferation, especially cancer, produce more heat as determined by liquid crystal plate thermography. The process does not diagnose cancer; it is only an extension of the physical examination and forewarns the physician that a woman with an abnormal thermogram, especially in the absence of a dominant lump, bears careful screening, more frequent examinations and mammography. As Gautherie pointed out, 'We must accept the concept that even with negative findings on physical examinations and mammography, an "isolated" abnormal thermogram may be the first sign of a "rapidly developing cancer".' His data show that 35% of women with abnormal thermograms develop cancer within 5 years[17]. Thus two methods, aside from mammography, may direct the physician's attention to ominous changes that may be taking place in what appears to be benign breast disease.

In the discussion following the formal presentations, controversy arose over the role of prolactin in both benign and malignant breast disorders. This emphasized the need for continuing studies in breast endocrinology so that breast hormonal pathophysiology may become clearer, hopefully leading to a decreased risk and improved prognosis for carcinoma of the breast.

REFERENCES

1. Vorherr, H. (1980). *Breast Cancer. Epidemiology, Endocrinology, Biochemistry, and Pathobiology.* (Baltimore and Munich: Urban & Schwarzenberg)
2. Burton, A. C. (1977). Why do human cancer death rates increase with age? A new method of analysis of the biology of cancer. *Perspect. Biol. Med.*, **20**, 327
3. Gambrell, R. D. Jr., Maier, R. C. and Sanders, B. I. (1983). Decreased incidence of breast cancer in postmenopausal estrogen-progestogen users. *Obstet. Gynecol.*, **62**, 435
4. Hoover, R., Gray, L. A. Sr., Cole, P. *et al.* (1976). Menopausal estrogens and breast cancer. *N. Engl. J. Med.*, **295**, 401
5. Ross, R. K., Paganini-Hill, A., Gerkins, V. R. *et al.* (1980). A case control study of menopausal estrogen therapy and breast cancer. *J. Am. Med. Assoc.*, **243**, 1635
6. Hulka, B. S., Chambless, L. E., Deubner, D. C. *et al.* (1982). Breast cancer and estrogen replacement therapy. *Am. J. Obstet. Gynecol.*, **143**, 638
7. Kaufman, D. W., Miller, D. R., Rosenberg, L. *et al.* (1984). Noncontraceptive estrogen use and the risk of breast cancer. *J. Am. Med. Assoc.*, **252**, 63
8. Anderson, D. E. (1977). Breast cancer in families. *Cancer*, **40**, 1855–60
9. Lynch, H. T., Albano, W. A., Danes, B. S., Layton, M. A., Kimberling, W. J., Lynch, J. F., Cheng, S. C., Costello, K. A., Mulcahy, G. M., Wagner, C. A. and Tindall, S. L. (1984). Genetic predisposition to breast cancer. *Cancer*, **53**, 612–22
10. Dupont, W. D. and Page, D. L. (1985). Risk factors for breast cancer in women with proliferative breast disease. *N. Engl. J. Med.*, **312**, 146–51
11. Bland, K. I., Buchanan, J. B., Mills, D. L., Kuhns, J. G., Moore, C., Spratt, J. S. and Polk, H. C. Jr. (1981). Analysis of breast cancer screening in women younger than 50 years. *J. Am. Med. Assoc.*, **245**, 1037–42
12. Bland, K. I., Kuhns, J. G., Buchanan, J. B., Dwyer, P. A., Heuser, L. F., O'Connor, C. A., Gray, L. A. Sr. and Polk, H. C. Jr. (1982). A clinicopathologic correlation of mammographic parenchymal patterns and associated risk factors for human mammary carcinoma. *Ann. Surg.*, **195**(5), 528–94
13. Wolfe, J. N. (1969). Xerography of the breast. *Cancer*, **23**, 791–6
14. American Cancer Society (1981). *Cancer*, **33**, 255
15. Dodd, Gerald D. (1984). Mammography: state of the art. *Cancer*, **53** (Suppl.), 652–7
16. Greenblatt, R. B., Chaddha, J. S., Teran, A. Z. *et al.* (1983). Fibrocystic breast disease: pathophysiology, hormonology, treatment. *Contemp. Surg.*, **24**, 49
17. Gautherie, M. (1983). Thermobiological assessment of benign and malignant breast disease. *Am. J. Obstet. Gynecol.*, **147**, 861
18. Dupont, W. D. and Page, D. L. (1985). Risk factors for breast cancer in women with proliferative breast disease. *N. Engl. J. Med.*, **312**(3), 146–51

FURTHER READING

Coffer, A. I., Lewis, K. M., Brockas, A. J. and King, R. J. B. (1985). Monoclonal antibodies against a component related to soluble estrogen receptor. *Cancer-Res.*, **45** (In press)

Coffer, A. I., Spiller, G. H., Lewis, K. M. and King, R. J. B. (1985). Immunoradiometric studies with monoclonal antibody against a component related to human estrogen receptor. *Cancer Res.*, **45** (In press)

Jensen, E. V., Greene, G. L., Closs, L. E., DeSombre, E. R. and Nadji, M. (1982). Receptors reconsidered: a 20-year perspective. *Recent Prog. Res.*, **38**, 1–40

King, R. J. B., Coffer, A. I., Gilbert, J., Lewis, K., Nash, R., Millis, R., Raju, S. and Taylor, R. W. (1985). Histochemical studies with a monoclonal antibody raised against a partially purified soluble estradiol receptor preparation from human myometrium. *Cancer Res.* (In press)

King, W. J., DeSombre, E. R., Jensen, E. V. and Greene, G. L. (1985). Comparison of immunocytochemical and steroid-binding assays for estrogen receptor in human breast tumors. *Cancer Res.*, **45**, 293–304

Leis, H. P. Jr. (1979). Breast cancer: patients at risk. In Strax, P. (ed.) *Control of Breast Cancer Through Mass Screening.* pp. 75–88. (Boston: PSG Publishing Co.)

Workshop 2

The aging male

Chairman: **A. Vermeulen** (Belgium)
Co-chairman: **M. Genderini** (Italy)

M. Featherstone (UK)
M. Hepworth (UK)
C. Zauner (USA)
H. Nankin (USA)
J. M. Davidson (USA)
A. Vermeulen (Belgium)
J.-P. Deslypere (Belgium)

'The aging male' was the theme of workshop 2. In their review of the history of the male menopause **Mike Featherstone** and **Mike Hepworth** pointed out that the current popularity of the term andropause can partly be explained by a number of threats to the status of men epitomized in the strength of the women's movement, which is creating a more independent economic and sexual status for women. This situation is reminiscent of the situation of women in post-revolutionary France, where changes in the social structure brought a vulnerability to those women in midlife who depended for their social status on their physical appearance: the effects of aging on physical appearance created an intense sexual anxiety which was seen as one of the chief characteristics of the menopausal syndrome. The 19th-century literature on the menopause was explicitly designed to dispel this aura of anxiety and to encourage women and their husbands to regard it as a transitory phase through which one should pass to a higher and more fulfilling state. The authors pointed out that in a similar fashion, the term 'male menopause' has become popular precisely at the moment when *men* are beginning to experience the pressures of a culture which places a high value on physical appearance and the sexual expression associated with it. The history of the male climacteric reflects an increasing preoccupation in contemporary society with appearance and sexuality during midlife, when for the first time the outward and visible signs of the aging process become visible.

In the second paper **Zauner** dealt with the changes in the parameters of physical fitness in aging men. He showed that from the age of 20 on, there is a continuing decrease in fitness parameters, such as forced ventilatory capacity, peak expiratory flow, maximum oxygen consumption, maximal heart rate and the like. Blood pressure, on the other hand increases with age, a consequence of increased vascular resistance. It appears, however, that the major factor in this decline is being sedentary, and that in physically trained elderly males the fitness parameters do *not* show much difference relative to younger subjects. Fifty-six middle-aged male joggers ($\bar{x}$ age = 43.3 years) were studied by Zauner; 38 were measured for maximal oxygen uptake ($\dot{V}O_{2max}$) and 18 for cardiac output at a heart rate of 170 bpm ($\dot{Q}170$). Each $\dot{Q}170$ was divided by subject body surface area to yield cardiac index ($CI170$). A treadmill protocol was used to elicit maximal exercise during measurement of $\dot{V}O_{2max}$. The bicycle ergometer was employed when measuring $\dot{Q}170$. In subjects measured for $\dot{V}O_{2max}$, heart rate at 3.5 mph and 5% treadmill grade (HR_{submax}) as well as heart rate at maximal exercise (HR_{max}) were noted. Data were grouped according to age (43 years and older; 42 years and younger). There were significant ($p < 0.05$) positive relationships between $\dot{V}O_{2max}$ and HR_{max} and between HR_{submax} and age. Significant negative relationships existed between HR_{max} and HR_{submax}, and between $CI170$ and 10 km running time. There were no significant differences ($p > 0.05$) between means achieved by the age groups. These findings suggest that men who remain physically active retain youthful characteristics of cardiorespiratory function. So it seems that the larger part of the age-related decline could be prevented by adequate physical training.

Nankin next discussed fertility in the aging male. The picture he described is a complex one: on the one hand aging is characterized by decrease in testicular volume, in number of tubules, in sperm production and in the number of tubules with normal sperm. It seems moreover that target tissues may become *less sensitive to androgens*. On the other hand, although there is no doubt that fertility decreases progressively with age, the sperm count in the ejaculate appears to increase with age and, albeit the percentage of motile sperm is decreased, if an elderly man has motile spermatozoa, he probably is *fertile*.

Davidson discussed the relation between hormones and sexuality. He showed that in *hypogonadal* males, testosterone decreases the frequency of hot flushes, illustrating the role of the androgens in this phenomenon. In elderly males, frequency of orgasm and morning erections decrease but frequency of sexual thoughts and enjoyment, in other words libido, is much less affected. It appears that in the aging male there is a much sharper decline in physical sexual processes (such as erection and orgasm), than in mental processes. The response to sexual stimuli such as erotic films remains normal in hypogonadal or castrate men, though the frequency of spontaneous erections is increased. The rate of response to sexual stimuli is, however, much lower in the elderly. There appears to exist a correlation between sexuality and plasma sex hormone levels in aging men, but the correlation is weak. The data cannot be explained simply by decreased androgen sensitivity of the tissues, because of the qualitative differences between sexual effects of aging and hypogonadism. As to results of hormonal treatment in male *hypogonads*, testosterone treatment improves undoubtedly sexual function, erection and orgasm, but few reliable data concerning its effects in *elderly* males are available.

Vermeulen discussed testicular endocrine function in elderly males. Recently several authors have questioned the previously generally accepted view that free plasma testosterone levels, that is the concentration of androgens available to target tissues, decrease in old age. They suggest the reported apparent decline to be a consequence of a bias in the selection of elderly subjects, the latter being often ambulatory consultants to geriatric outpatient clinics, often affected by minor illness, or living in homes for the elderly.

Vermeulen reported the results of a study in a carefully selected population of normal healthy males living under identical environmental conditions, namely monks living in a monastery; he observed a clearcut age-associated decrease in either total or free testosterone, resulting in a decrease of the T/E_2 ratio and an increase in plasma gonadotropin levels. Extension of this study to 300 normal males of all social classes and education level living in a semi-rural suburb of a middle-sized industrial town confirmed these results.

It appeared, however, that nycthemeral variations in elderly males are less pronounced than in younger men, and hence the age-associated decrease in plasma T levels is less apparent in the late afternoon. As to environmental factors affecting T levels, smokers of any age appear to have higher T levels than non-smokers, but diet, moderate physical activity, or type of residence does not affect T levels.

Vermeulen observed, moreover, that elderly subjects are less sensitive to stress as far as their pituitary-gonadal axis is concerned, as their T levels do not vary during hypoglycemia or the stress of myocardial infarction, whereas in younger males, these stress factors do decrease T levels significantly! These findings explain, at least in part, the conflicting data in the literature on influence of age on plasma T levels, another factor being adequate representation of the elderly males in many studies.

The workshop was very stimulating. Further research will have to elucidate the biochemical substrate of the decreased sensitivity of tissues to androgens, as eluded to by several speakers, the neurohormonal basis for the change in the feedback setpoint of gonadotropin secretion, the influence of androgen substitution or other therapy on sexual behavior of the aging male.

We do hope that in 3 years from now, at the next congress, many of these questions will have found their final answer!

FURTHER READING

Bruce, R. A. (1984). Exercise, functional aerobic capacity and aging – another viewpoint. *Med. Sci. Sports Exerc.*, **16**, 8–13

Davidson, J. M., Chen, J. J., Craps, L., Gray, G. D., Greenleaf, W. J. and Catania, J. A. (1983). Hormonal changes and sexual function in aging men. *J. Clin. Endocrinol. Metab.*, **57**, 71–7

Deslypere, J. P. and Vermeulen, A. (1984). Leydig cell function in normal men; effect of age, lifestyle, residence, diet and activity. *J. Clin. Endocrinol. Metab.*, **59**, 955–61

Harman, S. M. and Nankin, H. R. (1985). Alterations in reproductive and sexual function: male. In Andres, R., Bierman, E. L. and Hazzard, W. R. (eds.) *Principles of Geriatric Medicine*. pp. 337–53. (New York: McGraw-Hill)

Hayflick, L. (1979). Cell biology of aging. *Fed. Proc.*, **38**, 1847–50

Hepworth, M. and Featherstone, M. (1982). *Surviving Middle Age*. (Oxford: Blackwell)

Johnson, L., Petty, C. S. and Neaves, W. B. (1984). Influence of age on sperm production and testicular weights in men. *J. Reprod. Fertil.*, **70**, 211–18

Kwan, M., Greenleaf, W. J., Mann, J., Craps, L. and Davidson, M. (1983). The nature of androgen action on male sexuality. *J. Clin. Endocrinol. Metab.*, **57**, 557–62

Lakatta, E. G. (1979). Alterations in the cardiovascular system that occur in advanced age. *Fed. Proc.*, **38**, 163–7

MacLeod, J. and Gold, R. Z. (1953). The male factor in fertility and infertility: VII. Semen quality in relation to age and sexual activity. *Fertil. Steril.*, **4**, 194–207

Mineau, G. P. and Trussel, J. (1982). A specification of marital fertility by parents' age, age at marriage and marital duration. *Demography*, **19**, 335–49

Nieschlag, E., Lammers, U., Freischem, C. W., Langer, K. and Wickings, E. J. (1982). Reproductive functions in young fathers and grandfathers. *J. Clin. Endocrinol. Metab.*, **55**, 676–81

Vogel, R. B., Books, C. A., Ketchum, C., Zauner, C. W. and Murray, F. T. (1985). Increase of free and total testosterone during submaximal exercise in normal males. *Med. Sci. Sports Exerc.*, **17**, 119–23

Zauner, C. W. and Benson, N. Y. (1981). *Give Us This Day Our Daily Run*. (Ithaca, NY: Mouvement Publications)

Workshop 3

Lifestyles; coping with life events and stress at the climacteric

Chairman: L. Severne (Belgium)
Co-chairman: J. G. Greene (Scotland)

J. Resnick (USA)
A. Holte (Norway)
J. G. Greene (Scotland)
S. Ballinger (Australia)
C. S. Berkun (USA)
E. Olbrich (West Germany)

For many years a medical model of the climacteric prevailed. Wilson, followed by many others, saw the menopause as a 'deficiency disease', for which hormone replacement therapy (HRT) was *the* cure, as well as the best recipe for everlasting 'femininity'[1].

However, anthropological and sociological evidence called for a broader view of the life situation and complaints of climacteric women, revealing a vast variety of experiences at this stage of life. Obviously, a whole range of external and internal factors were playing a very important role in the etiology of many climacteric symptoms. This led to a reassessment of the 'true' menopausal complaints, i.e. those directly associated with estrogen deprivation and reaction to HRT: hot flushes, perspiration, vaginal dryness and dyspareunia[2].

Other symptoms came to be considered as the consequence of interacting social, cognitive, emotional and physiological factors: it was imperative to obtain a better insight into these factors and the intricate way they operate. This is what an ever-increasing body of scientific research has attempted to do in the past 10–15 years. The contributions to the workshop 'Coping with life events and stress in the climacteric' show to what extent the instruments to do this have improved. The use of non-clinical populations, of control groups, of more sensitive tests, of new statistical methods and of course of computers, are of paramount importance in sorting out the complex factors interplaying at midlife and in finding answers to important questions such as:

(1) Are climacteric women effectively confronted with an increase of significant life events and changes at midlife? If so which events are more stressful and under which conditions?
(2) Are women at greater risk to suffer from stress at the climacteric? Can this eventually be related to the premenopausal, perimenopausal or postmenopausal complaints?
(3) Can predisposing factors – or protective factors – for increased vulnerability at the climacteric be recognized?
(4) If one can identify the women at risk, what are the implications for a better management of the climacteric phase?

The participants of this workshop emphasized from the start how important it is to differentiate better between the *incidence* of life events – be it the menopause or a change in other areas – and the *perception* of the change and the distress caused by these events. Stress was seen as a function of life events in the present or past, which reflect change, be it welcomed or undesirable, expected or unexpected, sudden or extended over a long period.

The middle years and the climacteric are a time of social as well as physiological change, requiring psychological adjustment. To investigate to what extent this change can be associated with a higher level of stress. Resnick et al.[3] examined self-report measures of stress and significant life events in a cross-sectional study of biological and psychological adaptation of women to aging. The design of the study, which was conducted over a 3-year period with a sample of 145 Caucasian healthy women (volunteers aged between 36 and 76 years), permitted comparisons across chronological age and hormonal status groups[4].

The results did not show any significant relationship between the total stress scores (which were obtained on a modified Holmes and Rahe Social Adjustment Rating Scale[5]) and the biological or chronological age (Table W3.1). In a factor analysis, stress proved to be independent of the factors functional age/climacteric status and psychological adjustment. In view of the limitation introduced by preselected categories and weights in the rating scale, three open-ended questions were added regarding the happiest, the saddest and the most important times or personal events occurring during the year. Menopause was mentioned by none of the women as a significant change. The frequent comments relating to children, rarely referred to children leaving home. Work-related and

Table W3.1 Means and standard deviations of stress scores by age groups

Source		Age groups				
		Menstruating		Non-menstruating		
		36–45	46–55	46–55	56–65	66–75
Total stress	M	235.6	199.5	224.7	248.8	193.2
	SD	115.5	82.9	93.6	148.4	97.6
Marital status	M	13.8	2.5	6.1	9.8	3.7
	SD	38.0	13.6	18.8	26.6	19.2
Family	M	50.5	81.2	64.2	76.2	76.9
	SD	41.8	53.1	38.9	63.7	45.8
Work	M	48.3	23.8	36.9	37.3	11.7[a]
	SD	48.8	27.1	43.4	59.8	25.0
Personal	M	84.8	58.8	80.4	92.2	82.8
	SD	65.0	34.8	54.8	54.7	57.2
Money	M	34.7	28.6	36.7	30.4	17.7[b]
	SD	25.7	22.5	25.9	25.7	17.5

[a] Spearman non-parametric correlation with age: $r = -0.29$, $p < 0.004$.
[b] Spearman non-parametric correlation with age: $r = -0.25$, $p < 0.002$.
From ref. 4

Table W3.2 Sources of significant life events and sample excerpts

Source category	Type of event	Sample excerpt
Interpersonal	Happiest	Seeing my grandchildren
	Saddest	Would like my relationship with my hunsband to be different
	Most important	Having the family home and happy together at Christmas
Intrapersonal	Happiest	Winning teacher of the year at my school
	Saddest	When I was conflicted about leaving my husband for a while because of a better job in another community
	Most important	Choosing to return to the work force and having the guts to do it
Health	Happiest	My husband's recovery from surgery
	Saddest	Spent time with my brother who has cancer
	Most important	My husband's heart attack caused us to think and change our lives a bit
Death	Happiest	(Not mentioned)
	Saddest	The recent death of my mother
	Most important	The death of my father – now both my parents are gone
Vacation	Happiest	Enjoyed my vacation – getting away, feeling free, and returning refreshed
	Saddest	(Not mentioned)
	Most important	Taking a month's trip north in our camper

From ref. 4

other 'mastery' experiences were often brought up as important life events, especially by the younger women. Not surprisingly, illness and death often came up as the saddest of life events, but no significant differences were found in life events in relation to age or menstrual status (Table W3.2).

Essentially, then, the results for this particular population do not point to a higher level of stress at any age. However, the panel agreed that the experience of the climacteric is very heterogeneous, needing a differential approach in which mediating or modifying social and psychological processes must be taken into account.

For **Olbrich**, these processes are to be seen in a biographical perspective. Our experience depends on the cognitive appraisal of an event (which is in part culturally determined) and on coping styles developed through life. Work by Lehr[6,7] in Germany, revealed marked differences in outlook, opinions, and coping styles in cross-sectional groups of premenopausal and postmenopausal women, the latter appearing to have developed a stronger sense of self-reliance and more satisfaction with their life.

Pursuing this line of investigation, Olbrich, Wohlfart and Hedrich explored in a small homogeneous group of women teachers (mean age 50.6), the impact of a set of life events on their lifestyles and coping skills. Using semi-structured biographical series of interviews they found that normative events – i.e. expected events occurring 'on time', such as becoming a grandparent at middle age – were considered as of little significance and dealt with effectively. In particular, the menopause was a time of trouble only for a minority: most women had thought about it before, had shared information and did not view it as a starting point in aging.

On the other hand, non-normative events were very frequently experienced as dramatic and frightening, especially when implying sudden loss such as death in the family or loss of work. In such cases little or no anticipatory coping was possible. It was necessary to develop new attitudes and new emotional or palliative processes, a situation which was often felt as ambiguous and possibly threatening.

The coping style will reflect the nature of the life event. For non-normative events, reflexive–cognitive behavior was frequently encountered: get all possible information concerning the event; understand its causes and effects and adapt own behavior rather than try to change the situation. On the contrary, in the case of more foreseeable events, problem-focused and active styles of coping emerged, aiming rather at changing the environment.

Of particular interest was the influence of historical and social events on the attitudes of these German women. This generation had experienced many hardships during and after the Second World War and, through adversity, had developed coping skills which gave them self-confidence and enhanced their capacities, also in looking for new solutions. In general, the less traditionally oriented women, professionally active, who had female friends and were relatively autonomous, proved to cope best in the climacteric.

The influence of less traditional – or rather quite untraditional life styles – also appears in a preliminary study by **Berkun**, comparing heterosexual and homosexual women. In the two groups the perceptions of aging and of attractiveness, and of course the relationship with men, differed widely.

The lesbians were more comfortable with their aging bodies; not being preoccupied with male relationships, they did not feel obliged to live up to certain standards of attractiveness, and consequently felt no guilt at not being able to do so. They did not expect their bodies to feel the same way all the time; changes – such as the menopause – were not distressing when they were understood as normal and were expected[8, 9].

Having come to terms with being 'different' – often in a lonely and painful way – they have learned to rely on themselves and were living lifestyles they had designed. This also reflects feelings of mastery and strength in coping: they have worked themselves out of trouble and know 'I can do it again'. Thus, certain personality, cognitive and experiential traits have a predictive value for effective coping at the climacteric.

The tendency of a person to react to stresses in a consistent repeated way, independent of their origin, is seen by **Holte** as '*psycho-biological response specificity*'. His hypothesis is that past menstrual coping style may be predictive of later climacteric coping style. In a large prospective longitudinal study, known as the Norwegian Female Climacteric Project, Holte and Mikkelsen examined the relationships between certain psychosocial factors, response to menstruation in earlier life and current climacteric symptoms[10].

Factor analysis yielded four symptom-patterns factors: mood lability, vague somatic symptoms, vasomotor symptoms and urinary problems. Only the vasomotor symptoms (flushes, perspiration and vaginal dryness) were found to be related to menopausal status, although they were not widely distributed in this population of women. These symptoms were found to appear most frequently 3–12 months and 2–5 years after the menopause.

An interesting finding was the relation between the amount of current cigarette smoking and a higher frequency of vasomotor symptoms. Multiple regression analysis showed further that the remaining factors: mood lability, vague somatic symptoms and urinary problems, were not related to the biological changes of the menopause, but to the woman's earlier pre-established pattern of coping with the menstrual cycle. Explanatory variables were mainly feelings of depression and irritation at menstruation, expectations and perceptions of the change at menopause, the number of close female friends (i.e. the social network) but only a few social background variables[11].

So far, the studies presented in this report are all concerned with healthy women and showed results which seem to be in several respects contrary to those obtained with clinical populations, i.e. women consulting menopause clinics or other clinics. What then are the differences between women presenting themselves for medical treatment and those who do not?

Ballinger, in a very carefully designed study, tested the hypothesis that climacteric women asking for help, suffer from more psychosocial stress that those who do not consult. 123 postmenopausal patients (mean age 54.4) attending a menopause clinic were compared on a number of parameters with a control group of 164 postmenopausal women from the general population (mean age 55.1), matched on geographic and socioeconomic parameters.

Depression, anxiety and life events were assessed by the Hamilton Rating Scale for Depression[12] and Ballinger's Life Events Questionnaire for Middle Aged Women, based on a modified Tennant-Andrews scale[13]. Psychosocial stress was measured not only in terms of current life events, but also in terms of ongoing or long-term stress (such as living with an invalid parent or an alcoholic partner) by a stress/coping rating scale, based on clinical judgement. Symptoms and their frequency were assessed by open-ended questions at interviews as well as by a set of symptom scales. Multivariate analysis of variance and stepwise discriminant function analysis were performed to discover how symptoms, clinical stress measures and life events distinguished between the two groups.

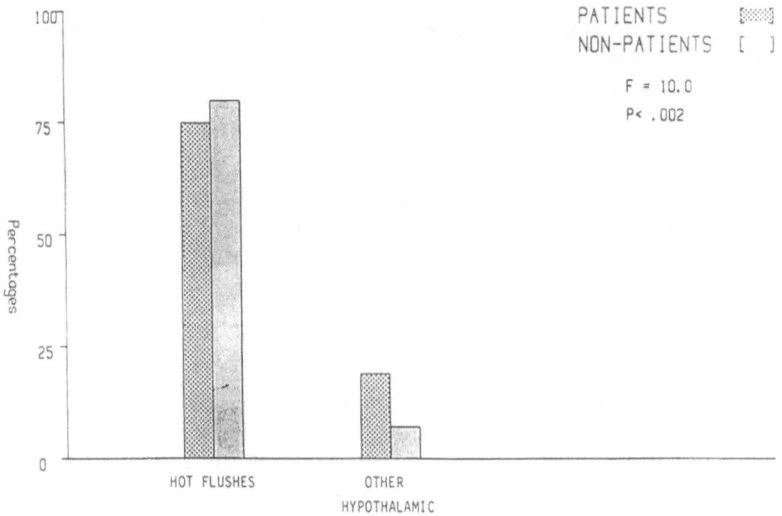

Figure W3.1 Hyperthalamic symptoms

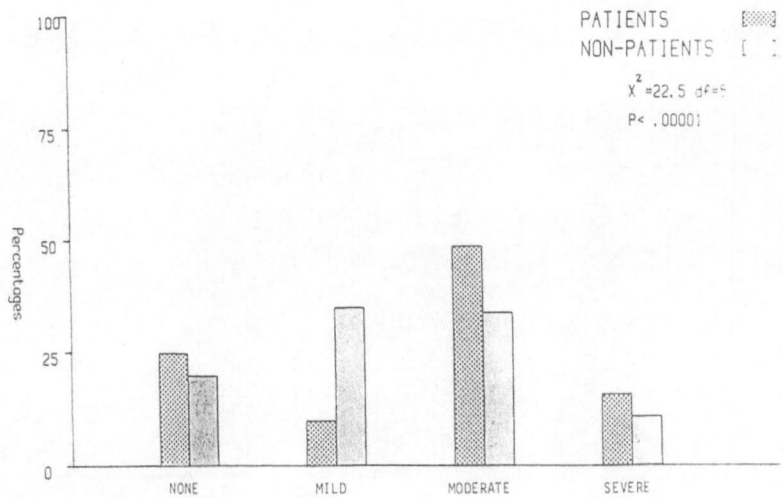

Figure W3.2 Hot flushes – severity

No significant difference was found between the 'patient' and 'non-patient' groups concerning the occurrence of the classic symptoms of the menopause – i.e. flushes and perspiration (70–80%) and vaginal atrophy (10%) (Fig. W3.1). However, in the 'patient' group, flushes were much more severe (Fig. W3.2) and there was a significantly higher incidence of psychological symptoms (Fig. W3.3). 'Patients' had not only higher scores on all clinical measurements of stress (Fig. W3.4) and a higher total number of life events too (Fig. W3.5), but they also perceived

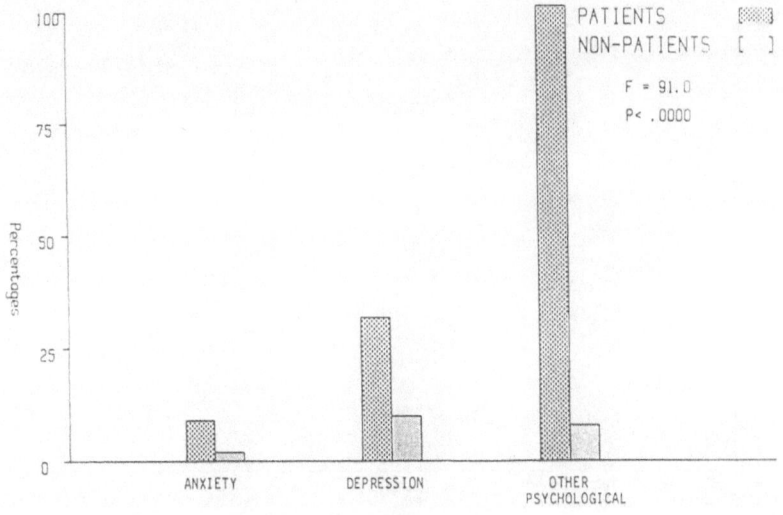

Figure W3.3 Psychological symptoms – self-reported

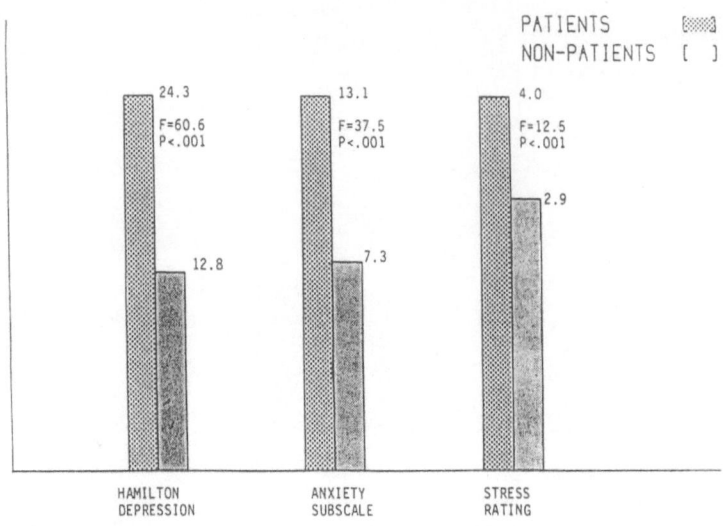

Figure W3.4 Clinical stress scores

their impact, i.e. the change these events caused in their lives and the distress they felt about them, as significantly greater. For example, in case of an extramarital affair, the reaction of a woman 'patient' could be 'I feel guilty' or 'frightened of being found out', and that of a non-patient 'it's marvellous'.

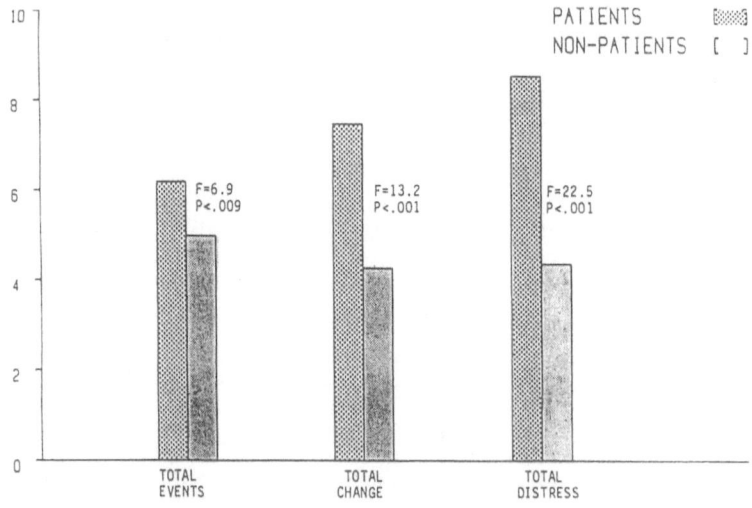

Figure W3.5 Life events between patients and non-patients

More specifically, Ballinger found few differences between the 'patient' and 'non-patient groups with respect to 'entrance' - and 'exit' events, involving people coming into, or leaving, the social field of a person (Table W3.3). However, the 'patients' reported significantly more undesirable events (such as a husband losing work). They seemed to cope less well in a period of heightened vulnerability and were more prone to enter into a vicious circle. Another finding was that significantly more of the patients suffered from depression prior to the climacteric.

Table W3.3 Analyses of variance comparing entrance and exit, desirable and undesirable events and impact between patients ($n = 88$) and non-patients ($n = 158$) with means and standard deviations

	Variate		Patients		Non-patients	
Events	$F^{1,244}$	$p<$	M	SD	M	SD
Entrance	0.1	N.S.	0.24	0.50	0.22	0.55
Exit	1.9	N.S.	0.64	0.97	0.49	0.68
Desirable	0.6	N.S.	1.0	0.86	1.1	0.93
Undesirable	10.2	0.002	1.8	2.0	1.1	1.4
Impact	25.4	0.001	2.3	1.1	1.6	1.1

These findings are consistent with many other more general studies on illness behavior, showing that people with more life stress report more symptoms (particularly psychological symptoms such as depression and anxiety), and are more likely to seek medical help[14-16]. They point to the necessity of considering the role of stress as well as hormonal factors in the etiology and severity of menopausal symptoms[17]. Moreover, consideration of stress factors should include not only the number and the impact of life events, but also personality differences - such as how women perceive these events - and coping style.

A significant contribution to the study of the relationship between life events and climacteric symptoms was made by **Greene**, based on the results of his survey among a general population of Scottish women aged 25–65 years[15]. In this study, once again only vasomotor symptoms proved to be directly associated with the perimenopause. The non-specific symptoms increased before the menopause, and life events scores also rose significantly in the early part of the climacteric. The increase in non-specific symptoms, both somatic and psychological, was shown by statistical analysis to be, at least in part, a response to a higher level of stress arising from life events, in which the perimenopause itself was not an important factor[18, 19].

Of particular interest was the subsequent finding that various types of life events have a differential effect on different types of symptoms[21].

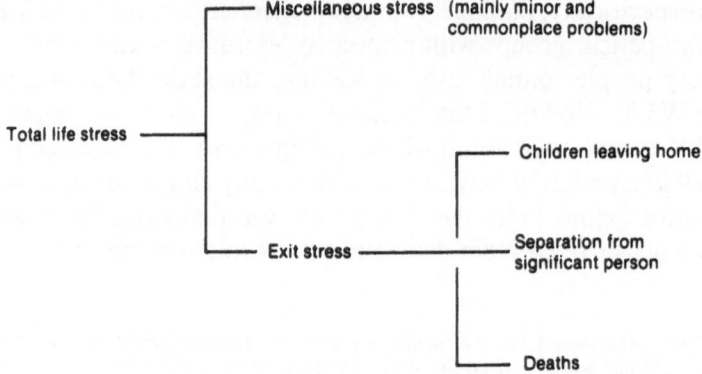

Figure W3.6 Schematic diagram of the main categories of life stress during the climacteric (from ref. 19)

Greene considered two main groups of life events as sources of stress scores in the various age groups of his sample: 'exits' (i.e. departures from the social field of a person) and 'miscellaneous events' (i.e. a mixed group of rather commonplace problems; work, financial minor illness, housing,

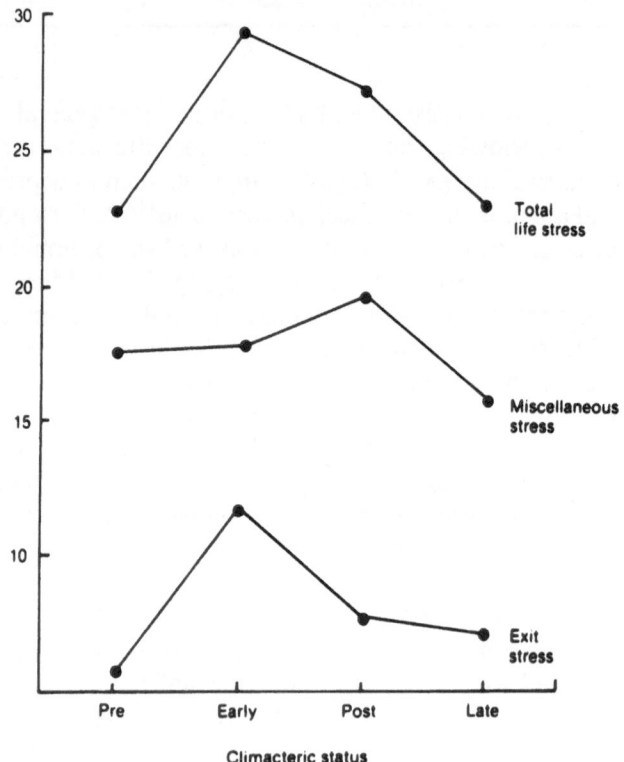

Figure W3.7 Mean scores for total life stress and its two main subcategories in relation to climacteric status (from ref. 21)

etc.) (Fig. W3.6). Analysis of the results showed that the significantly higher level of total life stress at the early climacteric was accounted for by stress from exits (Fig. W3.7). These were due to children leaving home, to separations and above all to deaths of a family member or other close persons. The latter accounted for some 60% of all exits amongst climacteric women, as opposed to only 10% in pre-climacteric women (Fig. W3.8).

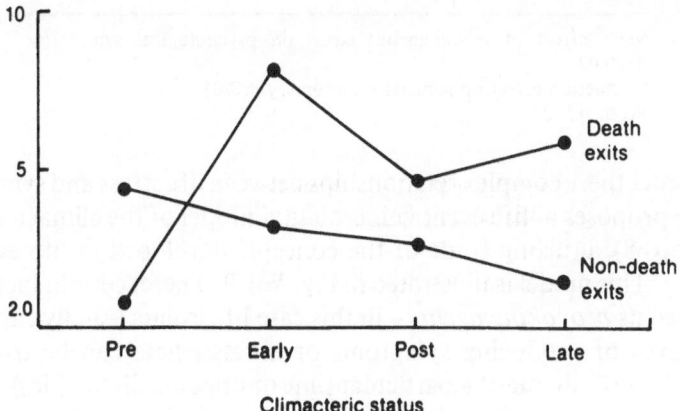

Figure W3.8 Mean stress scores for two subcategories of exits in relation to climacteric status (from ref. 22)

Miscellaneous stress remained fairly constant in the different age groups but climacteric women experiencing a high level of miscellaneous stress reported a higher degree of symptomatology than did preclimacteric women experiencing equally high levels of such stress. This effect was heightened in those climacteric women who had experienced a recent bereavement. In contrast, bereavement had no additional effect for women reporting low levels of miscellaneous stress. These results refer to total symptoms scores. When somatic and psychological symptoms were examined separately, significant differences appeared[22]. There was a direct relation with the level of miscellaneous stress only for psychological symptoms, which suggests the existence of a climacteric vulnerability to commonplace problems. Somatic symptoms, however, are affected only when a high level of miscellaneous stress is coupled with a death exit (Table W3.4). A tentative explanation for this somatization of stress is that the symptoms behavior is in some way linked to the health problem of the deceased. This effect may be enhanced in women who are already experiencing age- or hormone-related physical changes or discomfort. Since most of the deaths were of persons with whom the woman had a close, supportive relationship, the bereavement reactions of the women could have been aggravated by the consequent loss of the social and family support, needed to cope with their other current problems[23].

Table W3.4 Mean scores on the psychological and somatic symptom scales in relation to miscellaneous stress and deaths

	Miscellaneous stress			
Death	High	Low	High	Low
Yes	14.45	7.5	8.03	3.83
No	11.67	8.5	3.58	3.25
	(Psychological)		(Somatic)	

Main effect of miscellaneous stress on psychological symptoms, $p < 0.025$
Interaction effect on somatic symptoms, $p < 0.05$
From ref. 22

To order these complex relationships between life stress and symptoms, Greene proposes a 'life event vulnerability' model of the climacteric (ref. 19, chap. 8), utilizing some of the concepts developed in life event research[24]. This model is illustrated in Fig. W3.9. There, certain factors are classified as *provoking agents* – in this case life events usually capable in themselves of producing symptoms or illness (these can be traumatic happenings occurring at a particular time or ongoing difficulties). Others are classified as *vulnerability factors* which by definition do not have an effect in themselves but increase the risk of illness or the severity of symptoms but only in the presence of a provoking agent. Being climacteric is classified as a vulnerability factor since, as found in the study, life events provoke symptoms to a greater degree at that time of life than they do during the preclimacteric. A third set of factors included in this model are *symptom formation factors*, such as in this case the illness of the deceased person, which can influence the nature of the symptoms experienced or the form the stress reaction takes.

Many of the factors researched by other participants in this workshop can also be considered as vulnerability or symptom formation factors. These include low socioeconomic status (Severne), loss of social support through deaths of relatives (Greene and Resnick), previous menstrual

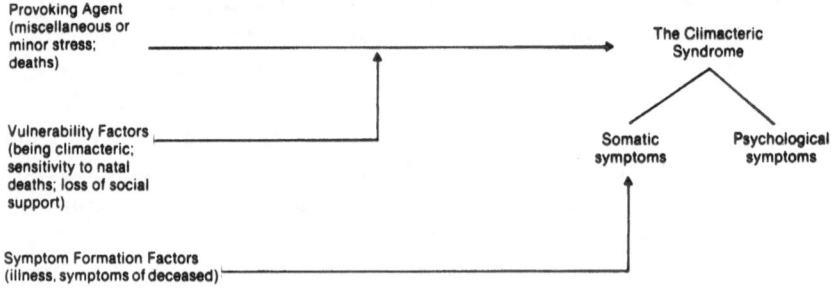

Figure W3.9 Schematic diagram of relationship between life events and climacteric symptoms (from ref. 19)

coping style (Holte), lack of self-confidence and of coping skills (Olbrich), event perception (Ballinger), over-strong traditional or dependent lifestyles, fear of aging and lack of control over life (Berkun).

In this model, therefore, vulnerability and symptom formation factors can be viewed as intervening variables which determine the severity and form of the woman's reactions to life stress during the climacteric.

In the general discussion, the workshop concluded on certain practical implications of the material presented.

(1) When confronted with climacteric complaints, other than the vasomotor symptoms directly linked to the menopause, the role of stress has to be assessed; the more so since the possibility of a vicious circle exists: stress produces symptoms, but the latter also produce or increase stress.

(2) The role of different types of stress on symptomatology was emphasized, more particularly that of stress resulting from bereavement. However, less dramatic events may also be the source of miscellaneous stress or of ongoing stress. They can play an important role, especially in concomitance with other stress factors.

(3) Predisposing factors – such as personality traits and earlier coping style – influence the perception and the experience of the menopause. Cognitive behavior modification therapy can be helpful for women experiencing a problematic climacteric, not only to help in acquiring a less negative perception of events felt as threatening, but also in enhancing coping capacities.

(4) Elementary prevention at the approach of midlife should comprise: individual information and de-briefing; advice on the use of available resources; ego-strengthening and counselling for a better handling of stress, for improving relationships, or for maintaining and extending the social network. The latter has been shown to be of particular importance and in this connection the rapid extension of self-help groups for climacteric women, is a very positive factor[20].

(5) Finally, rather than construing the climacteric as a deficiency disease, it should be seen as a life phase with its own possibilities for further development, but which for too many women remain as yet unexploited.

REFERENCES

1. Wilson, R. A. (1966). *Feminine Forever*. (New York: Mayflower-Dell)
2. Utian, W. H. and Serr, D. (1976). The climacteric syndrome. In Van Keep, P. A. *et al.* (eds.) *Consensus on Menopause Research*. pp. 1-4. (Lancaster: MTP Press)

3. Resnick, J. L., Dougherty, M. C. and Notelovitz, M. (1983). Stress measurement and aging in women. Paper presented in poster session at the meeting of the American Psychological Association, Anaheim, CA
4. Notelovitz, M., Dougherty, M. C., Resnick, J. L. and Cunningham, W. (1982). Psychological and biologic adaptation of women to aging: final report (Grant No. ROI AGOO 796). Washington, DC: National Institute on Aging
5. Holmes, T. H. and Rahe, R. H. (1967). The social readjustment rating scale. *J. Psychosom. Res.*, **11**, 213–18
6. Lehr, U. (1961). Veränderungen der Daseinsthematik der Frau im Erwachsenenalter. *Vita Humana*, **4**, 193–228
7. Lehr, U. (1977). Zur Problematik des Menschen im reifen Erwachsenenalter – eine sozialpsychologische Interpretation der 'Wechseljahre'. In Thomae, H. and Lehr, U. (eds.) *Altern: Probleme und Tatsachen.* pp. 227–34. (Frankfurt: Akademische Verlagsgesellschaft)
8. Berkun, C. S. (1983). Perceptions of changing appearance for women in the middle years of life: trauma? In Markson, E. (ed.) *Older Women.* (Lexington MA: Lexington Books)
9. LaTorre, R. and Wendenburg, K. (1983). Psychological characteristics of bisexual, heterosexual and homosexual women. *J. Homosexuality*, **9**(1), 87–97
10. Mikkelsen, A. and Holte, A. (1982). A factor-analytic study of climacteric symptoms. *Psychiatry Soc. Sci.*, **2**, 35–9
11. Holte, A. and Mikkelsen, A. (1982). Menstrual coping style, social background and climacteric symptoms. *Psychiatry Soc. Sci.*, **2**, 41–5
12. Hamilton, M. (1960). A rating scale for depression. *J. Neurol. Neurosurg. Psychiatry*, **23**, 56–62
13. Tennant, C. and Andrews, G. (1976). A scale to measure the stress of life events. *Austr. N.Z. J. Psychiatry*, **10**, 27–32
14. Ilfield, F. W. (1977). Current social stressors and symptoms of depression. *Am. J. Psychiatry*, **134**(2), 161–6
15. Greene, J. G. and Cooke, D. J. (1982). Psychosocial factors in women during the climacterium: a community study. In Main, C. J. (ed.) *Clinical Psychology and Medicine.* pp. 131–52. (New York: Plenum)
16. Craig, T. J. and Van Natta, P. A. (1983). Disability and depressive symptoms in two communities. *Am. J. Psychiatry*, **140**(5), 598–601
17. Coulam, C. B. (1981). Age, estrogens and the psyche. *Clin. Obstet. Gynaecol.*, **1**, 219–29
18. Greene, J. G. and Cooke, D. J. (1980). Life stress and symptoms at the climacteric. *Br. J. Psychiatry*, **136**, 486–91
19. Greene, J. G. (1984). *The Social and Psychological Origins of the Climacteric Syndrome.* (Aldershot UK and Brookfield USA: Gower)
20. Severne, L. (1984). The view of the woman. In van Herandael, B. *et al.* (eds.) *The Climacteric an Update.* pp. 19–29. (Lancaster: MTP Press)
21. Cooke, D. J. and Greene, J. G. (1981). Types of life events in relation to symptoms at the climacteric. *J. Psychosom. Res.*, **25**, 5–11
22. Greene, J. G. (1983). Bereavement and social support at the climacteric. *Maturitas*, **5**, 115–24
23. Miller, P., Ingham, J. G. and Davidson, S. (1976). Life events, symptoms and social support. *J. Psychosom. Res.*, **20**, 515–22
24. Brown, G. W. and Harris, T. (1978). *The Social Origins of Depression: a study of psychiatric disorder in women.* (London: Tavistock)

FURTHER READING

Ballinger, S. E. (1981). A comparison of possible effects of acute and chronic stresses on post-menopausal urinary oestrogen levels. *Maturitas*, **3**, 107–13
Ballinger, S. E. and Cobbin, D. (1981). Biochemical correlates of depression in the post-menopause. In Sheppard, J. L. (ed.) *Advances in Behavioural Medicine*, vol. 1, pp. 45–56

Black, S. M. and Hill, C. E. (1984). The psychological well-being of women in their middle years. *Psychol. Women Q.*, Spring, pp. 282–93

Channon, L. D. C. and Ballinger, S. E. (1982). Women as therapists: a menopause clinic. *Bull. Br. Psychol. Soc.*, **35**, 236–7

Rich, A. (1980). Compulsory heterosexuality and the lesbian experience. *Signs*, **5**(1), 631–60

Workshop 4

Genital tract and other target tissues

Chairman: **S. Campbell** (UK)
Co-chairman: **J. Semmens** (USA)

R. Goswamy (UK)
M. Whitehead (UK)
J. Studd (UK)
L. Cardozo (UK)

Goswamy presented a major prospective study of the peri- and post-menopausal ovary as studied by ultrasound. Patients were more than 45 years old, unselected, and were typical of the United Kingdom mature female population. The object of the study was to determine:

(1) if ultrasound screening could detect ovarian cancer in Stage I which has a 90% 5-year survival as opposed to Stage III which is the usual stage of diagnosis and which has a 14% 5-year survival;
(2) if yearly scanning was the correct time interval for this new screening test;
(3) if identification and removal of tumors with a potential for malignancy such as serous cystadenomas would reduce the incidence of ovarian carcinoma.

The study is now in its second year. Over 5500 women over 45 have been recruited, and these women will be scanned yearly for at least 5 years. At the end of this time we would expect 15 cancers hopefully all diagnosed in Stage I. The number of cancers may be less due to the removal of ovarian neoplasms with a potential for malignancy. The findings so far are:

(1) About 4% of peri- and postmenopausal women have a morphologically atypical ovary on the first scan or an ovarian volume more than 2 standard deviations greater than the normal range. The incidence in subsequent years is 1% per annum.

(2) The vast majority of such tumors cannot be detected clinically.

(3) Ultrasound cannot distinguish which tumors are innocent and which are malignant – the definitive diagnosis as with cervical screening has to be made by biopsy.

(4) Ultrasound screening can detect Stage I cancers: five Stage I cancers have been detected so far, three primary and two secondary. There have been no advanced cancers and no missed cancers.

(5) It is too early to say whether yearly intervals are correct but a hopeful sign is that two of the cancers were detected in the second year of scanning, normal ovaries having been found in the first year

This brief summary cannot do justice to a unique study of major importance. One interesting snippet: in the normal population, ovarian volume was found to have a negative correlation with menopausal age but a positive correlation with patients on hormonal therapy.

Studd made a plea to Americans to stop using the word 'flash' (which was incorrect) as opposed to 'flush', which was logical and etymologically correct.

He described a new technique called thermal entrainment which uses a photoplethysmograph on the finger to measure fluctuations in blood flow. As this only measures to a depth of 3 mm he assumes that the blood flow changes come from the dermal microcapillaries. The premenopausal woman shows fine oscillations in blood flow which do not change with external stimuli, such as heat or cold. All premenopausal women show a loss of fine vascular control following a hot or cold stimulus with wide swings of flow, but estrogen therapy restores control to that of the premenopausal state. The message is that all postmenopausal women lose the fine control of their skin microcirculation and that a flush is merely an extension to a total loss of vascular control. Most women can eventually adapt to these changes which is why flushes are self-limiting.

Dr Studd's other theme concerned measurement of skin thickness by an adaptation of a soft tissue mammography technique. He and his team have shown:

(1) Skin thickness can be simply and cheaply measured by this method.

(2) If initial skin thickness is low then significant increases can result from estrogen therapy. Skin thickness is inversely related to menopausal age.

(3) Forearm skin thickness is highly significantly related to thigh collagen content.

(4) There is a significant correlation between skin thickness/collagen content and the metacarpal index.

Dr Studd and his team have demonstrated mathematically that there is a relationship between skin and bone collagen and believe that by measuring skin thickness an index of bone collagen content can be derived. This is of great significance especially as evidence was produced suggesting the primary defect in postmenopausal osteoporosis may be the loss of collagen bone matrix and not of minerals. Clearly the anxiety is that just as CT-scan studies have shown regional variation in bone mineral content, so there may be similar regional changes in tissue collagen content. If this is not true and skin thickness measurements represent the status of collagen throughout the body, an important new cheap screening technique for bone collagen status will be readily available. If bone mass at the start of the menopause is an important factor in determining which woman will get osteoporosis, then screening for skin thickness may also become an important part of this assessment.

Cardozo made a plea for proper urodynamic evaluation of women with urinary symptoms. These studies include the 60 min pad test, uroflowmetry, cystometry and urethral pressure profile (UPP) studies. Clinical evaluation cannot reliably distinguish between genuine stress incontinence (GSI), destrusor instability (DI) and urethral instability (UI). The last two conditions are not cured by surgery and indeed are likely to be made worse by this treatment.

The postmenopausal woman has an increased incidence of urological symptoms. In the perimenopausal years GSI increases dramatically and in the late postmenopause (70+ years). DI is the major problem.

Dr Cardozo's studies show that 50% of postmenopausal women have an incompetent bladder neck and a shortened proximal urethra under stress. However the majority compensate by moving their maximal urethral closure pressure to the distal one-third of the urethra by use of their perineal muscles and thus maintain continence.

The importance of not performing bladder neck operations on women who complain of incontinence just because they have an incompetent bladder neck was stressed. The incontinence may be due to DI or UI, and operation would be inappropriate.

Dr Cardozo found that 7% of postmenopausal women have the condition called UI with fluctuations of urethral pressure >25 cmH$_2$O. This may cause incontinence on stress. If not properly diagnosed by UPP studies surgery may be undertaken inappropriately.

Finally, Dr Cardozo addressed the question as to whether estrogen therapy can help stress incontinence. She found that in those patients who had moved their urethral closing pressure distally, their skin collagen was low. She asked the question: could bladder neck competence be collagen/elastic fiber in origin and could it be that estrogen therapy would not only increase (skin) collagen in patients with low starting levels but the collagen of the bladder neck as well? In other words, skin thickness measurements may define a group of GSI patients that would respond to estrogen therapy. This important question will be answered in the next conference.

Whitehead described the development of our current belief that postmenopausal women on estrogen therapy require 12 days of progestin each month to protect fully the endometrium against the development of adenomatous hyperplasia and carcinoma. The addition of a high dose of progestin for 12 days each month caused anxiety among many clinicians in view of the well-known side-effect of progestins on HDL cholesterol and the potential adverse effect on arterial disease and symptomatology.

He then described studies on the endometrium which were performed in collaboration with Roger King which will profoundly change the pattern of postmenopausal therapy. These studies on endometrial ultra-structure, DNA synthesis, receptor machinery and enzymatic activity have demonstrated that the dosage of progestin currently available for addition to postmenopausal estrogen therapy is grossly in excess of that required to suppress mitotic activity. For example, an endometrium primed with Premarin® 0.625 mg requires only 0.7 mg of norethisterone (norethindrone) or $150 \mu g$ of dl norgestrel for protection – dosages that are 3–7 times less than currently prescribed. This will hopefully permit therapeutic regimens that will suppress mitotic activity but not disturb lipid metabolism or cause significant symptomatology. There is already evidence that this is the case.

These sophisticated endometrial studies will hopefully identify a continuous/combined regimen that will have a good antimitotic effect without induction of enzymatic activity and secretory change. In this way perhaps even smaller dosages of progestin may be given with total suppression of mitotic activity, no bleeding, no adverse symptomatology and no lipid changes.

Another approach presented by Dr Whitehead is the 'all natural' oral therapy – natural estrogen and natural progesterone, which, at a 300 mg dosage, has a good antimitotic effect and apparently no adverse lipid changes.

The perfect safe therapeutic regimen for the postmenopausal woman does not seem to be far off.

FURTHER READING

Goswamy, R. K., Campbell, S. and Whitehead, M. I. (1983). Screening for ovarian cancer. *Clin. Obstet. Gynecol.*, **10**, 621–43

Moyle, J. W., Rochester, D., Sider, L., Shrock, K. and Krause, P. (1983). Sonography of ovarian tumors: predictability of tumor type. *Am. J. Rad.*, **141**, 985–91

Ostergard, D. R. (ed.) (1985). *Gynecologic Urology of Urodynamics: theory and practice*, 2nd edn. (Baltimore and London: Williams & Wilkins)

Workshop 5

Hormones and metabolism

Chairman: **G. Samsioe** (Sweden)
Co-chairman: **V. Upton** (USA)

G. Samsioe (Sweden)
G. Silfverstolpe (Sweden)
M. Notelovitz (USA)
J. Mehta (USA)
A. Basdevant (France)

The topic of this workshop was to sum up some areas of special interest regarding hormones and metabolism.

When considering the epidemiological background of the problem – hormonal replacement therapy and cardiovascular disease **Silfverstolpe** noted it is essential to be aware that according to several epidemiologists[1,2], a spontaneous menopause at the normal time *per se* does not imply an increased risk for cardiovascular disease. On the other hand it is no longer controversial that an association exists between a premature menopause and an increased risk for cardiovascular disease.

Because of the high incidence of cardiovascular disease in the age categories given hormonal replacement therapy (HRT) in the climacteric period, a very modest increase in the relative risk for cardiovascular disease under therapy would result in an unacceptable number of cases attributable to the drug therapy. As the incidence of myocardial infarction among women 50–55 years old is in the order of 100 per 100 000 women per year a relative risk of 1.4 would give 40 cases of myocardial infarction per 100 000 women per year attributable to the drug therapy. Such a small increase in the relative risk (1.4) under a drug therapy is investigatively almost impossible to reveal.

The information available about hormonal replacement therapy and cardiovascular disease is very scarce compared to what we know about oral contraception and its effect in this context. The limited number of studies undertaken does not, however (with few exceptions), reveal either an increased or a decreased relative risk for cardiovascular disease when women are given exogenous estrogens as HRT. Most women on HRT are presently given a progestogen along with their estrogen. This might imply a completely new situation as regards HRT and cardiovascular disease. From the experience with oral contraception (OC) we now know that progestogens are correlated to cardiovascular morbidity[3, 4.] To the best of my knowledge there are presently no studies available about the effects on cardiovascular morbidity and mortality from estrogen–progestogen combinations given postmenopausally.

Through delineation of the effects on the pathogenetic intermediary factors for cardiovascular disease should be carried out before new estrogen–progestogen regimens or new steroidal compounds are introduced into clinical practice as HRT. Estrogen–progestogen combinations or new steroidal compounds[5] which have clear and substantial adverse effects on these systems should not be accepted.

The concept of lipoprotein was further discussed by **Samsioe**, who described the complexity of this task. Indirect as well as direct effects exist and the latter can be subdivided into receptor-mediated and non-receptor-mediated ones. As all effects either parallel or oppose one another it is more or less impossible to predict the metabolic response by a hormone or by a hormonal combination. In addition, intra- as well as interindividual variations are great.

A crude schematic presentation would, however, suggest natural as well as synthetic estrogens to increase HDL possibly to decrease LDL and for ethinyl estradiol also usually an increase in VLDL. Progestins in many respects have opposite effects with a decrease in HDL concomitant with a small increase in LDL. This is most marked for progestins belonging to the 19-nortestosterone derivatives which, in addition to their anti-estrogenic properties, also carry clear-cut androgen qualities, which also reduce HDL and VLDL, possibly through stimulation of hepatic lipase.

Notelovitz reviewed the controversial topic of coagulation, noting that the formation of a blood clot involved the interaction of the factors in the coagulation cascade, the inhibitory blood clotting system incorporating anticoagulant factors such as antithrombin III, and fibrinolytic activity of plasminogen and plasmin antagonists such as α_2 antiplasmin. The least researched area is that of platelet activity: aberrations in this parameter are often responsible for triggering the coagulation cascade and for the synthesis of the procoagulant prostaglandin derivative – thromboxane A_2 – which causes increased platelet adhesiveness and vasospasm. This activity is counterbalanced by prostacyclin I_2 produced by the vascular intima; the vasodilatation and decrease in platelet adhesiveness

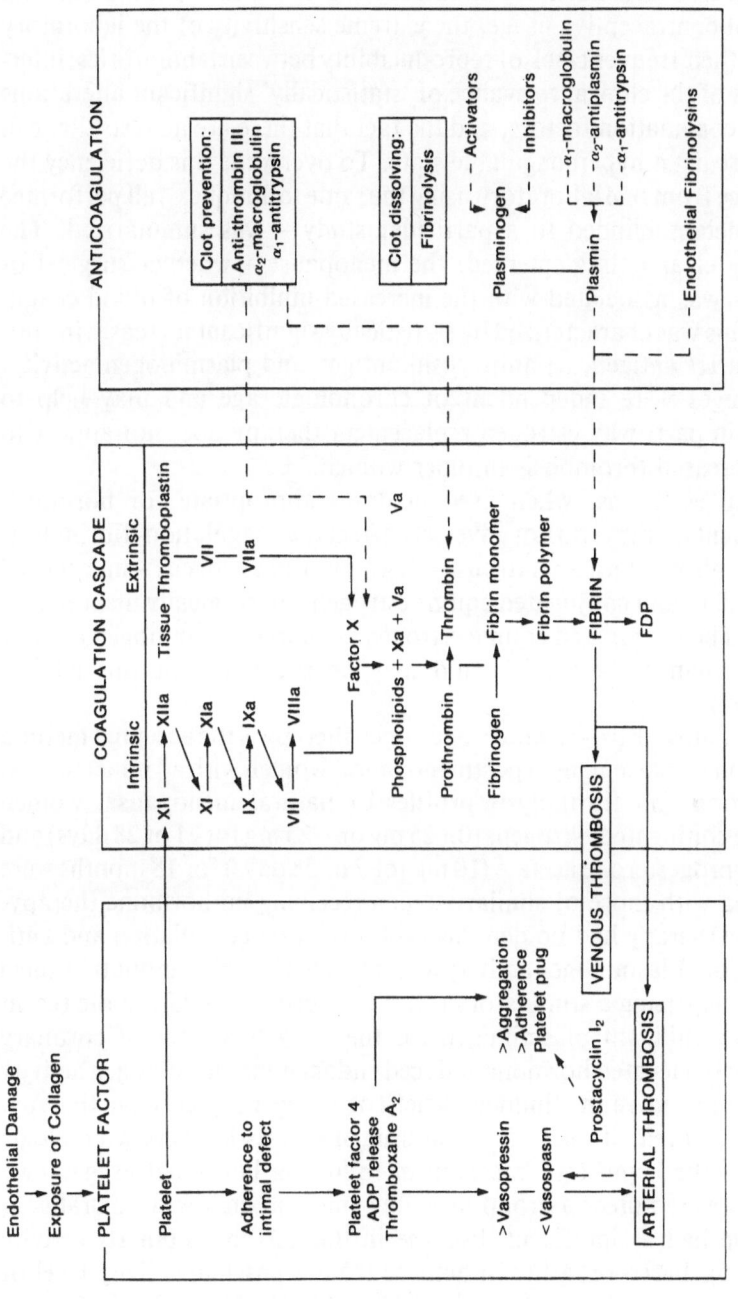

Figure W5.1 Integration of the platelet factor, coagulation cascade and anticoagulation mechanisms in the pathogenesis of arterial and venous thrombosis (from Notelovitz, M. (1985). Oral contraception and coagulation. *Clin. Obstet. Gynecol.*, **28**, 73–83)

induced by prostacyclin serves as a check to thromboxane overactivity (Fig. W5.1).

Part of the confusion in the literature is due to the extrapolation of data from oral contraceptive usage; the extreme sensitivity of the laboratory tests and their frequent lack of reproducibility between laboratories; interpretation of the clinical relevance of 'statistically' significant alterations in blood coagulation factors; and the fact that there are no tests that can indeed predict a hypercoagulable state. To overcome this deficiency the experience from one laboratory using the same techniques – all performed by technicians blinded to a particular study – was summarized. The following clear points emerged: the menopause – whether surgical or natural – was associated with the increased inhibition of blood coagulation. This was characterized by statistically significant increases in anti-thrombin III antigen, α_1-antitrypsin antigen and plasminogen activity. The changes were independent of chronologic age and may help to explain, in part, why estrogen replacement therapy does not appear to cause increased thrombosis in older women.

Natural estrogens, when used in doses appropriate for hormonal replacement therapy, do not adversely affect the coagulation–fibrinolysis system. This was based on the use of two natural estrogens – micronized 17β-estradiol and conjugated equine estrogen – in surgically menopausal women. The conjugated equine estrogen enhanced plasminogen activity more so than 17β-estradiol, and may be preferred for this clinical population.

Combination estrogen and progestogen therapy is the accepted method of hormone replacement in postmenopausal women with an intact uterus. Coagulation and fibrinolysis profiles of natural menopausal women receiving conjugated estrogens (0.625 mg or 1.25 mg for 21 of 28 days) and medroxyprogesterone acetate (10 mg for 7 of 28 days) for 18 months were compared with those of similar women receiving no hormone therapy. Hormone therapy had no demonstrable effect on coagulation and anti-coagulation. Plasminogen activity was enhanced in the hormone treatment groups, suggesting a stimulatory effect on fibrinolysis. Given the recent use of recombinant plasminogen for the early treatment of coronary thrombosis, elevated hormone-induced endogenous plasminogen activity may be a preventive and 'hidden' benefit of estrogen replacement therapy.

Finally, Notelovitz addressed the issue of a statistical versus a biologic change in the hemostatic mechanism following hormonal usage. Two examples were noted: a group of young smokers on low-dose oral contraceptive had a significant decrease in the anti-thrombin III activity ($p < 0.005$), based on a fall in activity from a baseline activity level of $104.3 \pm 2.0\%$ to a 6-month nadir of $97.3 \pm 2.2\%$. Normal values range from 80% to 100%; clot formation will only occur with values $< 50\%$ of normal. The biologic significance of this observation is therefore in doubt.

Another group of older premenopausal women (mean age 35) on the same low-dose oral contraceptive had a decrease in α_2-antiplasmin activity from $95.2 \pm 6.5\%$ of normal to a 6-month level of $73.2 \pm 4.8\%$. In this instance the value was below the reference range (80–120%) and thus likely to produce a biologic effect. Low levels of α_2-antiplasmin are associated with increased plasmin and hence fibrinolytic activity – a potential beneficial side-effect of low-dose oral contraceptives in pre-menopausal women using steroid contraception.

Notelovitz concluded by cautioning against the extrapolation of data based on short-term studies involving small numbers of women, using sex steroids for purposes unassociated with hormone replacement therapy, or in doses inappropriate for their intended use – symptomatic relief or osteoporosis prevention.

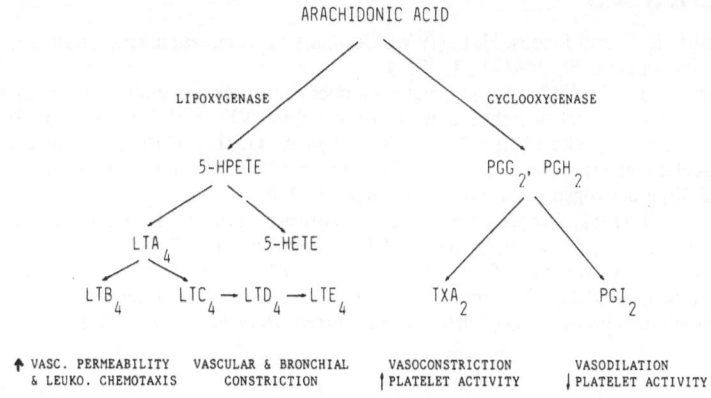

Figure W5.2

The fascinating field of prostaglandins was introduced by **Mehta**. Based on data mainly from animals it has been repeatedly reported that thromboxane A_2–prostaglandin I_2 balance is of importance in the regulation of the platelet homeostasis and maintenance of vascular tone (Fig. W5.2). This balance seems to be influenced by female gonadal hormones. However, some methodological problems exist and it is too early for a decisive opinion in this matter. Further information in large human series is highly warranted.

Basdevant described the differences between oral and parenteral administration of estrogens. He found that the liver response is more exaggerated by the oral route but emphasized that the explanation may not be as simple as bypass of the first liver passage. He stressed the influence on the hormonal balance in favor of estrone formation as part of the explanation (Fig. W5.3).

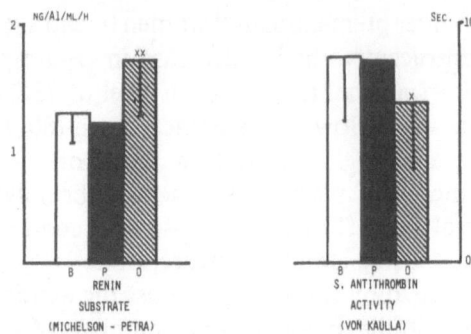

Figure W5.3 Renin substrate and serum antithrombin activity before (B) and following oral (O) and parenteral (P) estradiol replacement therapy

REFERENCES

1. Heller, R. F. and Jacobs, H. S. (1978). Coronary heart disease in relation to age, sex, and the menopause. *Br. Med. J.*, **1**, 472-4
2. Furman, R. H. (1968). Are gonadal hormones (estrogens and androgens) of significance in the development of ischemic heart disease? *Ann. NY Acad. Sci.*, **149**, 822-33
3. Meade, T. W., Greenberg, G. and Thompson, S. G. (1980). Progestogens and cardio-vascular reactions associated with oral contraceptives and a comparison of the safety of 50 and 30 μg oestrogen preparations. *Br. Med. J.*, **280**, 1157-61
4. Kay, C. R. (1982). Progestogens and arterial disease – evidence from the Royal College of General Practitioners' study. *Am. J. Obstet. Gynecol.*, **142**, 762-5
5. Crona, N., Silfverstolpe, G. and Samsioe, G. (1983). A double-blind cross-over study on the effects of ORG OD14 compared to oestradiol valerate and placebo on lipid and carbo-hydrate metabolism in oophorectomized women. *Acta Endocrinol.*, **102**, 451-5

FURTHER READING

Ali, M. B. and Williams, K. I. (1983). Influence of sex steroids on prostacyclin synthesis by rat aorta and myometrium. *Adv. Prost. Thromb. Leuk. Res.*, **12**, 437-41

Basdevant, A., de Lignieres, B. and Guy-Grand, B. (1983). Differential lipemic and hormonal responses to oral and parenteral 17β estradiol. *Am. J. Obstet. Gynecol.*, **147**(1), 77

Bygdeman, M. (1983). Endocrine effects of prostaglandins in fertility regulation. In Benagiano, G. and Diczfalusy, E. (eds.) *Endocrine Mechanisms in Fertility Regulation.* pp. 125-39. (New York: Raven Press)

Elekik, F., Gompel, A., Mercier Bodard, C., Kuttenn, F., Guyenne, P. N:, Corvol, P. and Mauvais-Jarvis, P. (1981). Effects of percutaneous estradiol and conjugated estrogens on the level of plasma proteins and triglycerides in post-menopausal women. *Am. J. Obstet. Gynecol.*, **143**, 888

Geola, F. L., Frumar, A. P. and Tartaryn, I. V. (1980). Biological effects of various doses of conjugated equine estrogens in post-menopausal women. *J. Clin. Endocrinol. Metab.*, **51**, 620

Lobo, R. A., March, C. M., Goebelsmann, U., Krauss, R. M. and Mishell, D. R. (1980). Subdermal estradiol pellets following hysterectomy and oophorectomy. *Am. J. Obstet. Gynecol.*, **138**, 714

Mammen, E. F. (1982). Oral contraceptives and blood coagulation: a critical review. *Am. J. Obstet. Gynecol.*, **142**, 781

Mandel, F. P., Geola, F. L., Meldrum, D. R., Lu, J. H. K., Eggena, P., Sambhi, M. P., Hershman, J. M. and Judd, H. L. (1983). Biological effects of various doses of vaginally administered conjugated equine estrogens in post-menopausal women. *J. Clin. Endocrinol. Metab.*, **57**, 133-9

Mehta, J. (1983). Prostaglandins: regulatory role in cardiovascular system. *Int. J. Cardiol.*, **4**, 249–59

Notelovitz, M., Kitchens, C., Rappaport, V. *et al.* (1981). Menopausal status associated with increased inhibition of blood coagulation. *Am. J. Obstet. Gynecol.*, **141**, 149–52

Notelovitz, M., Kitchens, C. and Ware, M. D. (1984). Coagulation and fibrinolysis in estrogen-treated surgical menopausal women. *Obstet. Gynecol.*, **63**, 621–5

Notelovitz, M., Kitchens, C., Ware, M. D. *et al.* (1983). Combination estrogen and progestogen replacement therapy does not adversely affect coagulation. *Obstet. Gynecol.*, **62**, 596–600

Notelovitz, M., Levenson, I., McKenzie, L. *et al.* (1985). The effect of low-dose oral contraceptives on coagulation and fibrinolysis in two high-risk populations: young female smokers and older premenopausal women. *Am. J. Obstet. Gynecol.*, **152**, 995–1000

Workshop 6

Technology and techniques

Chairman: **W. Utian** (USA)
Co-chairman: **N. Siddle** (UK)

J. Studd (UK)
P. Stumpf (USA)
B. Ettinger (USA)
R. Mazess (USA)
M. Brincat (UK)
P. Fottrell (Ireland)
L. Cardozo (UK)

The successful completion of a Workshop under the title 'Technology and techniques' bears evidence to the rapid development of research into the entire subject of the female climacteric, and the escalating complexity of some of the technologies being introduced to evaluate the subject. Indeed, the history of the International Menopause Congresses has reflected this development with the first Congress in 1976 being one of definition, the second Congress in 1978 reflecting the intense interest in estrogen-related uterine cancer problems, and the third meeting in 1980 being one of consolidation.

The current Workshop was divided into two subsections, the first concentrating on techniques for detecting and evaluating bone mass, and the second reviewing miscellaneous technologies.

The great improvement over the past decade in techniques for quantification of bone mineral was emphasized by **Ettinger**: whereas previously there was reliance on inexact and insensitive peripheral measurements such as radiogrammetry, photodensitometry, and single-energy photon absorptiometry, Ettinger felt we can now accurately measure mineral content of the spine, which is the site of clinical osteoporosis. In his comparison of spinal dual photon absorptiometry (DPA) versus quantitative computed tomography (QCT), he examined the following areas: (1) availability, (2) practical considerations, (3) precision, (4) accuracy, (5) validation by clinical usefulness.

Unlike DPA, QCT does not require a dedicated machine but is simply a low-cost modification of present-generation CT scanners. The only additional item required is a standard phantom which is scanned with each patient. About 250 centers have had no difficulty in adopting the QCT technique and inter-center comparisons have shown close correlations. The corrections and calibrations are especially easy for the General Electric and Siemens scanners, about 75% of CT scanners in use today. On the other hand, the DPA machine is relatively small and inexpensive with an initial cost of about $30 000 and monthly isotope costs of about $500. Some users have had difficulty with corrections and calibrations but newer software programs may help.

QCT is performed in 10 min and the analysis presently takes another 10 min. DPA usually takes 25 min but some centers feel that better precision is obtained by 40-min scanning. Analysis takes 20 min. The average charge for both studies is $150.

The patient must remain still for 1 min then 3 min to obtain a QCT scan, but for 20 min to allow a DPA scan. The QCT machine is frightening for some patients, whereas DPA is not.

The minimum radiation exposure for QCT is 150 mrem but some scanners require 400 mrem. This is still about one-tenth the dose of standard abdominal CT and there is virtually no dose to the gonads because of a very narrow beam width. DPA radiation is 10–15 mrem with negligible gonadal dose.

QCT has a precision of between 2% and 4% depending upon the methodology used. DPA, with a 2–3% precision, is especially good in younger women who do not have distorted anatomy, i.e. no crush fractures, no disc abnormalities, no arthritis.

With increasing age, red marrow is replaced by yellow marrow; between ages 20 and 80 the average fat content of the vertebra increases 50%. Both methods are affected by this change, but since DPA measures total spinal bone mass, it is less affected. The error introduced by fat will result in an underestimation of bone mineral. For QCT this is approximately 5% in younger women and 10–15% in older women. This error can be partially adjusted away, but about a 7% degree of uncertainty persists. The fat error of DPA is about one-third that of QCT. QCT correlates well with vertebral histomorphometry and ash weight. Using dual-energy QCT to accurately assess the error introduced by fat it has been shown that the biologic variation in spinal mineral is much greater than the uncertainty due to fat. Under the worst of conditions the underestimation due to fat is 15% while postmenopausal bone loss is approximately 25% per decade.

While QCT measures only the highly active trabecular bone within the vertebral body, DPA is a measurement of both the trabecular and the slowly turning over cortical elements. DPA measures all the mineral scanned – cortical shell, posterior elements, transverse processes. The result of mixing equal parts of slow-turnover bone with high-turnover bone is a reduction in DPA's sensitivity by two-thirds. Inaccuracies due to inclusion of extraneous calcifications can add to the problem when hypertrophied articular facets, calcified ligaments, disks, aorta or osteophytes are included in the spinal mineral result.

The ultimate value of any test resides in its ability to provide useful clinical information – to discriminate those subjects who are or who will be affected by disease. **Genant** and co-workers have found that the degree and number of vertebral fractures correlated better with QCT than with DPA. The QCT is usually 50% or more reduced in patients suffering from osteoporosis, while DPA shows reductions of only 25–35%. Women studied at the time of menopause have showed an average annual loss of 7% for QCT but only 2–3% for DPA. Whereas QCT has proved to be of use in several clinical research studies, prospective studies using DPA are just beginning and it will be some time until its value as a research tool will be known. Neither test is presently acceptable for mass screening; cost, time and complexity are excessive and neither test has yet been shown to have predictive value.

Mazess addressed the subject from a different perspective. He stated that in the past decade it has become evident that various radiologic indices (spine biconcavity and Singh index) are useless clinically. The inaccuracies and insensitivity of radiogrammetry, and of the particular photodensitometry methods used in the USA, preclude their clinical application. Aside from several research methods, with limited availability, this leaves computed tomography and single- and dual-photon absorptiometry for use in osteoporosis. Only the latter two methods are suitable for widespread application because of cost, availability and radiation dose.

Dual-photon absorptiometry (DPA) using ^{153}Gd has been shown to be a useful diagnostic aid in crush–fracture osteoporosis since 50–70% of patients fall at the 90th percentile compared to age-matched controls. Almost every case lies at least 3 SD below the mean value in young normals. DPA also is useful in monitoring; relatively large positive responses have been seen in the spine with various forms of therapy. On the other hand DPA scans of the femoral neck (as practiced in Europe) are of limited diagnostic value for fracture, and in fact radius scans may be superior.

Technical problems with DPA are minor when proper procedures are followed. Calibration on standards must be done to minimize influences of system drift and source changes. If appropriate correction factors are not used results can vary with patient thickness or position in the beam. Proper baseline and edge determinations are essential for both precision and accuracy. Finally data must be normalized for bone and body size to achieve meaningful diagnostic application.

Major advances have been made in single-photon absorptiometry (SPA) over the past several years including (a) use of rectilinear scanners and (b) use of computers for control and data acquisition. The former step has halved the precision error by averaging out anatomical variation (3–15%). Use of computers has allowed scanners to be more flexible – different bones of both infants and adults can be measured. The use of computers also has extended the useful source life to 6 months or more by obviating the need for tin filtration on ^{125}I sources.

It is now recognized that the usual radius shaft site does not provide a good indication of spinal state in bone disease, but there have been unverified suggestions that sites on the distal radius are more sensitive for both diagnosis and monitoring. They examined the relationship between spinal density in over 150 women with absorptiometry at various radius sites and found that these speculations were not supported. The predictive error for L2-L4 BMD was similar (0.1 g/cm^2 or about 1 SD) at all sites; the correlations were 0.3–0.5. Even though the radius is not a good indicator of axial bone it can serve as a useful approach to mass screening.

An indirect method of detecting postmenopausal women at risk of osteoporosis was described by **Brincat**. He emphasized that a simple-to-use, cheap, and reliable mass screening technique is needed to identify the population at risk of osteoporosis. He felt that some methods are too expensive and too complicated to be practical, for example, dual-photon absorptiometry and quantitative computer tomography, and have not as yet been shown to be reliable as predictors.

He also emphasized that simple radiological methods, on the other hand, have been shown to be unreliable in predicting the at-risk population. Since bone is composed of *both* collagen and mineral, and since collagen constitutes an important structural element of bone, any method that could suggest the performance of bone collagen with years since menopause would provide a useful diagnostic tool.

Brincat and co-workers have shown that skin collagen correlates well with skin thickness (Sk T) as measured by a radiological method that they have developed.

Because metacarpal index (MI) is mostly representative of the mineral component of bone and only indirectly indicates what the bone collagen is, they improved the correlation of MI to MA by putting a collagen 'element' into the equation. By adding skin thickness with MI and looking at the mean values ($\pm$SD) of 124 postmenopausal women at various ranges past the menopause, nomograms of cross-sectional data were constructed.

The performance of a group of postmenopausal osteoporotics on the graph was then compared to their performance on a MI nomogram and a skin thickness nomogram, both of which had been plotted in the same way.

They suggest that a (Sk T) (MI) index is a more accurate way of detecting women at risk than MI alone, and that when further developed this method would provide a cheap, effective, simple mass screening technique that will enable them to pick out the women who are starting with a low reserve of both bone matrix (collagen) and bone density (MI) and are most at risk of developing osteoporosis.

Despite the urgent need for an accurate, cheap and easily available method for evaluating bone mass and differentiating the patients at risk of osteoporosis, it is obvious from the above discussion that none of the current techniques is yet ideal. Nonetheless, the application of computer science to radiology, or to radioisotopic densitometry, has enhanced the ability to differentiate the situation more accurately, and does offer hope for effective screening methods in the future.

The measurement of hormones in the urine and blood have been the traditional approaches but the increasing accuracy of assays and the greater need for the results obtained have stimulated a research for alternate and perhaps simpler techniques. **Fottrell** described a rapid method of measuring steroids in saliva. The use of saliva as a biological fluid for steroid analysis is a new and exciting development in clinical endocrinology. Saliva is easily collected in the patient's home, and samples can be mailed or transported to the laboratory for analysis. This non-invasive procedure allows multi-sampling regimens for long-term intensive studies of hormone secretion. Such studies are very relevant to monitoring estrogen and progesterone profiles during the climacteric. Steroid concentrations in saliva are independent of flow rate and reflect the plasma 'free', non-protein bound and biologically active moiety.

Saliva therefore offers a new potential for assessing the endocrine status of subjects. The problem, however, is that existing techniques for measuring steroids in saliva usually involve extraction with organic solvent followed by radioimmunoassay. Serial saliva sampling generates large numbers of assays and it is necessary therefore to have rapid direct assays to cope with the additional work load. Radioimmunoassay procedures require specialized laboratory facilities, relatively expensive counting equipment and are not suitable for smaller laboratories.

The object of the research done by Fottrell and his colleagues was the development of rapid non-isotopic immunoassays for salivary steroids such as progesterone and estrogens. They have recently developed the first enzyme immunoassay for salivary progesterone. The accuracy, precision and specificity together with the applications of this assay were discussed. The assay is very suitable for monitoring premenopausal fertility and hormonal replacement therapy. Similar assays for estrogens are being developed and these assays will have important applications in monitoring steroids such as 17β-estradiol and estrone during the climacteric.

In summary, the measurement of steroids in saliva by rapid non-isotopic methods will be of considerable benefit for endocrinological studies during the climacteric. Cost-effective methodology such as the enzyme immunoassay described here will greatly extend the applications of these assays.

The different methods of administering estrogen, other than pellets, was described by **Stumpf**. He emphasized that the inherent advantages of parenteral administration included avoidance of the intestinal metabolism component, avoidance of a bolus response by the liver cells, a reduction in gallbladder disease, and the ability to use 17β-estradiol itself.

Various sustained release systems have been developed with specific advantages. These include the ability to avoid bolus administration and to enhance the simplicity of measuring resultant levels in the serum, and an ability to maintain preselected levels for long periods of time.

One area of development has been that of steroid-containing vaginal rings. The history of siloxane release characteristics and the development of contraceptive vaginal rings was presented by Dr Stumpf and this has led to estradiol and progesterone vaginal rings. The characteristics of these rings and preliminary patient experience were presented, and the suggestion made that they offer significant potential value in the future.

Some reference was made to transdermal delivery of estradiol by skin patches.

The various routes of administration for exogenous estrogen were also reviewed by **Studd**. He was particularly enthusiastic about percutaneous implants. He emphasized that oral estrogen therapy is straightforward and will doubtless remain the most frequently used. However, there are theoretical metabolic problems associated with the first-pass liver response. These will include high levels of plasma estrone with unphysiological ratios of estrone to estradiol, induction of liver enzymes and clotting factors, and abnormal glucose tolerance. Patients receiving oral estrogen therapy may also have an inadequate symptomatic response or develop gastrointestinal complaints. Percutaneous estrogen bypasses the enterohepatic circulation and probably avoids these problems. Estradiol 50 mg implants with or without testosterone 100 mg pellets are the most frequently used route of estrogen administration at Dulwich Hospital. During the past 10 years the incidence of pellet implantation has increased from 7% to 85%. The indications in climacteric patients are inadequate oral therapy, gastrointestinal symptoms with oral therapy, severe depression, loss of energy and libido, patients who have had a hysterectomy and, increasingly, patient preference. Physiological levels of estradiol and estrone and FSH are maintained with repeated implants every 6 months with minimal cumulative effect over 10 years.

There is no extensive weight gain nor change in blood pressure. All patients with a uterus must have cyclical progestogen each month to prevent endometrial hyperplasia. Thirteen days of progestogen each month will eliminate this risk but progestogenic symptoms are often unacceptable for this time. Seven days of progestogen each month seems to be a workable compromise associated with a Vabra curettage every 3 years.

A larger dose of estradiol (1100 mg) is anovulatory and can be used in perimenopausal patients who have severe cyclical symptoms such as premenstrual tension and menstrual migraine. Such a dose is also con-traceptive and it is likely that this therapy is an ideal form of birth control in the 40-year-old woman for whom conventional oral contraception is contraindicated and who may be experiencing problems of the premen-strual syndrome, cyclical headaches and the approaching symptoms of the climacteric.

The information presented by **Cardozo** on the urodynamic evaluation of the perimenopausal patient is presented elsewhere in this book.

The subjects discussed represent only a few areas in which modern technology is enhancing the recent research information acquired about the climacteric, as well as enhancing the ability to improve preventive care in the perimenopausal woman. The rate of introduction of new tech-nology into medicine is so rapid that at future menopause meetings it is certain that more than one Workshop will be required to present the information that is forthcoming.

FURTHER READING

Cann, C. E., Genant, H. K., Kolb, F. O. and Ettinger, B. (1985). Quantitative computed tomography for prediction of vertebral fracture risk. *Metab. Bone. Dis. Rel. Res.*, **6**, 1–7

Genant, H. K. and Boyd, D. P. (1977). Quantitative bone mineral analysis using dual-energy computed tomography. *Invest. Radiol.*, **12**, 545–51

Genant, H. K., Cann, C. E., Ettinger, B. and Gordan, G. S. (1982). Quantitative computed tomography of vertebral spongiosa: a sensitive method for detecting early bone loss after oophorectomy. *Ann. Intern. Med.*, **97**, 699–705

Richardson, M. L., Genant, H. K., Cann, C. E., Ettinger, B., Gordan, G. S., Kolb, F. O. and Reiser, U. J. (1985). Assessment of metabolic bone disease by quantitative computed tomography. *Clin. Orthop. Rel. Res.*, **195**, 224–38

Tallon, D. F., Gosling, J. P., Buckley, P. M. *et al.* (1984). Direct solid-phase enzyme immuno-assay of progesterone in saliva. *Clin. Chem.*, **30**, 1502–11

Workshop 7

Sexuality in the climacteric

Chairman: **L. Dennerstein** (Australia)
Co-chairman: **R. Good** (USA)

> **G. Bachmann** (USA)
> **P. Sarrel** (USA)
> **R. Good** (USA)
> **E. Brecher** (USA)
> **J. Davidson** (USA)
> **M. Hepworth** (UK)
> **M. Featherstone** (UK)

INTRODUCTION

Loss of interest and responsivity in sex are complaints frequently expressed by women attending menopause clinics. These complaints are also expressed frequently by women during their reproductive years. There are many issues of importance to the clinician.

Is there a deterioration in sexual functioning associated with the climacteric? What is the specific nature of any changes in sexuality? Do such changes reflect biological factors, such as chronological aging or the hormonal changes associated with the declining ovarian function, or psychosocial changes? Finally there are the problems of diagnosis and intervention.

During the Workshop these issues were addressed by the speakers, whose background varied from non-medical writer to psychiatry, gynecology, physiology and sociology. Despite the diversity of discipline some consensus was achieved on these important issues.

CHANGES IN SEXUALITY WITH THE CLIMACTERIC

Previous studies of sexual behavior during the climacteric years and beyond have been cross-sectional in nature. In Kinsey's study[1] 48% of women who had experienced a natural menopause believed that their sexual response had decreased at this time. Interestingly, these changes were attributed by Kinsey either to the male's declining interest in socio-sexual activities or to the opportunity for women to use the excuse of menopause for discontinuing sexual relationships. Conflicting evidence was provided in later studies. Pfeiffer *et al.*[2] showed a dramatic decline in the sexual interest of women between the years of 45 to 55. Hallstrom[3] also found dramatic declines in sexual interest, capacity for orgasm and coital frequency of women in the middle years of life.

At this Workshop the results of the first detailed longitudinal study of sexuality in women were reported by **McCoy and Davidson**. They followed normal women through the climacteric for up to 6 years. Subjects had not been ovariectomized or hysterectomized, had not begun estrogen replacement therapy and had a sexual partner or partners. All women kept calendars on which they recorded menstrual and coital information and were interviewed at 4-monthly intervals. Analysis of results found a significant decline in the number of sexual thoughts and fantasies and decreased vaginal lubrication following the last menstrual cycle. Coital frequency also declined. The decline was found to be already evident 24 to 12 months before the last cycle. When menstrual calendars were examined the number of menstrual cycles had also decreased, indicating that hormonal changes were present. These findings are of interest as studies of psychological symptomatology also demonstrated an increase in incidence of such complaints in the 1–2 years prior to the menopause[4].

TYPES OF CHANGES IN SEXUALITY

Davidson also presented psychophysiological studies which confirmed a decrement in sexual responsivity associated with the menopause. Vaginal pulse amplitude in response to erotic film and fantasy were measured in young cycling women, premenopausal women (mean age 50.6 ± 0.9 years) and postmenopausal women (mean age 57.4 ± 1.8 years). There were no differences in the response of young cycling women or premenopausal women to film or fantasy despite a 20-year or more age difference between the two groups (Fig. W7.1). There was a significant difference in response to film (but not to fantasy) when the pre- and postmenopausal women were compared. The nature of changes in sexuality by women with specific menopausal complaints was explored by **Sarrel and Whitehead**. One hundred and eighty-five women attending a menopause clinic were interviewed for 1–3 hours. One hundred and fifty-four (86.5%)

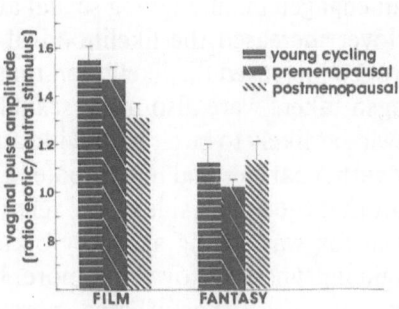

Figure W7.1 Age, menopause and sexual response

were found to have sexual problems. In 33 the problems had been long-standing. Of the 24 women whose sex lives were unchanged or improved, one-third had new sexual partners, all of whom were younger than the women. Only two of the 154 women with problems had new partners.

When the nature of the problems experienced was examined, deterioration was found in most aspects of sexual response. Forty-five percent had loss of interest in sex and 10% had developed a sexual aversion. Fifty-five women (36%) had touch impairment, 36% had vaginal dryness and 20% loss of clitoral sensation. All 55 women having touch impairment had elevated gonadotropins and decreased estradiol levels. These, however, found the touch of clothing irritating and almost all had sensations of numbness and tingling in the hands and feet. There were orgasmic phase problems in 37% of the women and dyspareunia in 43%. On examination, about half of the women with dyspareunia were found to have developed vaginismus. The role of the partner was emphasized either in possible causation of some problems or as having developed associated problems.

ETIOLOGY OF CHANGES

The work of McCoy and Davidson suggests a biological origin for declining sexual functioning. **Backmann** studied 22 postmenopausal women in good health and not taking estrogen therapy. Fifty-four percent reported a decrease in sexual interest or desire. Decreased sex interest was not related to FSH, LH or androstenedione or estradiol levels.

Brecher carried out an analysis of 1764 postmenopausal respondents to a Consumers Union questionnaire. The women were aged between 50 and 90. There were 408 estrogen users and 1356 estrogen non-takers. Estrogen takers were more likely to be in their 5th decade, from homes with family incomes over $50 000, better educated, married, or even more likely unmarried but engaged in an ongoing sexual affair. It was unclear whether having a lover increased the likelihood of taking estrogen or whether taking estrogen increased the likelihood that such a woman will take a lover. Estrogen takers were also more sexually active than non-takers. They were twice as likely to be either having an extramarital affair or to both have sex with a partner and masturbate. Estrogen takers were more likely to report that the sexual side of the relationship was important. Their interest in sex was strong and they became easily aroused, experienced less vaginal dryness, enjoyed sex more, had sex more often, experienced climax more often, masturbated more often and reported more nocturnal sexual experiences. There was no difference between estrogen takers and non-takers in overall enjoyment of life, experience of loneliness and perception of happiness in their marriage. Concern was expressed about the possible biasing effects of age and the need for further statistical analysis to clarify the effects of such variables.

Three hundred of the 764 women experienced a surgical menopause. Surgical menopause women not on estrogen were even less sexually active and interested than women with natural menopause not taking estrogen.

Sarrel reported that many of the adverse changes in touch impairment could be effectively reversed by estrogen therapy.

Davidson reported Dennerstein's study of oophorectomized women[5]. In this study 49 women were administered an estrogen, a progestin, a combination of both hormones and a placebo in a double-blind crossover study. Estrogen had a more beneficial effect on all aspects of female sexuality (desire, arousal, enjoyment, orgasm) than the other medications.

Thus the consensus of opinion was that there was a deterioration in sexual functioning occurring in the climacteric and continuing into the menopause, which was related to the decline in hormone production, particularly that of estrogen. Although many women experienced a decline in sexual functioning not all became dysfunctional. This suggests that hormonal factors may provide a vulnerability but other factors, particularly intrapsychic or interpersonal, may determine the severity of the changes.

MANAGEMENT – PROBLEMS OF DIAGNOSIS AND INTERVENTION

Good then addressed the 'real-world' problem of the patient in her middle years who has a sexual problem but seeks medical care presenting multiple complaints. He noted that irritability, tiredness, backache, sleep disturbances, decreased libido and similar non-specific symptoms may be due not only to a marital–sexual problem but might also be due to estrogen lack, a specific affective disorder, or be indicative of maladjustment to midlife changes.

It requires clinical expertise to make a differential diagnosis in order to plan meaningful, specific therapeutic intervention. He suggested that the family physician, internist and gynecologist can obtain a gross evaluation of the patient's psychosocial status by the use of the 'simple palindrome', HATAH, which stands for 'How are things at home'.

It is not unusual for the history, physical findings, and indicated laboratory tests to reveal multiple causes for the symptomatology requiring an integrated approach to management. Adequate treatment may require combining estrogen replacement, antidepressant medication, counseling and specific sexual therapy.

With regard to specific therapies **Bachmann** studied the effects of a weekly exercise program and found no effects on sexuality. The role of androgen therapy was discussed. Clinical reports of favorable effects on both sexuality and drive or energy were noted. Davidson emphasized the need for further studies to delineate how androgens produce such effects in women.

CONCLUSION

Sex as a sociological concept was introduced by **Featherstone** and **Hepworth**. In their review of social aspects of male sexuality they noted that while there is no conclusive empirical evidence that the *majority* of men undergo a hormonal 'change of life' equivalent to that found in women, a significant number do experience psychological and social difficulties at some point in middle age. In certain respects these negative experiences resemble those typically associated with a traumatic menopause in middle-aged women. Amongst the various symptoms reported, of particular interest was the recurring expression of male sexual anxiety and/or dissatisfaction with sex life. A comparative analysis of professional and lay publications which appeared in the UK and USA, 1930–83, was carried out to locate the expression of sexual anxiety in the context of a changing conception of middle age in the Western world. The main focus was on the influence of contemporary models of sexualized lifestyle on sexual expectations and relations between the sexes during mid-life. In this context therapists will need to be mindful of the complex interaction between objective events, physically determined symptoms and the subjective quest for personal meaning.

REFERENCES

1. Kinsey, A. C., Pomeroy, W. B., Martin, C. E. and Gebhard, P. H. (1953). *Sexual Behaviour in the Human Female.* (Philadelphia: Saunders)
2. Pfeiffer, E., Verwoerdt, A. and Davis, G. C. (1972). Sexual Behaviour in Middle Life. *Am. J. Psychiatry*, **128**, 1262

3. Hallstrom, T. (1977). Sexuality in the climacteric. In Greenblatt, R. B. and Studd, J. (eds.) *Clinics in Obstetrics and Gynaecology: The Menopause Vol. 4*. pp. 227–39 (London: Saunders)
4. Dennerstein, L. and Burrows, G. D. (1978). A Review of the Studies of the Psychological Symptoms found at the Menopause. *Maturitas*, **1**, 55–64
5. Dennerstein, L., Burrows, G. D., Wood, C. and Hyman, G. (1980). Hormones and Sexuality: Effect of Estrogen and Progestrogen. *Obstet. Gynecol.*, **56**, (3)

FURTHER READING

Featherstone, M. (1982). The body in consumer culture. *Theory, Culture and Society*, 1(2), 18–33
Gould, R. L. (1972). The phases of adult life: a study in developmental psychology. *Am. J. Psychiatry*, **129**(5), 521–31
McCoy, N. and Davidson, J. M. (1985). A longitudinal study of the effects of menopause on sexuality. *Maturitas*, **7**(3), 203–10
McCoy, N., Cutler, W. and Davidson, J. M. (1985). Relationships among hot flashes, sexual behaviour and hormone levels in perimenopausal women. *Arch. Sex. Behav.*, **14**(5) (In press)
Morrel, M. J., Dixon, M. J., Carter, S. and Davidson, J. M. (1984). The influence of age and cycling status on sexual arousability in women. *Am. J. Obstet. Gynecol.*, **148**, 66
Nadelson, C. C. *et al.* (1978). Marital stress and symptoms formation in mid-life. *Psychiat. Opin.*, September
Neugarten, B. L. and Kraines, R. J. (1965). 'Menopausal symptoms' in women of various ages. *Psychosom. Med.*, **27**(3), 266–73
Pratt, J. (1982). The sexual landscape. *Theory, Culture and Society*, 1(1), 65–82
Pfeiffer, E. *et al.* (1972). Sexual behavior in middle life. *Am. J. Psychiatry*, **128**(10), 82–7
Sarrel, P. and Whitehead, M. (1985). Sex and menopause: defining the issues. *Maturitas*, **7**(3), 217–24
Sarrel, P. (1982). Sex problems after menopause. A study of fifty married couples. *Maturitas*, **4**, 231–7
Winokur, G. (1973). Depression in the menopause. *Am. J. Psychiatry*, **130**(1), 92–3

Workshop 8

Nutrition

Chairman: **L. Reimer** (USA)
Co-chairman: **L. Ellenbogen** (USA)

E. B. Feldman (USA)
C. Gallagher (USA)
R. Rivlin (USA)
P. Wagner (USA)
C. Nagant de Deuxchaisnes (Belgium)
L. Reimer (USA)

There were several common threads that came through as each presenter discussed different aspects of midlife nutritional well-being. These were:

(1) *Nutritional influences middle year health.* However, it is not the only factor. We know, for an example, in osteoporosis that calcium and vitamin D are important, but we also recognize that exercise genetics and hormones are contributing factors. We also know with cancer risks that diet is a factor, but we recognize that there are other environmental chemical and perhaps viral and genetic factors.

(2) *Risk factors for developing deficiencies in midlife include:*
    (a) Sedentary lifestyle – as people decrease their activity, they also decrease their caloric intake. This decreases the likelihood that they will consume enough calories to provide adequate vitamins, minerals and trace elements. One example of this is the fact that menopausal women, despite not having monthly menstrual loss, develop anemia due to low intake of iron.
    (b) Lack of variety – as people become more set in their ways and perhaps only cook for one, there is a lack of variety in the diet.

This contributes to vitamin, mineral and trace element deficiencies. For example, a tea and toast diet would be deficient in vitamins. A diet eliminating meat would lose a good source of trace elements and iron. A diet without milk would lose a good source of calcium.

(c) Alcohol use – frequent and social use of alcohol is a major contributor to vitamin deficiencies. In addition the use of over-the-counter drugs and prescriptions can interfere with absorption or utilization of vitamins.

(3) *Moderation is important* – all the speakers pointed out in different ways that this age group is prone to deficiencies; moderation correction is important. Most of the speakers stressed the need for a correction of deficiencies through the diet and not through supplementary pills. In fact, there are problems with taking high-level supplements. Excess amounts are not used and are wasted. In addition overdose syndromes can mimic diseases (with lymph node, liver enlargement, symptoms of increased intracranial pressure).

(4) *Dietary interactions exist* – for example, fiber is important and is protective against development of cancer, particularly in the GI tract, but a very high fiber diet may interfere with mineral absorption. Meat is a good source of iron and trace elements and also protein; however, it is also a high source of fat in the diet. A high-protein diet can contribute to decreased calcium absorption. From these examples of interaction we note that it is important to keep the diet varied and not eliminate elements out of the diet or become extreme in focusing on one or two elements in the diet.

(5) *Doctor or professional monitoring is needed* – with estrogens, **Feldman** pointed out that checking lipids after estrogen and hormone supplementation is important. With vitamin D, **Gallagher** pointed out that checking calcium in the serum and urine is important. **Rivlin** pointed out that professional monitoring of vitamin supplementation is important. **Wagner** pointed out that taking trace elements pills can easily lead to toxic levels.

RECOMMENDATIONS

From these common threads that came forth from the Nutritional Workshop the recommendations would be:

(1) Nutrition is an important element in the health of middle-aged people and it is indeed one factor that contributes to preventing certain problems.

(2) Nutrition should be provided by the diet and not by pills, except that calcium supplements may be needed.
(3) An adequate diet can be insured by maintaining an active life so that adequate calories can be consumed.
(4) A monotonous diet would not provide the variety necessary for nutrients.
(5) Keeping alcohol at a minimum – less than two drinks per day.
(6) Having professional monitoring and guidance for dietary review.

NUTRITION AND CANCER – A BRIEF OVERVIEW

Major points

(1) Nutrition is one factor in the risk profile of cancer.
(2) Epidemiological evidence of diet factors is reviewed.
(3) Dietary factors are: excesses, deficiencies, additives.
(4) General recommendations based on information and guidelines from the Director of Cancer Prevention, M. D. Anderson Hospital and Cancer Institute, and the National Cancer Institute will be translated into practical tips.

Epidemiological evidence

Reimer: Two hundred years ago a British surgeon, Potts, noticed a rare form of cancer (scrotal) in chimney sweeps. Since then, many other relationships between environmental factors and cancer have been recognized: vinyl chloride and liver cancer; and asbestos and certain types of lung cancer (mesothelioma) are two examples. This led some researchers to suspect that environmental factors could include diet. The incidence of cancer does indeed vary between communities based on differences in diet.

The incidence of cancer often changes as people move to new countries and adapt to new diets. An example is the change in mortality of stomach and colon cancer is Japanese who migrate to the United States (Fig. W8.1). Cancer incidence also changes over time with dietary alterations in the same community. Stomach cancer has decreased over the past 50 years. This is thought to be due to increased use of refrigeration, which inhibits the reduction of nitrate, and a decrease in the need for salt as a preservative (Fig. W8.2). Trends suggested by community studies (epidemiologic), when investigated in the laboratory, allows for a calculation of the degree that diet influences cancer formation. It is estimated that 35% of cancer is potentially preventable by diet (Table W8.1).

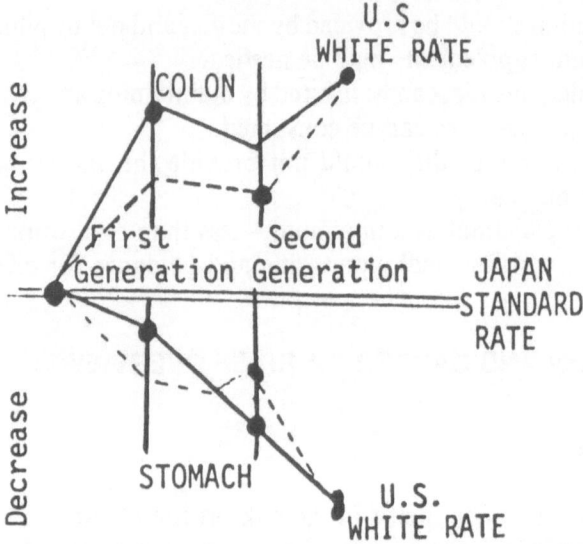

Figure W8.1 Mortality trends of Japanese migrants to US - cancer of the stomach and colon: ●——●, male; ●- - -●, female (adapted from *Cancer Detection and Prevention*, **3**, 367–417; 1980)

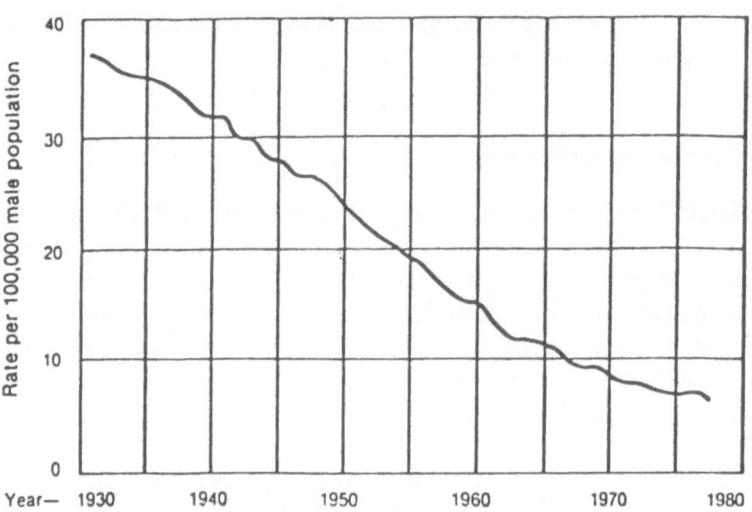

Figure W8.2 Age-adjusted cancer death rates - males (stomach cancer) US, 1930–1978. (From *CA - A Cancer Journal*, **33**(1), 000–00; 1983)

Table W8.1 Cancers potentially preventable by diet

Stomach and large bowel	90%
Endometrium, gallbladder, pancreas, breast	50%
Lung, larynx, bladder, cervix, mouth, pharynx, esophagus	20%
Other types	10%
Overall	35%

Responsible dietary factors

Potential carcinogenic factors include dietary excesses, deficiency of nutrients in the diet, and certain additives and contaminants.

Dietary excesses

An excess of total calories, fat, salt and *alcohol* has been linked to cancer. Lean and underfed animals have a decreased incidence of spontaneous and induced neoplasms (tumors) when compared to animals of greater body weight.

Similar data for humans are suggested by insurance statistics which show that overweight, middle-aged, or older persons have a higher cancer mortality than do those of comparable age who are of average weight. High caloric consumption/obesity has been correlated with the incidence of endometrial (uterus lining) and breast cancer in women.

Dietary excess is correlated with breast and colon cancer and perhaps that of the ovary, uterus and prostate. Fat intake parallels gross national product; people in affluent countries consume more fat. The average United States citizen consumes four times more fat than natives of Asia, Africa and Central and South America. Carroll's 1975 study showed a direct correlation between the mortality rate for breast cancer and per capita fat intake in 39 countries.

Salt seems to act in combination with other factors. Countries with a high incidence of hypertension also report a high incidence of gastric cancer. This form of cancer has decreased in the past 40 years, as refrigeration has become more available and the need for salt has diminished. Exceptions are in Japan, mountainous areas of Latin America, northern and eastern Europe and Iceland. In these countries salt and pickling are still used extensively and may be the reason why the high incidence of gastric cancer persists. Another possible contributing factor in Iceland is the practice of smoking food. This produces polycyclic hydrocarbons, which have been shown to cause stomach cancer in rodents.

Alcohol contributes invisible calories which are not reported in national surveys. Alcohol excess is linked to certain forms of cancer.

Dietary deficiencies

The *fiber* content of Western diets decreased as more fat was incorporated into the diet. Fiber is defined as the plant wall residues resistant to animal digestive enzymes, and is found in vegetables, fruits and grains. Populations consuming a high-fiber diet, such as Seventh Day Adventists and Africans, have a low cancer incidence. Low-fiber diets are associated with higher colon cancer rates in Great Britain and rectal cancer in Finland and

Denmark. The frequency of this form of cancer varies inversely with the amount of fiber. This epidemiological finding is confirmed by experimental studies. Animals fed a carcinogen with increased fiber in their diet developed cancer less frequently than animals with a lower-fiber diet.

A USDA report (1947–58) and the Hanes study (Health and Nutrition Survey, 1971–72) cited that some children and adults had *low vitamin C and A level*. These vitamins have a potential role in cancer prevention. Vitamin C is a 'reducing' agent that prevents the formation of chemicals known as nitrosamines from certain foods. Reduction of nitrosamines will decrease gastric and perhaps esophageal cancer. Vitamin C may also have a protective role in colon and lung cancer. Vitamin C's antioxidant effect has been shown to decrease tumor growth in animals.

Vitamin A is necessary for normal cell function and development. Population studies have shown that vitamin A intake in humans was associated with a lower risk of lung, esophagus, stomach, large bowel and bladder cancer. Since vitamin deficiency may contribute to cancer development, it is important to obtain adequate vitamins from fresh fruits and vegetables.

Dietary additives and contaminants

Additives are used to flavor, color, or preserve food. Contaminants are compounds that are not intentionally added to food (e.g. certain types of fungi). Certain additives and contaminants may contribute to cancer formation.

Of the nearly 2700 additives that have been tested for their potential cancer-producing activity, some have been banned (sweetener – cyclamate, butter yellow – thiourea), some are used sparingly (sodium nitrate to cure meat and prevent fatal botulism), while others have been shown to decrease cancer growth (BHA and BHT – antioxidant preservatives). Nitrate is an additive that has been studied in detail.

Summary

Cancer has multiple causes, diet being only one factor. Recommendations, such as the National Cancer Institute's 'prudent diet', will contribute to lessening the risk of certain types of cancer. Decrease dietary fat, decrease salt intake, reduce your alcohol intake, minimize additives and increase your dietary fiber. Finally – easier said than done – achieve and maintain your ideal body weight.

VITAMINS IN MIDDLE AGE

Major points

(1) Vitamins are viewed by the public as a way of keeping young, and have an extra edge against aging.
(2) The people in middle-aged and elderly populations are at risk of becoming deficient in certain vitamins.
(3) This same population also uses vitamin supplements to a high degree, consuming 'overdose at times and also non-vitamins'.

The elderly and deficiencies

Rivlin: The elderly are at risk of becoming deficient because of decreased caloric consumption, decreased variety in the diet, increased use of alcohol and increased use of drugs that interfere with vitamin absorption.

In different studies, different vitamins have been found to be low. Some of these include B1, B2, B3, A and C. In one study 25% of people at 60 years of age were found to consume less than 75% of the RDA for B6, B12, vitamins D and E, folic acid, calcium and zinc. This decreased consumption is due to a decreased caloric intake as lifestyle becomes more sedentary. Some studies have shown iron deficiency in the elderly and the menopausal. This may be surprising since there is no monthly menstrual loss with women at this age. However, the decreased caloric intake decreases the amount of iron available. In addition, there may be a decrease in variety in the diet. For instance, if meat is decreased, which is a good source of iron, then iron deficiency can occur.

Increased use of alcohol is also a risk factor for developing vitamin deficiencies. B1 is very sensitive to alcohol use and the steady consumption of daily amounts of alcohol will lead to thiamine deficiency more than binge drinking.

The other contributing factor to deficiencies in this age group is use of prescription and over-the-counter drugs. For example, some laxatives cause an increased loss of vitamin A.

The elderly and supplement use

It has been estimated that a third to a half of the public use supplementary vitamins, the most common being vitamins C and E. Oral supplements may not be consumed in excessive amounts. In a recently published study from our laboratory in a group of healthy well-nourished elderly women, doubling of vitamin B2 increased B2 urine excretion. (B2 riboflavin nutriture, as assessed by means of the erythrocyte glutathione reductase activity coefficient, was not improved under these circumstances.)

Vitamin status should be assessed more frequently in elderly persons than is done at present, therapy should be supervised by a qualified health professional.

In addition, people use non-vitamins such as vitamin B15 and vitamin B17, neither of which have been adequately documented as true vitamins. Some people develop overdoses which can mimic diseases; for example, high levels of vitamins A or D can cause the syndrome of pseudomotor cereberi (with symptoms of increased intracranial pressure) and enlargement of lymph nodes and sometimes liver enlargement.

In conclusion, this age group may attempt to fight off advancing years by taking supplementary vitamin pills. They are at increased risk of developing deficiencies; however, unsupervised use of vitamin supplements can lead to problems. A varied diet, increased activities so that adequate calories can be consumed, and decreased use of alcohol would help many deficiencies in this age group.

TRACE ELEMENTS IN MIDLIFE HEALTH

Major points

(1) The science of trace elements is presently in its infancy.
(2) Guidelines for adequate and safe levels of trace elements in the diet are being established presently.
(3) A mixed varied diet from plant and animal sources is important.
(4) Adequate calories to supply trace elements are important.
(5) Decreased use of refined foods and fabricated foods would help increase the trace element density in the diet.

History of trace elements

Wagner: The science of trace elements is presently in its infancy. It was not until the 1970s, with the use of total parenteral nutrition (TPN), that induced deficiencies were found in man. On TPN without consumption of food orally for long periods, different deficiencies became obvious. Before this the deficiencies were studied in animals, particularly poultry, swine and cattle.

The establishment of RDAs for trace elements

In the most recent 1980 edition of the National Research Council's *Recommended Dietary Allowances*, a specific RDA amount of only three trace elements is suggested – iron, iodine and zinc. The group of scientists on the NRC-RDA committee for the first time also tentatively suggested ranges of daily dietary intakes for six other trace elements including copper, manganese, fluoride, chromium, selenium and molybdenum. These ranges are referred to as estimated safe and adequate daily dietary intakes.

It is suggested that the upper levels for trace element intake should not be habitually exceeded, since toxic levels may only be several times the usual intakes. Other newer elements are being studied to develop guidelines and include silicon and nickel.

A mixed and varied diet is needed to supply trace elements, particularly with an adequate calorie intake. It is estimated that on average only 5 mg of zinc are contained in 1000 calories of food. Therefore, if the RDA of zinc is 15 mg, foods of high zinc density should be selected. A high consumption of calories is necessary to supply this. The use of fat, sugar, alcohol and highly refined fabricated food lowers the trace element density in the diet. These foods supply a lot of calories without trace elements. Also, the reduced energy intake accompanying the sedentary lifestyles of many people increases the risk of trace element deficiency.

Awareness of the importance and complexity of the role of trace elements in nutrition in health leads to an appreciation of such simplified dietary recommendations as 'variety', 'balance' and 'moderation'. Selection of a variety of foods from plant and animal sources helps to insure an adequate trace element intake. Many patients ask questions about monitoring and measuring trace elements, particularly hair analysis. Hair analysis is at present a research tool and is not really usable in a clinical setting.

In conclusion, as we learn more about trace elements, we will be better able to define recommended daily allowances for a wider spectrum of trace elements and define their role in health. Presently, the advice to give our patients includes a mixed and varied diet, of high nutrient density and with adequate calories.

LIPIDS AND ESTROGEN IN MIDDLE AGE

Major points:

(1) The lipid levels in any individual are affected by many factors. In an individual, therefore, the lipid levels cannot be predicted and must be measured periodically.
(2) Estrogen supplementation has many effects on lipids and depends on the combination of hormones given, the preparation, the dose and the route.

Factors that affect lipids

Feldman:
(1) Lipids vary with age (Fig. W8.3). In the female, cholesterol levels remain lower than males until menopause at which time cholesterol

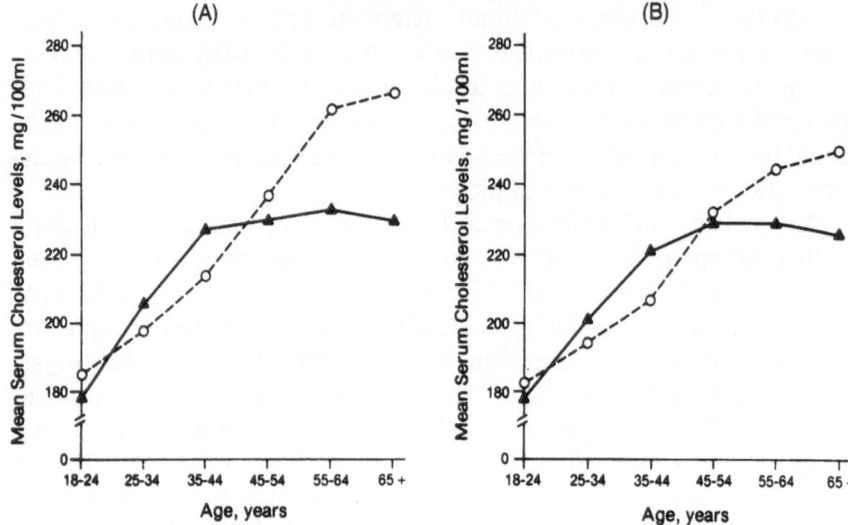

Figure W8.3 Circulating cholesterol levels in men and women with age: A in 1961, B in 1975; O– – –O women, ▲——▲ men

levels in females increase to levels higher than males. In females, HDL levels exceed those of males at all ages, pre- and postmenopausally. Triglyceride levels remain lower in females until about age 70 when they exceed male levels (see also Table W8.2).

(2) Carrier proteins affect lipids. HDL is higher in females and thereby has a protective effect on myocardial infarction risk. If LDL levels are higher, then the risk for MI is increased. Therefore, when

Table W8.2 Average levels of circulating lipids[a]

Age (years)	White males				White females			
	Total C	LDL C	HDL C	TG	Total C	LDL C	HDL C	TG
15–19	152	93	46	68	157	93	51	64
20–24	159	101	45	78	165	102	51	80
25–29	176	116	44	88	178	108	55	76
30–34	190	124	45	102	178	109	55	73
35–39	195	131	43	109	186	116	53	83
40–44	204	135	43	123	193	122	56	68
45–49	210	141	45	119	204	127	58	94
50–54	211	143	44	128	214	134	62	103
55–59	214	145	46	117	229	145	60	111
60–64	215	143	49	111	226	149	61	105
65–69	213	146	49	108	233	151	62	118
70+	214	142	48	115	226	147	60	110

[a] 50th percentile
C = Cholesterol; LDL = low-density lipoprotein; HDL = high-density lipoprotein; TG = triglyceride
Adapted from Lipid Research Clinics Prevalence Study

measuring cholesterol levels in patients it is important not only to measure total cholesterol, but also to get HDL levels and triglyceride levels.
(3) Diet affects lipid levels but will not be reviewed in detail during this Workshop.

Estrogen effects on lipids

(1) Estrogen increases triglycerides, increases chylomicrons and thereby increases incidence of pancreatitis in type 5 hyperlipidemias. Cholesterol synthesis and oxidation is increased in addition to HDL increase. There is a decrease in cholesterol esters via LCAT. In general all hyperlipidemias are made worse by estrogen use with the exception of type 3 which is helped by estrogens.
(2) Progesterones affect lipids. They increase HDL removal and also increase hepatic lipase.
(3) The dose of estrogen may have an effect on lipid levels.
(4) The type of preparation depending on the form of estrogen may have an effect.
(5) The route of estrogen administration such as orally vs. subcutaneously will have an effect on lipid levels.
(6) Combination of hormones also has an effect.

In conclusion: the effect of hormones on lipids depends on the combination of hormones, the preparation, the dose and the route. Since there are multiple factors that affect lipids in addition to estrogen it is important that, with hormone use, *lipid levels be checked 3 months after they are initiated and also every year thereafter*.

THE USE OF VITAMIN D SUPPLEMENTS

(1) The use of vitamin D supplements between age 20 and 65 years is unnecessary in most women in the USA. However, their use in northern European countries where sunlight exposure is decreased may be necessary.
(2) All elderly people may need vitamin D supplementation once they reach the age of 70 years. This is because of the inability of the kidney to produce 1,25-dihydroxyvitamin D, as well as the decreased exposure to sunlight that occurs in sedentary elderly people.

Factors that affect vitamin D

Gallagher: About 80% of circulating vitamin D is derived from sunlight and about 20% from diet. All of the circulating vitamin D that is derived from sunlight is vitamin D3, whereas the circulating vitamin derived from the diet may be either D2 or D3 depending on which vitamin preparation has been added to the diet. In northern European countries, exposure to vitamin D is limited by cloud cover and the decreased number of months when sunlight is most effective in forming vitamin D in the skin. It is not uncommon in elderly people in northern Europe to find serum 25-hydroxy D levels which are barely detectable. In North America, however, the finding of such low 25-hydroxy D levels is uncommon, although age-related measurements of serum 25-hydroxy D in North American individuals show a decrease with age. This may be related to decreased exposure to the sun as one gets older, impaired production of vitamin D3 in the skin or conversion to 25-hydroxy D in the liver. The net result is reduced levels of serum 25-hydroxyvitamin D and 1,25-dihydroxyvitamin D.

Extreme vitamin D deficiency can produce osteomalacia in elderly people. In Northern Europe, osteomalacia, as a cause of hip fracture, is more common than one might think; however, its role in the pathogenesis of hip fractures in the North American continent has not yet been evaluated.

How much vitamin D supplementation is necessary?

We are not sure how much supplementation of vitamin D2 or D3 is necessary *in elderly people* since serum 1,25-dihydroxyvitamin D levels have never been measured after supplementation in elderly people. It is suggested that a supplementation of vitamin D2 or D3, not exceeding 2000 units/day, be used. An additional problem in elderly people is the decrease in calcium absorption that occurs with increasing age. This can probably be explained by the decline in vitamin D levels that occurs with age, but the possibility that the gut ages in its ability to absorb calcium is also a possibility.

Complications of vitamin D therapy

As mentioned previously, vitamin D supplementation in normal people below the age of 65–70 is probably not warranted. In the younger population it is possible that vitamin D supplementation may lead to higher levels of circulating vitamin D and its metabolites, resulting in hypercalciuria or hypercalcemia. If routine supplementation is going to be used in normal people, then a dose greater than 400 units/day is probably unnecessary. In elderly people it is unlikely that 2000–3000 units/day of vitamin D2 or D3 would lead to significant elevations in serum calcium or urine calcium unless the patient had pre-existing renal failure, but it would be good clinical practice (in elderly people who are being supplemented with vitamin D) to perform a measurement of serum and urine calcium twice a year.

In patients with osteoporosis, treatment with vitamin D is more complicated. There is a possibility that the active metabolite of vitamin D, namely 1,25-dihydroxyvitamin D3, is a more effective agent than either vitamin D2 or D3 given separately. However, because of its potential toxicity and the ease with which it can cause hypercalcemia and hypercalciuria more frequent monitoring of serum and urine calcium is necessary if patients with established osteoporosis and fractures are to be treated with this active metabolite. In our experience the use of 0.5 μg/day of 1,25-dihydroxyvitamin D3 is useful in the prevention of further vertebral fractures in patients with established spinal osteoporosis. In patients on this dose we measure serum and urine calcium every 6 weeks. Because of its potency in increasing calcium absorption we do not recommend adding calcium supplements to a patient's regime when they take 1,25-dihydroxyvitamin D3, and we usually estimate that a calcium intake of 600–700 mg/day is adequate for patients so treated.

NUTRITIONAL FACTORS IN OSTEOPOROSIS

Nagant de Deuxchaisnes: Nutritional factors represent one of the significant determining factors of osteoporosis. *Calcium* is the main operative nutritional factor, and therefore I will focus the attention on calcium intake. Before this, I want to point out that *phosphate* has attracted too much of the attention of nutritionists, because in growing animals it produces secondary hyperparathyroidism. Recent balance studies in humans have failed to show any adverse effect of phosphate on the Ca balance. *Protein* intake, when high, does induce excess Ca excretion in the urine and a negative Ca balance. It therefore increases the Ca requirements in the diet. Most experiments on protein have been conducted by offering purified protein products. The obtained information thus only pertains to the proteins tested, and cannot be extrapolated, for example, to meat, which is often done. Indeed meat also provides high amounts of phosphate, which by decreasing Ca output in the urine, offsets the effect of the additional protein contained in meat. Thus, when providing extra protein as meat, no adverse effect is seen on Ca balance or urinary Ca excretion.

Other factors in the diet are also important, such as a high-*fiber* diet, or a high-*phytate* diet (as in unpolished rice or unleavened bread), both of which decrease the intestinal absorption of Ca and therefore increase the Ca requirements in the diet. High *caffeine* does the same, by increasing the urinary losses of Ca. *Tobacco*, and especially *alcohol*, have adverse effects on the bone mass, but these cannot be considered as nutritional factors, and therefore fall outside the scope of this review. Finally, one should also draw attention to the *total caloric intake*, since obesity is known to protect the skeletal mass from decreasing, as was shown in an observation by Paul Saville[1]. In Saville's experience the dividing line between osteoporotic and non-osteoporotic postmenopausal women lies around 140 lb. Above this weight there were more normals than osteoporotics, and osteoporosis disappeared at 180 lb. Below 140 lb there were more osteoporotics than normals, and the normals disappeared below 100 lb. If one is fat, one gets osteoarthritis; if one is slender, one gets osteoporosis. The reason why excessive fat exerts a protective role is dual: first, fat transforms androstenedione of adrenal origin into estrone, and estradiol results from peripheral conversion of estrone (the role of gonadal hormone does not need to be stressed in a Congress on the Menopause). Second, fat adds extra weight, and more physical stress and strains result from such common activities as rising from a chair, climbing stairs, or simply walking. This is forced physical activity.

Having considered these important nutritional factors, I will now deal with by far the most important one: the *calcium* intake. Two decades after the Albright theory[2] of hormonal imbalance, it was Nordin who in 1960[3] put the emphasis on the role of Ca deficiency which has been re-emphasized recently through the magnificent studies performed by Heaney and co-workers[4]. First, let us consider the role of calcium *in the elaboration of adult peak bone mass*. In this respect, calcium may indeed play a crucial role, according to the studies of Matkovic in Yugoslavia[5], comparing a high-Ca district (Podravina) and a low-Ca district (Istra), which were otherwise comparable. The adult peak bone mass, as measured by radiogrammetry, was significantly higher in the high-Ca district, and accordingly the fracture frequency was significantly lower than in the low-Ca district. This, however, was true only for hip fractures, and not for wrist fractures. More recently, Sandler and her co-workers[6] in Pittsburgh studied self-reported milk consumption. Those women who retrospectively did report drinking milk with every meal had significantly higher bone density in the radius, whether considered in childhood, adolescence or during pregnancy or lactation. Only in adulthood (non-pregnant, non-lactating group) was the difference not statistically significant. Finally, Kanders *et al.*[7], studying adult women by means of dual photon absorptiometry (L2–L4) found significantly lower values in those women taking less than 0.75 g/d of dietary Ca. These three studies therefore point out the importance of calcium in the elaboration of the bone mass. Since having a high peak bone mass may be one of the major factors protecting from fracturing later, these observations are of utmost importance.

Calcium, however, is also of crucial importance *as far as bone loss* is concerned. Bone loss is of paramount importance since spontaneous fractures occur when one is below a certain bone mass, which is considered as a fracture threshold. The aim is never to reach the fracture threshold as far as bone mass is concerned. To do so, one should avoid being in a negative Ca balance. The magnificent studies by Heaney[4] should be quoted here. They were performed on perimenopausal nuns flown in every 5 years and studied repeatedly on self-selected diets. Several interesting points emerged. First, the group as a whole had an average Ca intake of 0.6 g/d, well below the US recommended daily allowance (RDA) of 0.8 g/d. Second, the group was in negative Ca balance, and there was a positive correlation between Ca intake and Ca balance. Third, the menopause affected the Ca balance adversely, but the correlation between intake and balance remained positive. To be at neutral Ca balance the intake had to be on average 1.0 g/d before the menopuase and 1.4 g/d after the menopause. The increased requirement after the menopause was equally due to less efficient Ca absorption from the gut and less efficient Ca conservation of the absorbed Ca by the kidney. These studies therefore pointed out that the Ca requirements are 25% higher than the RDA before the menopause, and 75% higher than the RDA after the menopause. This difference in Ca requirement can be abolished by the administration of estrogens. In any event, the Ca intake in the diet should be greatly increased, the more so that the average intake of Ca by postmenopausal women is 0.45 g/d in the US. It is quite similar in Belgium (0.49 g/d). Unfortunately, the Ca intake decreases with age. Calcium absorption is further decreased by certain drugs, like the aluminum-containing antacids, or in certain states, like achlorhydria. Furthermore, some groups of the population have an even lower Ca intake, for example the patients on sodium-restricted diets, the strict vegetarians, the alcoholics, and those who suffer from lactase deficiency.

One of the most striking abnormalities in postmenopausal osteoporosis, now called osteoporosis type I, is diminished Ca absorption in the group as a whole. If we could overcome this diminished Ca absorption by giving Ca supplements, we might hope that through a mass action these Ca supplements might be able to suppress postmenopausal bone loss. Recent studies by Nordin[8], performed in Adelaide, South Australia, introduce a distinction, based on radiocalcium absorption, between osteoporotics with normal Ca absorption and those with Ca malabsorption, both groups being approximately equally represented. When giving Ca (1 g/d) to normal Ca absorbers, the fasting hydroxyproline/creatinine ratio can be significantly reduced, whether measured after 8 days or after 8 weeks. After 8 weeks the serum alkaline phosphatase level is also significantly reduced. These modifications cannot be obtained with Ca alone in the group of Ca malabsorbers unless calcitriol (0.25 μg/d) is added. In so far as these changes reflect an inhibition of bone resorption (and later also of bone formation) it was anticipated that Ca supplements would only influence those patients without Ca malabsorption. This of course remains to be proven, since the exact mechanism of action of Ca supplements remains to be shown. They probably act through a diminution of the endogenous production of parathyroid hormone, to which postmenopausal women are more sensitive. The subtle distinction between normal absorbers and malabsorbers of Ca is impracticable to the clinician. It is impossible to test with labeled ^{45}Ca or ^{47}Ca all the population at risk for its Ca absorption. Therefore, we have to deal with groups of postmenopausal patients on the whole and see how they fare on Ca supplements.

In this respect the longitudinal study of Nordin et al.[9], performed in Leeds, England, showed that by giving 1.2 g/d of supplemental Ca (elemental Ca, that is), the cortical area of the metacarpals (measured by radiogrammetry) could be maintained, whereas there was a significant loss in the control group, and in the group on Ca + vitamin D, as well as in the group on 1α-hydroxyvitamin D. Furthermore, there was no deterioration in the 'spine score', in contrast to the deterioration observed in the control population. Another longitudinal study was performed by Recker and his co-workers[10] in Omaha, Nebraska, following both the metacarpals by radiogrammetry (cortical bone), and the distal radius by single photon absorptiometry (trabecular and cortical bone). The treatment group was given 1.0 g/d of Ca supplements. This group fared better than the control group, although this was only statistically significant as far as the metacarpals were concerned. Finally, in a recent study by Nilas et al.[11] in Denmark, during the early postmenopausal period the loss of bone, as measured by single photon absorptiometry on the distal part of the forearm (containing significant amounts of trabecular bone), no significant difference was found between three groups of patients with respectively a low, a medium, and a high Ca intake, all supplemented with Ca 0.5 g/d. This study contrasts with the previous ones, but immediate postmenopausal years, as well as the exclusive use of single photon absorptiometry on the distal forearms, may have been determining factors. If women lose bone more rapidly during the immediate postmenopausal period it should be stressed that they continue to lose bone, especially at the distal radius (as we have shown), all their life, and this is what makes them osteoporotic. Therefore, studies should not be restricted to the immediate postmenopausal years.

Longitudinal studies are of course more useful than cross-sectional ones. Nevertheless, the retrospective study performed by Riggs et al.[12] at the Mayo Clinic should be quoted. They found that the vertebral fracture rate decreased significantly on Ca therapy (Ca as calcium carbonate 1.5–2.5 g/d), and fell to half of the rate observed in untreated patients; an encouraging observation.

Finally, the *estrogen-sparing* action of calcium, which has only very recently been demonstrated, should be stressed. Whereas the dose necessary to maintain bone mass after the menopause is 0.625 mg/d of conjugated equine estrogens, lower doses such as 0.3 mg/d, perfectly inadequate when given alone, are effective when given in addition to Ca supplements (1.5 g/d), as demonstrated by Genant et al.[13] in San

Francisco. The method used was quantitative computed tomography scanning of the lumbar vertebral bodies, and selectively measuring trabecular bone loss. Therefore, women who do not tolerate the higher dose of estrogens, for example as far as their breasts are concerned, may fare well on lower doses provided they take Ca supplements.

In conclusion, Ca is essential in building up an adequate peak bone mass, as are other factors like physical activity and the genetic and racial background[14]. As far as bone loss is concerned, Ca probably retards cortical bone loss, which is so important as far as the cervical hip fractures are concerned. Ca possibly is effective in preventing or slowing down trabecular bone loss, but in this regard more work needs to be done with different measuring devices, on different parts of the skeleton, and at different times after the menopause.

REFERENCES

1. Saville, P. (1970). Observations on 80 women with osteoporotic spine fractures. In Barzel U.S. (ed.). *Osteoporosis*. pp. 38–46. (New York: Grune & Stratton)
2. Albright, F., Bloomberg, E. and Smith, P. H. (1940). Post-menopausal osteoporosis. *Trans. Assoc. Am. Physicians*, **55**, 298–305
3. Nordin, B. E. C. (1960). Osteomalacia, osteoporosis and calcium deficiency. *Clin. Orthop*, **17**, 235–57
4. Heaney, R. P., Recker, R. R. and Saville, P. D. (1978). Menopausal changes in calcium balance performance. *J. Lab. Clin. Med.*, **92**, 953–63
5. Matkovic, V., Kostial, K., Simonovic, L., Buzina, R., Broadarec, A. and Nordin, B. E. C. (1979). Bone status and fractures rates in two regions of Yugoslavia. *Am. J. Clin. Nutr.*, **32**, 540–9
6. Sandler, R. B., Laporte, R., Sashin, D., Cauley, J., Bayles, C., Slemenda, C., Petrini, A. and Schramm, M. (1984). The epidemiology of physical activity and postmenopausal bone loss: first year of a clinical trial. In Christiansen, C., Arnaud, C. D., Nordin, B. E. C., Parfitt, A. M., Peck, A. W. and Riggs, B. L. (eds.) *Osteoporosis*. pp. 317–22. (Copenhagen: Aalborg Stiftsbogtrykkeri)
7. Kanders, B., Lindsay, R., Dempster, D., Markhard, L. and Valiquette, G. (1984). Determinants of bone mass in young healthy women. In Christiansen, C., Arnaud, C. D., Nordin, B. E. C., Parfitt, A. M., Peck, A. W., Riggs, B. L. (eds.) *Osteoporosis*. pp. 337–40. (Copenhagen: Aalborg, Stiftsbogtrykkeri)
8. Nordin, B. E. C., Peacock, M., Need, A. G., Horowitz, M., Hartley, T. F. and Philcox, J. C. (1984). The relationship between calcium absorption and fasting urinary calcium and hydroxyproline excretion in postmenopausal women in Leeds and Adelaide. In Christiansen, C., Arnaud, C. D., Nordin, B. E. C., Parfitt, A. M., Peck, A. W. and Riggs, B. L. (eds.) *Osteoporosis*. pp. 513–5. (Copenhagen: Aalborg Stiftsbogtrykkeri)
9. Nordin, B. E. C., Horsman, A., Crilly, A. G., Marshall, D. H. and Simpson, M. (1980). Treatment of spinal osteoporosis in postmenopausal women. *Br. Med. J.*, **1**, 451–4
10. Recker, R. R., Saville, P. D. and Heaney, R. P. (1977). Effects of estrogens and calcium carbonate on bone loss in postmenopausal women. *Ann. Intern. Med.*, **87**, 649–55
11. Nilas, L. Christiansen, C. and Rodbro, P. (1984). Calcium supplementation and post-menopausal bone loss. *Br. Med. J.*, **289**, 1103–6
12. Riggs, B. L., Seeman, E., Hodgson, S. F., Taves, D. R. and O'Fallon, W. M. (1982). Effect of the fluoride/calcium regimen on vertebral fracture occurrence in postmenopausal osteoporosis: comparison with conventional therapy. *N. Engl. J. Med.*, **306**, 446–50
13. Genant, H. K., Cann, C. E., Ettinger, B., Gordan, G. S., Kolb, F. O., Reiser, U. and Arnaud, C. D. (1984). Quantitative computed tomography for spinal mineral assessment. In Christiansen, C., Arnaud, C. D., Nordin, B. E. C., Parfitt, A. M., Peck, W. A. and Riggs, B. L. (eds.) *Osteoporosis*. pp. 65–72. (Copenhagen: Aalborg Stiftsbogtrykkeri)

14. Nagant de Deuxchaisnes, C. (1983). The pathogenesis and treatment of involutional osteoporosis. In Dixon, A. St. J., Russell, R. G. G. and Stamp, T. C. B. (eds.) Osteoporosis: a Multi-disciplinary Problem. pp. 291–333. (London: Academic Press)

FURTHER READING

Anron, J. E., Gallagher, J. C., Anderson, J. *et al.* (1974). Frequency of osteomalacia and osteoporosis in fractures of the proximal femur. *Lancet*, **2**, 229–33

Corless, D., Gupta, S. P., Sattar, D. A., Switala, S. and Bouches, B. J. (1979). Vitamin D status of residents of an old people's home and long-stay patients. *Gerontology*, **25**, 350–5

Feldman, E. B. (ed.) (1983). Nutritional factors in cardiovascular disease. In *Nutrition in the Middle and Later Years*. pp. 107–26. (Littleton, Mass.: Wright-PSG)

Feldman, E. B. (ed.). Diet and plasma lipids and lipoproteins. In *Nutrition and Heart Disease. Contemporary Issues in Clinical Nutrition*, vol. 6, ch. 3. (New York: Churchill Livingstone)

Lipid Research Clinics Prevalence Study (1979). *Circulation*, **60**, 433

Mertz, W. (1981). The essential trace elements. *Science*, **213**, 1332–8

Nordin, B. E. C., Heyburn, P. J., Peacock, M. *et al.* (1980). Osteoporosis and osteomalacia. *Clin. Endocrinol. Metab.*, **9**, 177–205

Parfitt, A. M., Gallagher, J. C., Heaney, R. P., Johnston, C. C., Neer, R. and Whedon, G. D. (1982). Vitamin D and bone health in the elderly. *Am. J. Clin. Nutr.*, **36**, 1014–31

Workshop 9

Self-help groups at middle age

Chairman: R. Schmid-Heinisch (West Germany)
Co-chairman: M. Flint (USA)

M. Flint (USA)
C. Rector (USA)
G. Myrberg (Sweden)
K. MacPherson (USA)

In the first phase of congress planning the title of this Workshop was a bit different – namely: consumer support groups – an expression which includes a more passive attitude. Now, speaking about 'Self-help groups' means introducing the idea of activity, independence and self-determination as distinguishing characteristics and it is exactly this delicate difference between the two terms, which illustrates a central point of our topic in approaching a subject with an enormous impact on almost every part of social life.

The fact that for the first time within the scope of a Menopause Congress this aspect of self-help and self-care is on the program certainly reflects a growing understanding of its meaning. Amazingly enough it took only about 10 years for the rapid growth of the self-help movement – a movement with a great variety of appearances and with about half a million groups throughout the world by now.

Though this workshop presented a very specific, limited field: self-help groups at middle age, it seemed useful to focus – with the introduction of **Schmid-Heinisch** on some general aspects:

(1) self-help groups are – in the first place – a social phenomenon, not a medical one;
(2) they are the reaction to a need;

(3)   they are an expression of dissatisfaction towards the medical and
      social system;
(4)   they are a new way of social learning, in situations and times where
      the networks of family, neighborhood and friendship have lost
      meaning or simply do not exist any more;
(5)   they want to find alternative models of health care, social care,
      social life.

The wide range of definitions of what self-help covers and causes, does
not fit into a strict paradigm, structure or system. No question whether
it concerns post-care groups (after an operation or serious illness), groups
with a common physical and/or emotional problem or encounter and
discussion groups; whether it concerns groups with a facilitator or those
without a guiding person – they all have at least one of the following aims:

(1)   to change behavior;
(2)   to change the individual mental attitude;
(3)   to change circumstances of individuals as well as of society.

This general openness is a symptom of the particular dynamism of self-
help groups and of their effectiveness. Fortunately this lively diversity
became obvious through the different contributions to the Workshop.
Reports were based on analytic as well as on empirical data.

Flint spoke about her work with a 'post-mastectomy self-help group'
for middle-aged patients. They were women in Essex County in the State
of New Jersey – aged 40–50 years – all referred by the American Cancer
Society, to whom Flint gave advice on self-help. She made clear that the
final goal is for the facilitator to leave the group. After an average
interaction of only 1 month, with a weekly group meeting of about
2 hours, she should turn her initially necessary role into a finally unnecessary one. In such a short time this seems to be a great success – for the
guide as well as for the group – if one thinks (beyond the personal
problems of these women) – how sensitive the process is that makes a
group a group.

Contrary to the intimacy of the post-mastectomy group work **Rector**
developed an overview of activities with the title 'Educational outreach
methods'. This presentation about the CLOUT community program –
CLOUT stands for Climacteric Outreach, an affiliate of the Center for
Climacteric Studies at the University of Florida – informed about 'terms
and time' of the program, about 'possible outcomes', about seminars,
discussion groups, brochures, clinics, health fairs, fitness units, mobile
units, private providers – in one phrase: public relations in its very best
meaning, for women at menopause as individuals or as a group.

How it is possible to integrate into a national public program something
as specific as 'Summer camps for women over 40' was presented by

Myrberg in a most vivid report. In Sweden summer camps have a long tradition; no wonder that with the growing women's movement there were camps formed also for and by women only – but the participants were young women! In 1982 the first camp for women over 40 was organized on the island of Gotland, one of Sweden's most popular vacation resorts. During the first summer three times as many women as could be accommodated on the campus wanted to come. There are still always more applications than can be accepted. Some of the rules in these camps seem extraordinary, and at the same time typical for what this Workshop tried to find out a bit more about: namely group procedures. One rule says: no drugs whatever, including psychotropics; no alcohol; smoking outdoors only. Another rule is called 'the trade secret'. That is: women are not allowed to speak among themselves about their profession. 'If I had known you were a dentist I would never have dared to talk with you', said a cleaning woman. 'I thought all social workers were supercilious', remarked another one who had been taken care of by the social authorities. Yet the difference between women with education and those without, still leads to problems: 50% were educated (25% of them with higher education), 50% had no or lower education. This means that the summer camps on Gotland attained one goal which is missed by so many other groups: to approach those women we speak of mostly but we meet so rarely – the underprivileged women.

Again – through the report of **MacPherson** – another perspective of menopause self-help groups got into shape. The review of historical origins, structures and purposes of menopause self-help groups in the United States led to a study on this subject, which was conducted by the Menopause Collective of Cambridge, Massachusetts and started in 1979. Based on social 'grass roots' movements, such as the self-help and women's health movement, two basic models have been developed specially for menopausal women, which are organized and guided by facilitators. The communal goal is that experiences of women defining and dealing with menopausal changes may bring up – also by debating this issue between self-helper and physicians – a new definition of menopause; a definition which could determine the way menopause is viewed and responded to by society in future.

Another model of supporting menopausal women was presented by **Vizzotto** from Italy. She described the work of 'a guided self-help center', which she is running with Elaine Antonucci, a gynecologist, in Milano. The special approach of this center differs from other menopause clinics in Italy not only by quantity but by the fact that the first person to talk with the woman is not a professional expert, nor a psychologist (experiences in this direction very often went wrong in Italy because of affinity to 'being crazy') the first contact is with a woman who is an expert on menopause – a 'menopausologist'. If necessary there is gynecological treatment as well as referral to other doctors, but the main goal is helping the women to overcome their mostly nonphysical problems by themselves. There are discussion groups of about 10–15 persons as well as so-called 'minigroups', with the family members or friends only. There is a direct exchange 'woman to woman' – by phone and by an information box where addresses and special interests are deposited quite informally. An atmosphere of intimacy and volunteer cooperation means this is a place where women find the confidence to make their own decisions.

Two main perspectives which illustrate the present situation regarding self-help and its various contacts with health care and medical service summarized the following discussion:

(1) Clichés and prejudices still have to be cleared up. Self-help groups are neither quackery nor rivalry for medical and/or psychological experts.
(2) The question is not whether self-help groups are necessary – the question is what they bring about.

We have to get involved deeply in why and where and how self-help groups work. We must realize that they are a new method for inducing change – for the individual as well as for societal structure. For self-help groups at middle age 'change' as a keyword has a distinctive meaning.

It is certainly not by chance that all presentations in this Workshop were concerned with projects for women at middle age, though the topic was mutual in regard to sexes. Therefore it was brought out once more here how desirable – no, necessary! – it seems that men at middle age also learn about self-help groups. To make another, further step towards groups of middle-aged couples it should be done under the condition of experiences of women with women only. Following a general consensus this demand must not mean demarcation inside the family or new forms of dependency outside the family. The fact that sometimes husbands and also children make the first connections for their wife, their mother, to participate in women groups (Myrberg) shows an improving understanding on their side. It is true that for women there are mostly rather concrete problems when joining a particular group; but physical complaints may be only part of it.

The fact that the 'greying societies' we are talking about are in reality 'greying societies of women', points out succinctly the bundle of far-reaching questions women at middle age are confronted with. In order to find the answers, we need individual efforts as well as understanding help by others – and, last but not least we will need courage.

FURTHER READING

Kickbusch, I. and Trojan, A. (1981). *Gemeinsam sind wir stärker.* (Frankfurt, aM: Fischer Alternativ)

Lehr, U. M. (1982). Intervention und Rehabilitation in der Gerontologie – die Herausforderung der Zukunft. *Notabene Medici,* **8**

Moeller, M. L. (1981). Anders helfen. *Selbsthilfegruppen und Fachleute arbeiten zusammen.* (Stuttgart: Klett-Cotta)

Myrberg, Gunilla (1981). Kvinnor över 40. *En Bok om Klimakteriet.* (Stockholm: Prisma)

WHO, Regional Office for Europe, Copenhagen (1984). *Self-Help and Health in Europe* (ed. Stephen Hatch and Ilona Kickbusch)

Workshop 10

Contraception in the premenopause

Chairman: **H.-D. Taubert** (Germany)
Co-chairman: **H. Tatum** (USA)

M. Breckwoldt (Germany)
V. Upton (USA)
A. Audebert (France)
P. Stumpf (USA)
E. Connell (USA)

INTRODUCTION

The problem of evaluating the contraceptive needs of the middle-aged woman or couple is a relatively recent phenomenon. The reasons for this are manifold, but the most obvious contributing factor is that the life-expectancy has greatly increased within the last century. Women used to live to their thirties or forties, and many died either in childbirth or with intercurrent infection even before reaching that age[1]. Today, women can expect to live to an age of 70 years or more, and there is some evidence that the expansion of the lifespan has been accompanied by a certain postponement of the menopause[2]. Moreover, the reproductive pattern has undergone deep changes within a few generations in that the number of pregnancies and the duration of lactational amenorrhea has decreased, whilst the number of years with menstrual cycles has greatly increased. As a consequence, women are exposed to the risk of pregnancy for longer periods of time than their ancestors.

Even though the risk of pregnancy is rather low during the years of the premenopause as compared to earlier phases of life, and decreases progressively until menopause, at which time it reaches zero, women over 40 years of age who want to avoid pregnancy must practice contraception, as a certain chance of becoming pregnant remains. The age-dependent decrease in fertility is not due simply to a reduction in the number of ovulatory cycles, and an increase in the number of cycles with an inadequate luteal phase. As the partner ages, his fertility may diminish, too. Moreover, the frequency of intercourse decreases with age, and that relates to the chance of pregnancy (**Stumpf**).

By the same token, as age advances, the dangers of adverse side-effects of certain types of contraceptives such as the oral contraceptives, and from pregnancy and delivery, increase. The latter tend to be more complicated in women over 40 years of age in that there is a higher maternal risk from complications due to obstetrical and concurrent medical problems. There is also a higher fetal risk, and there are more cytogenetic disorders and birth defects, which may even be passed on to the next generation.

A decision has to be made at what time these relative risks balance one another to the point that a particular method of contraception appears to be preferable to others (**Stumpf**). As an unwanted pregnancy in the premenopause is socially, economically, and also medically even more undesirable and unacceptable than in earlier years, the contraceptive method should offer adequate protection even though the chance of becoming pregnant is low. It should be pointed out in this context that the at times almost unrational fear of pregnancy in premenopausal women should not be summarily dismissed, although it may be out of proportion to the actual risk.

IS CONTRACEPTION STILL NEEDED?

As the decrease in fertility during premenopause is a rather variable phenomenon, it is not easy to predict in any individual woman at what point the risk of pregnancy becomes insignificant. Before recommending a particular method the further need for contraception should be determined and, if this should be the case, approximately for what period of time. There is as yet no single test which could be used to answer these questions reliably in all cases, but some guidelines evolved:

(1) When a woman over 40 years of age still menstruates regularly, she is likely to ovulate, too. As a consequence, she is at a risk of becoming pregnant and needs contraceptive protection even when the serum FSH level is already somewhat elevated.

(2) When a premenopausal woman menstruates irregularly the risk of pregnancy has decreased considerably, but ovulatory cycles may recur even after an episode of amenorrhea. The chance of becoming pregnant can therefore not yet be ruled out with certainty. When

such a woman seeks contraceptive advice, the therapeutic benefits of sex hormones have to be weighed with particular care against possible risks.

(3)   No further contraception is needed when a patient has not menstruated for 6 months or more, there is no withdrawal bleeding upon administration of a progestogen, and the serum FSH has reached a critical level. This level was set at 100 mIU/ml by **Stumpf**, but may of course differ in other laboratories.

THE CHOICE OF THE METHOD

When continuing need for contraception has been established, the choice of a suitable method will be guided by the following considerations:

(1)   Are there typical climacteric complaints and symptoms such as hot flushes, bouts of tachycardia and perspiration, insomnia, nervousness, and dyspareunia due to vaginal dryness requiring *estrogen replacement* therapy?
(2)   Are there menstrual irregularities and disturbances such as short cycles, irregular cycles, hypermenorrhea, dysmenorrhea, and premenstrual tension which could eventually require the administration of a *progestogen*?
(3)   Are there uterine abnormalities such as endometrial hyperplasia, leiomyomas, and adenomyosis which could necessitate treatment with *sex hormones*?

HORMONAL CONTRACEPTION IN THE WOMAN OVER 40

Upton's review stated that there is an ever-increasing awareness[3] that women over 40 years of age can suffer from symptoms typical of the menopause (Fig. W10.1). Still, these women are menstruating and sexually active[4, 5].

No-one would deny that some form of contraception is needed in these women over 40, particularly in view of the increased mortality due to childbirth in these older women[6, 7]. Equally true, today, no-one would deny hormone replacement therapy to these same women if their complaints were perceived as severe estrogen-deficiency symptoms[8].

If one weighs the risk of death due to childbirth in the older woman (Fig. W10.2; Table W10.1) versus the risk of death due to cardiovascular accidents or acute myocardial infarction, mortality due to childbirth in the woman over 40 far outweighs the dangers of death due to the use of the birth control pill in either smokers or non-smokers. The data shown in Fig. W10.2 and Table W10.1 suggest that women who smoke are best advised not to use hormonal contraception nor conceive after 40 years of

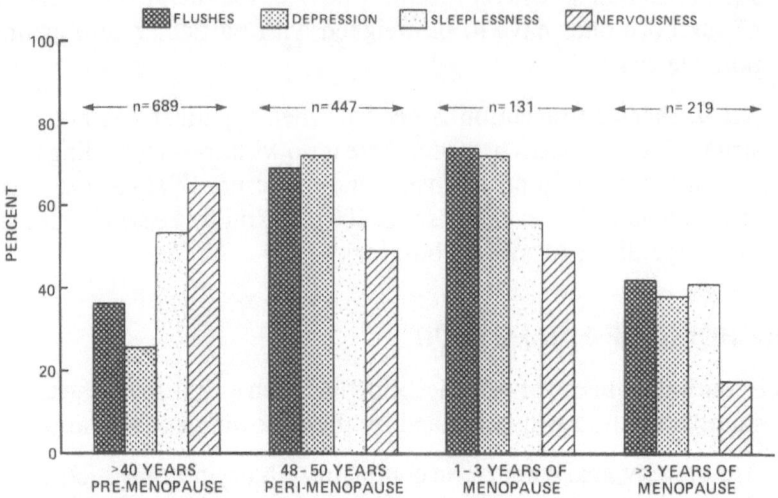

Figure W10.1 The incidence of various subjective symptoms at various ages after 40. These observations demonstrate that symptoms indistinguishable from menopausal complaints can occur in younger menstruating women. (Adapted from Lauritzen[3] with permission of the author)

age. In comparison, the mortality risk for non-smoking women over 40 due to oral contraceptive use is far less than the risks imposed by pregnancy itself in this older age group.

The available contraceptive methods do not adequately fulfill the needs of the woman over 40. A recent clinical study reported by Shargil[9] demonstrated the safe and beneficial effects of a triphasic (Triphasil®/ Trinordiol®) contraceptive in 100 women, age 40–49 years, over a 3-year period. The use of this triphasic contraceptive in older premenopausal

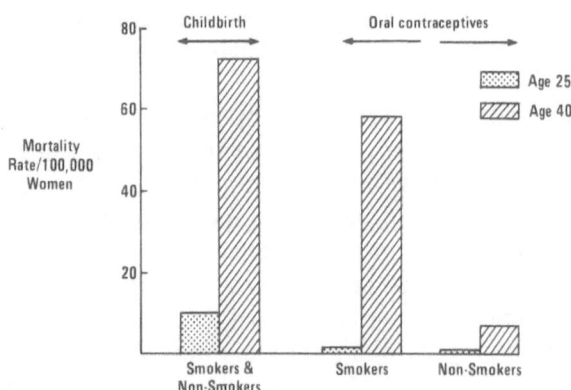

Figure W10.2 Comparison of mortality rates between women age 25 and age 40 or greater due to childbirth or cardiovascular complications associated with the use of oral contraceptives. (Adapted from Greenblatt[20] with permission of the publisher)

Table W10.1 Number and rate of maternal deaths,[a] by age, United States, 1974–78

Age group (years)	Number of deaths	Number of live births	Maternal mortality rate[b]	Relative risk[c]
15	11	59 326	18.5	1.7
15–19	312	2 838 992	11.0	1.0
20–24	645	5 579 344	11.6	1.1
25–29	663	4 863 648	13.6	1.2
30–34	469	2 061 560	22.8	2.1
35–39	319	596 282	53.5	4.9
40–44	114	125 324	91.0	8.3
45	18	7 379	243.9	22.2
Unknown	4	—		
Total	2555	16 131 855	15.8	

[a] Classified by CDC according to the ICD-9 definition of maternal death
[b] Maternal deaths/100 000 live births
[c] Based on an index rate of 11.0 deaths/100 000 live births for 15- to 19-year-olds.
Reproduced from Morbidity and Mortality Weekly Report, Maternal Mortality Surveillance[6].

women provided contraception, relief of symptoms and preservation of bone mass (Fig. W10.3) while maintaining an excellent lipid profile (Fig. W10.4). However, it would seem prudent during the perimenopause (45–55 years) to seek minimal dose products which provide both contraceptive protection and relieve symptomatology.

It is clear from the existing evidence that low-dose combination estrogen–progestogen therapy is strongly advised if any replacement therapy is to be given to the woman over 40, but whether these formulations will also provide effective contraception remains to be proven.

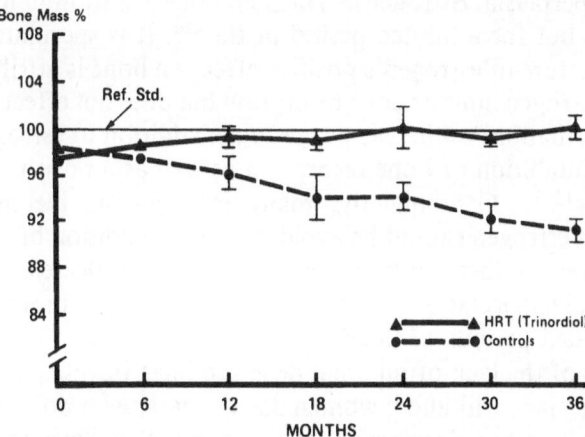

Figure W10.3 A comparison of bone mass measurements of 100 women treated with the triphasic oral contraceptive (Triphasil®/Trinordiol®) as HRT compared with 100 women age-matched controls during a 3-year study. (Reproduced from Shargil[9] with permission of the author and publisher)

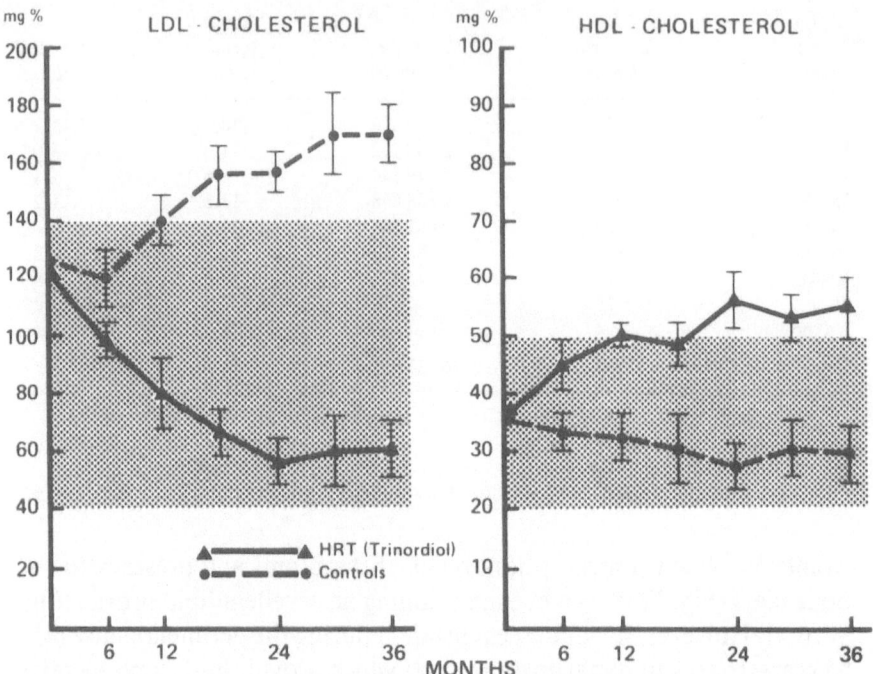

Figure W10.4 A comparison of plasma LDL-cholesterol and HDL-cholesterol values over 3 years in two groups of women; 100 women treated with the triphasic oral contraceptive (Triphasil®/Trinordiol®) as HRT and 100 women age-matched controls. The shaded area indicates the normal range for the laboratory. (Reproduced from Shargil[9] with permission of the author and publisher)

Estrogen alone will ensure tissue support but can also cause endometrial hyperplasia. Estrogen can prevent bone loss by inhibition of bone resorption but for a limited period of time[10]. It is speculated that this transient nature of estrogen's positive effect on bone is attributed to the fact that estrogen inhibits bone resorption but does not effect an increase in bone formation[11]; whereas progestogen addition to estrogen therapy results in inhibition of bone resorption as well as a positive increase in bone mass[12-14]. Consequently, many investigators recommend that unopposed estrogen should be avoided and the addition of progestogen is considered by them to be necessary in order to decrease the risk of endometrial hyperplasia and breast cancer, and to help prevent bone loss over extended periods of time[8, 9, 12-18].

Because of the lack of minimal dose products fulfilling such criteria, many physicians will allow women 35–45 years, who do not smoke, to continue with a low-dose oral contraceptive if they have no contraindications. Hopefully, future research will lead to a product close to ideally fulfilling both the contraceptive and therapeutic needs of women in the climacteric years.

RISKS OF HORMONAL CONTRACEPTION

In an overview on the risks of hormonal contraception, **Breckwoldt** emphasized that our present knowledge is almost exclusively based on epidemiological data which can be used to describe temporal events, but are not suitable to establish causal relationships. Moreover, most observations on side-effects of oral contraceptives were made at a time when preparations were used which contained higher dosages of sex hormones than today.

The first evidence for an association of oral contraceptive use and the incidence of ischemic heart disease, thrombosis, and thrombotic stroke, and a suggested relationship with hemorrhagic stroke which was related to oral contraceptive-induced hypertension, was provided as early as 1970 by Inman et al.[21] As the adverse side-effects appeared to be mainly caused by the estrogenic component and in a dose-related manner, the British Committee on Safety of Drugs recommended using only oral contraceptives containing 50 μg of estrogen or less.

Even though the use of oral contraceptives could not yet be associated with consistent changes in the wall of blood vessels, and there are no uniform and reproducible effects on platelet function (e.g. thromboxane production, prostaglandin release from the vessel wall, aggregation and dissociation of the platelets), the homeostasis of the clotting-system is altered. There is a dose-related increase in factor VII and factor X^{22}, a significant decrease in AT III, a shortened PAT, and an increase in resting fibrinolytic activity caused by the estrogen. It was, however, pointed out by Mammen[23] that all these assays measure only one aspect of coagulation, not the entire system. As a consequence it is not possible to extrapolate these laboratory data to the *in-vivo* situation. It has not even been proven that the observed changes are responsible for thromboembolic phenomena.

Epidemiological studies suggest an increased risk of myocardial infarction for users of oral contraceptives. This appears plausible as oral contraceptives increase the triglycerides and cholesterol in plasma depending on the dose. As high-dose contraceptives also decrease HDL, an acceleration of the arteriosclerotic process appears feasible in the presence of other risk factors. Knopp et al.[24] could show that the HDL level correlates directly with the dose of the estrogenic component, and indirectly with the dose of the progestogen; the arteriosclerotic risk appears to depend, however, both on formulation and dose. This was confirmed by Larsson-Cohn et al.[25] and Briggs[26], who could show that an oral contraceptive containing 30 μg of ethynyl-estradiol and 125 μg levonorgestrel had no adverse effect on the lipoproteins. Even though Slone et al.[27] had calculated a 2.5 risk of myocardial infarction in women between the ages of 40–49 years who had discontinued oral contraceptives years ago, after 10 years of continuous use no evidence could be established in the United Kingdom for the assumption that the mortality risk from ischemic heart disease in women between the ages of 35 and 44 years correlated with the use of oral contraceptives[28].

The rise in blood glucose and in plasma insulin associated with the use of oral contraceptives is usually of no clinical significance. The latter is due to peripheral increased insulin resistance brought about by the progestogen at the level of the insulin receptor. This effect is particularly noticeable when 19-nortesterone derivatives are used. The decreased glucose tolerance and the increased plasma insulin level caused by a combined preparation containing $30 \mu g$ ethyl-estradiol and $150 \mu g$ levonorgestrel suggest that the dose of the progestogen should be reduced[29]. This observation was confirmed in that triphasic preparations seem to have only a minimal effect on carbohydrate metabolism.

Oral contraceptives cause a slight yet significant rise in blood pressure in a dose-dependent manner. This effect seems to be mediated by changes in the renin–angiotensin–aldosterone system[30]. The report of the Royal College of General Practitioners showed, however, that in 1977 not only the dose of the estrogen but also the progestogen dose has to be considered as a causal factor. Low-dose preparations appear to have minimal or no effect[31].

Since Baum et al.[32] suggested that the use of oral contraceptives could be associated with benign liver tumors, more evidence has been presented that 17-alkylated steroids can induce such tumors, which appear histologically as focal nodular hyperplasia or adenomas, and very rarely as carcinomas. The incidence has been estimated to be 1 : 200 000 users. Even though they rarely cause symptoms and are difficult to detect, dramatic symptoms may develop due to rupture of the capsule with ensuing intra-abdominal bleeding. As premenopausal women on oral contraception are likely to have used synthetic steroids for extensive periods of time, the risk of developing a steroid-induced liver tumor should actually be higher than in younger women. Consequently, appropriate diagnostic steps, such as the use of ultrasound for scanning of the liver, should be part of the supervision of therapy when indicated.

Until 1983 no evidence for an increased cancer risk in users of oral contraceptives had been presented. Contrary to that, a reduction in the number of ovarian and endometrial cancers was shown to correlate with the dose and duration of use[33]. Even though Pike et al.[34] and Vessey et al.[35] reported on a higher incidence of breast cancer in young women who had used oral contraception, and a higher incidence of intracervical neoplasia and carcinoma in women using oral contraceptives as compared to intrauterine devices, no convincing evidence for such an association has as yet been presented. The studies were not corrected for important variables such as the number of sexual partners.

The data on adverse reactions towards oral contraceptives imply that the tenet cannot be maintained that the premenopausal woman should if possible not use any hormonal contraceptives. Quite to the contrary, health benefits seem to outweigh disadvantages and possible risks in many women. When an oral contraceptive is, however, prescribed, risk factors and contraindications should be carefully considered, the need for continuation of therapy should be re-evaluated at reasonable intervals, and the course of therapy should be carefully supervised.

INTRAUTERINE DEVICES

In the presence of contraindications against oral contraceptives, an intra-uterine device should be considered as a first alternative, even though there are as yet only sparse data on its performance in premenopausal women. **Audebert** reported that the present available intrauterine devices appear to be quite satisfactory with respect to efficiency, tolerance, acceptance, and reversibility. The clinician should be aware that copper-containing intrauterine devices increase the menstrual flow slightly, the Lippes loop even more, while progestogen-containing ones (progesterone and levonorgestrel) have the opposite effect and ameliorate menstrual cramps. Epidemiological studies indicate that the risk of death with the use of intrauterine devices is one of the lowest in comparison with other methods of birth control. Even though premenopausal women require efficient contraception because their fear of pregnancy is high, the decline in fertility makes a less efficient method such as the intrauterine device very acceptable. In addition, they are less apt to have multiple sexual partners or to get pelvic infection.

Menstrual disturbances such as dysfunctional uterine bleeding or hypermenorrhea, which at times may be associated with endometrial hyperplasia or uterine leiomyomas, may preclude the use of an intra-uterine device, except for a steroid-releasing one. As a consequence, the proper selection of the patients for the insertion of an intrauterine device should include the following steps:

(1) adequate counselling in regard to safety, adverse reaction, and the necessity of controls;
(2) evaluation of the menstrual cycle;
(3) assessment of the pelvic organs and of the uterine cavity.

Sonography is a useful tool to evaluate uterine morphology and the geometry of the uterine cavity, and to control fundal placement which is mandatory to obtain optimal performance. A progestogen may occasionally be administered to women over 40 years of age carrying an intra-uterine device to correct previous or secondary menstrual irregularities and to reduce bleeding, which is the main reason for the removal of an intrauterine device in this age group. Estrogen replacement may become necessary when vasomotor disturbances and other symptoms occur and become annoying.

The risk of pelvic inflammatory disease, cramping and bleeding, extra-uterine pregnancy, expulsion or perforation of the intrauterine device seems to be low in this age group as compared to younger women. The removal can become difficult when postponed until the postmenopause, as the intrauterine device can become trapped in the shrunken uterus. The available studies show that the all-over efficiency of intrauterine devices appears to be quite satisfactory in women over 40 years of age. This probably reflects to some degree the decreased fertility in that age group.

In summary, the intrauterine device appears to be a satisfactory method of contraception for selected pre-menopausal women who do not suffer from climacteric complaints and have normal and regular menstrual cycles.

STERILIZATION

There is a certain number of premenopausal women needing contraception who will not or should not use oral contraceptives, and who are not suitable candidates for the insertion of an intrauterine device. In such a situation, sterilization would be the method of choice unless there are contraindications even for minor surgery, or the patient is not comfortable with the aspect of permanency. Reversal of tubal occlusion should not, however, become an issue in women of that age group.

Sterilization is indicated in the presence of significant obstetrical and medical disease which would increase the risk for complications from oral contraceptives and intrauterine devices, and there are valid reasons against vasectomy of the partner.

The advantages of sterilization are the lower failure rate as compared to temporary methods of contraception, the non-recurring risk, and the possibility of evaluating and treating patients at the same time for other gynecologic disease. The main disadvantages are that it is relatively expensive, more difficult to perform than, e.g., the insertion of an intra-uterine device, and, albeit only once, more dangerous. It was emphasized by **Stumpf** that there is without doubt an increased risk of sterilization with age, mainly due to anesthetic death. Even though there is little information available as to what the actual risk is, it may be surmised that it is certainly less than the death risk from complications of pregnancy in women who do not practice contraception, and from vascular disease in smokers and non-smokers using oral contraceptives. When discussing the pro and con of sterilization with a woman suffering from climacteric symptoms, the continuing need for hormonal replacement therapy should be pointed out.

Sterilization can be done by laparotomy, laparoscopy, and vaginal or abdominal hysterectomy.

Tubal occlusion can be achieved either by laparotomy, mini-laparotomy, or colpotomy. Each method requires entering the peritoneal cavity, but this can be done by a very small suprapubic incision, and will require only a short hospital stay. The *Pomeroy* type of tubal ligation can be carried out by a vaginal or an abdominal approach. It involves tying off the Fallopian tube and removing one segment which can be used for histological verification. After dissolution of the sutures, the two segments of the tube separate, and scar tissue accomplishes the obliteration of the lumen. The *Yoshida* type of procedure is possibly even more effective, as the proximal end of the tube is buried between the two sheets of the mesosalpinx in order to protect it from the continuity of the peritoneal cavity. Less common is the *Kroner* type of procedure which involves amputation of the ampullary end to the tube. It is the least reversible type of tubal occlusion. This should, however, not pose a problem in this age group.

The advantages of laparoscopic sterilization are that the time required to stay in the hospital is, if anything, even shorter while the failure rate and the risks are equivalent to the laparotomy approach. It does, however, require special equipment and trained personnel, as the procedure can be more difficult and dangerous than other methods in the hands of the unskilled.

It is indicated when there is a need to limit surgical and recovery time as much as possible, and when the patient is concerned with the cosmetic effect of a suprapubic scar. Laparoscopy should not be performed in patients with past or present significant pelvic or abdominal disease, in very obese women, and in cases where it is difficult to examine the pelvic organs thoroughly. When there is a risk of peritoneal adhesions in patients who have previously undergone abdominal surgery, the opening of the abdominal cavity and the insertion of the laparoscope should be done under visual control. The obliteration of the lumen of the tube is achieved by electro-coagulation of one or two sections of the organ with a bipolar forceps which is either inserted through the laparoscope or a second puncture. It is disputed whether the effectiveness rate can be further improved by cutting the devitalized part of the tube. The occlusion of the tube can also be done by using clips and other mechanical devices. There is, however, no definite advantage using this approach, as patients of this age class are not likely to request reversal. The result of laparoscopic sterilization can easily be evaluated a few weeks later by performing a hysterosalpingography.

When there is concurrent gynecologic disease such as urinary stress incontinence, prolapse of the uterus, growing leiomyomas, or an adnexal tumor, and, in certain cases, a high risk for developing an endometrial carcinoma, hysterectomy may offer itself as an alternative to other forms of permanent contraception, even vasectomy.

Hysterectomy offers the advantage of being associated with the lowest failure rate. As it is more difficult to perform and more expensive, and involves a higher operative risk, it should not be carried out when there are contraindications for surgery, and in the absence of significant gynecologic disease. The need of contraception alone does not justify hysterectomy.

Vasectomy of the male partner should always be considered as an alternative, as it is cheaper, safer, and easier to perform than sterilization in the female.

CONCLUSION

There was unanimity amongst the members of the panel and the attendees of the Workshop that the premenopausal woman requires special attention with respect to contraception which sets her apart from other age groups, and that the presently available spectrum of contraceptive methods does not yet fulfill all needs. The workshop was brought to a conclusion by an overview on current contraceptive developments given by **Connell**, which showed some hopeful aspects at least with respect to new progestogens and delivery systems, although the recent decision against licensing medroxyprogesterone acetate was considered as a regrettable step in a wrong direction.

REFERENCES

1. Connell, E. B. (1984). Contraceptive needs of the middle-aged couple. *Contemp. Obstet. Gynecol.*, **95**, 115
2. Frommer, D. J. (1964). Changing age of the menopause. *Br. Med. J.*, **2**, 349
3. Lauritzen, C. (1981). The premenopause. In van Keep, P. A. *et al.* (eds.) *The Controversial Climacteric*. p. 9. (Lancaster: MTP Press)
4. Chez, R. A., Jaffe, R. B., Kase, N. G. *et al.* (1976). The sexually active premenopausal woman. *Dialogues in Oral Contraception*, 1(6), 000
5. Greenblatt, R. B., Nezhat, C. and McNamara, V. P. (1979). Appropriate contraception for middle-aged women. *J. Biosoc. Sci.* (Suppl.), **6**, 119
6. Kaunitz, A. M., Rochat, R. W., Hughes, J. M. *et al.* (1984). Maternal mortality surveillance, 1974–1978. *Mortality and Mortality Weekly Report*, **33**, 5SS
7. Tietze, C. and Lewit, S. (1977). Mortality and fertility control. *Int. J. Gynecol. Obstet.*, **15**, 100
8. Speroff, L., Glass, R. H. and Kase, N. G. (1983). The ovary from conception to senescence. In Speroff, L. *et al.* (eds.) *Clinical Gynecologic Endocrinology and Infertility*, 3rd edn, p. 101. (Baltimore: Williams & Wilkins)
9. Shargil, A. A. (1985). Hormone replacement therapy in perimenopausal women with a triphasic contraceptive compound: a three-year prospective study. *Int. J. Fertil.*, **30**(1), 15–28
10. Lindsay, R. (1982). The role of sex hormones and synthetic steroids in prevention of postmenopausal osteoporosis. *Clin. Invest. Med.*, **5**, 189
11. Gordon, G. S. (1978). Drug treatment of the osteoporosis. *Ann. Rev. Pharmacol. Toxicol.*, **18**, 253

12. Nachtigall, L. E., Nachtigall, R. H., Nachtigall, R. D. *et al.* (1979). Estrogen replacement therapy. I: A 10-year prospective study in the relationship to osteoporosis. *Obstet. Gynecol.*, **53**, 277

13. Upton, G. V. (1982). The perimenopause: physiologic correlates and clinical management. *J. Reprod. Med.*, **27**, 1

14. Upton, G. V. (1984). Therapeutic considerations in the management of the climacteric. A critical analysis of prevalent treatments. *J. Reprod. Med.*, **29**, 71

15. Gambrell, R. D. Jr (1984). Hormones in the etiology and prevention of breast and endometrial cancer. *So. Med. J.*, **77**, 1509

16. Whitehead, M. I., McQueen, J., Beard, R. J. *et al.* (1977). The effects of cyclical oestrogen therapy and sequential oestrogen/progestogen therapy on the endometrium of postmenopausal women. *Acta Obstet. Gynecol. Scand.* (Suppl.), **65**, 91

17. Whitehead, M. I., McQueen, J., King, R. J. B. *et al.* (1979). Endometrial histology and biochemistry in climacteric women during oestrogen and oestrogen/progestogen therapy. *J. R. Soc. Med.*, **72**, 322

18. Whitehead, M. I., McQueen, J., Minardi, J. *et al.* (1978). Clinical considerations in the management of the menopause: the endometrium. *Postgrad. Med. J.*, **54**, 69

19. Whitehead, M. I., Townsend, P. T., Pryse-Davies, J. *et al.* (1981). Effects of estrogens and progestins on the biochemistry and morphology of the postmenopausal endometrium. *N. Engl. J. Med.*, **305**, 1599

20. Greenblatt, R. B. (ed.) (1980). *A retrospective view of oral contraceptives in the development of a new triphasic oral contraceptive.* p. 9. (Lancaster: MTP Press)

21. Inman, W. H. N., Vessey, M. P., Westerholm, B. and Englund, A. (1970). Thromboembolic disease and the steroidal content of contraceptives. A report to the Committee on the Safety of Drugs. *Br. Med. J.*, **2**, 203

22. Bonnar, J. and Sabra, A. (1983). Comparative data on the effects of low-dose contraceptives on coagulation. In Elstein, M. (ed.) *Update on Triphasic Oral Contraception.* (Amsterdam: Excerpta Medica)

23. Mammen, E. F. (1982). Oral contraception and blood coagulation. A critical review. *Am. J. Obstet. Gynecol.*, **142**, 781

24. Knopp, R. H., Walden, C. E., Wahl, P. W., Hoover, J. J., Warnieck, R. G., Albers, J. J., Ogilvie, J. T. and Hazzard, W. R. (1981). Oral contraceptives and postmenopausal estrogen effects on lipoprotein triglyceride and cholesterol in an adult female population: relationship to estrogen and progestin potency. *J. Clin. Endocrinol. Metab.*, **53**, 1123

25. Larsson-Cohn, U., Wallentin, L. and Zador, G. (1979). Effects of three different combinations of ethynyl-estradiol and levonorgestrel on plasma lipids and high density lipoproteins. *Acta Obstet. Gynecol. Scand.* (Suppl.), **88**, 56

26. Briggs, M. (1982). Comparative investigations of oral contraceptives using randomized, prospective protocols. In Haspels, A. A. and Rolland, R. (eds.) *Benefits and Risks of Oral Contraception.* (Lancaster: MTP Press)

27. Slone, D., Shapiro, S. and Kaufman, D. W. (1981). Risks of myocardial infarction in relation to current and discontinued use of oral contraceptives. *N. Engl. J. Med.*, **305**, 420

28. Wiseman, R. A. and MacRae, K. D. (1981). Oral contraceptives and the decline in mortality from circulatory disease. *Fertil. Steril.*, **35**, 277

29. Wynn, V. (1982). Effect of duration of low-dose oral contraceptive administration on carbohydrate metabolism. *Am. J. Obstet. Gynecol.*, **142**, 739

30. Oelkers, W., Schöneshöfer, M. and Blümel, A. (1974). Effects of progesterone and from synthetic progestogens on sodium balance and the renin-aldosterone system in man. *J. Clin. Endocrinol. Metab.*, **39**, 882

31. Beral, V. (1977). Royal College of General Practitioners Oral Contraception Study. Mortality among oral contraceptive users. Lancet, **2**, 727

32. Baum, J. K., Holtz, F., Bookstein, J. J. and Klein, W. (1937). Possible association between benign hepatomas and oral contraceptives. *Lancet*, **2**, 926

33. Centers for Disease Control (1983). Cancer and steroid hormone study. Oral contraceptive use and the risk of ovarian cancer. *J. Am. Med. Assoc.*, **249**, 1596

34. Pike, M. C., Krailo, M. D., Henderson, B. E., Duke, A. and Roy, S. (1983). Breast cancer in young women and use of oral contraceptives: possible modifying effect of formulation and age of use. *Lancet*, **2**, 926

35. Vessey, M. P., McPherson, K., Lawless, M. and Yeates, D. (1983). Neoplasia of the cervix and contraception: a possible adverse effect of the pill. *Lancet*, **2**, 930

Workshop 11

Progestins

Chairman: **R. Sitruk-Ware** (France)
Co-chairman: **D. Gambrell** (USA)

C. Kitchens (USA)
R. Lindsay (USA)
M. Whitehead (UK)
J. Thijssen (Netherlands)
S. Sipinen (Finland)
L. Dennerstein (Australia)

The discovery of progesterone is relatively recent, being 50 years old in 1984. Butenandt and Westphal reported that in their first isolation in 1934, the ovaries of 50 000 sows were required to obtain approximately 20 mg of pure corpus luteum hormone[1].

Since that time research has come a long way. Progesterone, (P) the natural hormone, binds to its specific receptors to induce specific progestational effects. In addition to this binding, P is able to interfere with the binding sites of other steroids. Therefore the natural hormone exhibits an anti-estrogenic activity, and anti-androgenic activity and also exerts anti-mineralocorticoid effects[2]. For a long time progesterone could not be used in clinical applications because of a rapid liver inactivation after oral administration. Different types of orally active progestins have now been synthesized and derived from progesterone or 17α-hydroxy-progesterone or from 19-nortestosterone. The latter derivatives have to be converted to norethisterone (NET) to act at the target level. However, it must be kept in mind that all the progestins available on the market differ from the natural hormone. They mimic some of its actions through the progesterone receptor and exert other effects according to the molecule from which they derive and their binding capacities to other steroid receptors. The majority of synthetic progestins are active orally and possess substituted groups that aid bioavailability by delaying metabolism. They are absorbed from the gastrointestinal tract with considerable individual variations, bind to plasma proteins and are metabolized and excreted in urine, bile and feces.

Some progestins (19-norsteroids) interact with the androgen receptor and can produce androgenic effects. In parallel they exert a strong anti-gonadotropic activity and exert the highest anti-estrogenic activity[3]. Other molecules (pregnane derivatives) can inhibit or potentiate the action of androgens. Similar interactions with the glucocorticoid and mineralocorticoid receptors have also been described[2, 4].

More recently, micronized progesterone has been available and has been proved to be active after oral administration. Indeed, after oral ingestion of 200 mg of this drug, the plasma P levels increase at a peak level of 15 ng/ml at the third hour. Then the levels decrease, but remain over 5 ng/ml at the eighth hour (Fig. W11.1). After several days of treatment the plasma levels reach a plateau at about 8 ng/ml.

Since the first retrospective studies indicated that the risk of endometrial carcinoma from estrogen replacement therapy (ERT) was increased 3–10-fold, a 10–13-day course of progestins has been advocated for routine usage with estrogen therapy.

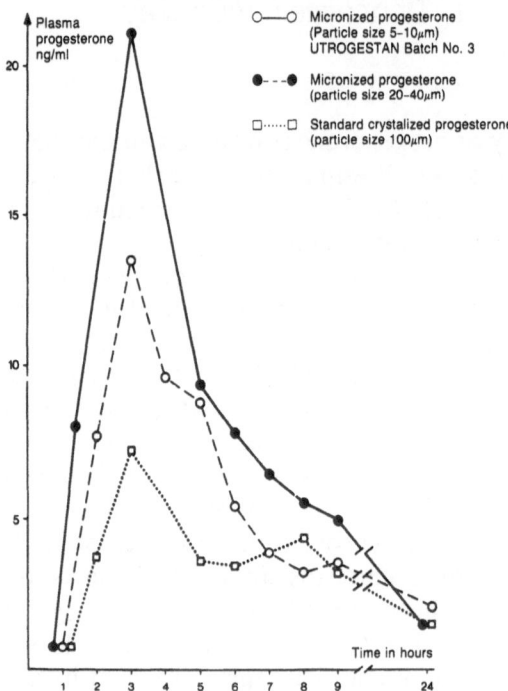

Figure W11.1 Mean plasma progesterone levels obtained with three different forms of oral progesterone in the same four postmenopausal women at 7 days interval

PREVENTION OF ENDOMETRIAL CANCER

Gambrell presented an update of the continuing studies at Wilford Hall USAF Medical Center. The incidence of endometrial cancer continues to decrease each year as more postmenopausal women are treated with progestins (Table W11.1). By 1983 the overall incidence of endometrial cancer declined to 29.1:100 000 women per year. Since the duration of added progestin to ERT was increased to 13 days for the past 2 years, there have been no new cases of adenocarcinoma and the incidence of this cancer for this group for the 9 years was 49.0:100 000 women. Endometrial cancer incidence remains high in the unopposed estrogen users at 390.6:100 000. Not only was the incidence of endometrial adenocarcinoma significantly lower in the estrogen–progestogen users than in the unopposed estrogen users, with $p \leqslant 0.0001$, but it was also significantly lower than that observed in the untreated women, which was 245.5:100 000 women, with $p \leqslant 0.005$.

Table W11.1 Incidence of endometrial cancer at WHMC, 1975–83

Therapy group	Patient-years observation	Patients with cancer	Incidence (per 100 000)
E + P	16 327	8	49.0
Unopposed E	2 560	10	390.6
EVC users	2 716	2	73.6
P or A users	1 160	0	—
Untreated women	4 480	11	245.5
Total	27 243	31	113.8

Incidence of endometrial cancer according to hormonal treatment: E = estrogens, P = progestins, EVC = estrogen vaginal creams, A = androgens

To identify those postmenopausal women who are at increased risk for endometrial cancer, the progestin challenge test should be administered to all postmenopausal women with an intact uterus, said Gambrell. If the patient has withdrawal bleeding then the progestin should be continued for 13 days each month as long as withdrawal bleeding follows.

He also presented some data on the effect of different progestins on serum lipoproteins. With medroxyprogesterone acetate 10 mg there is a good induction of HDL with corresponding reduction in both LDL and VLDL from baseline values. With norgestrel 25 mg, a moderate increase in HDL, no change in LDL, and a good reduction in VLDL was observed. When norethindrone acetate 5 mg was prescribed, there was only a slight increase in HDL, moderate decrease in LDL, and basically no change from baseline levels in the VLDL fraction.

PROGESTERONE RECEPTORS IN TARGET ORGANS

Steroid hormones are supposed to induce their specific effects after binding to specific intracellular proteins, called receptors. In all target organs these receptors have been demonstrated. Only the complex of receptor and the steroid is able to induce the effects.

Binding of progesterone to its receptor results in a change in the apparent localization of the receptor from the cytoplasm to the nucleus of the cell (translocation). The concentration of progesterone receptors (PR) in an organ is thought to be related to the sensitivity of an organ toward stimulation by progestins.

Thijssen pointed out that the regulation of the receptor concentration is not completely understood. In uterine tissues estrogens clearly stimulate the induction of PR. The variation in their endometrial concentration during the menstrual cycle can largely be explained by the effects of estrogens and progesterone on the PR. In non-uterine tissues this relation between estrogenic milieu and induction of the PR is less clear. In a number of these tissues the causal relation between estrogenic influence and the receptor has not been established.

In malignant breast tumors progesterone receptors can be detected usually in combination with estrogen receptors. However, the concentrations of PR do not appear to be regulated simply by the influence of estrogens because in postmenopausal women he found that the levels of PR were higher than in younger women.

Also in other non-uterine tissues the PR levels are not in accordance with the straightforward estrogenic stimulation theory, and their regulation seems to be more complicated.

It must be kept in mind that the breast tissue is different from the endometrium as it is a permanent tissue throughout genital life, and does not shed monthly as does the endometrium.

However, progestins have been shown to be able to act at the breast level just as in the endometrium. Kuttenn et al.[5] have shown that in human breast fibroadenomas, lynestrenol, a potent norsteroid derivative, was able to induce the translocation of the PR from the cytosol to the nucleus. This progestin was also able to induce the increase of 17β-dehydrogenase activity considered to be the marker of the PR action[6]. Percutaneous progesterone applied topically on the breast was also demonstrated to stimulate this enzyme activity[6].

Finally Vignon et al.[7] have reported that R5020, a potent progestogen derived from progesterone, decreased DNA synthesis and cell multiplication in human carcinoma breast cells in culture. The same observation was also reported in human normal breast cells in culture[8].

These data, together with the data of Gambrell[9] indicating a decreased breast cancer risk in estrogen–progestogen users, led us to recommend the addition of progestogens to ERT also in women who had an hysterectomy. It has also been shown that the nortestosterone derivatives, the most potent anti-estrogenic progestins (namely lynestrenol) were able to correct breast symptoms in premenopausal women[10]. Therefore, women with previous benign breast disease, or with breast intolerance while on ERT, could require the use of these potent derivatives to return to a normal state.

EFFECTS OF PROGESTINS ON THE ENDOMETRIUM

In prospective histologic studies the two menopause clinics at King's College and Dulwich Hospital have reported that the addition of progestogens to estrogen therapy reduces the incidence of endometrial hyperplasia, and that these beneficial effects are dependent upon the duration of progestogen administration. Thus, the incidence of hyperplasia, which is 25–30% with estrogen therapy alone, is reduced to 4% with 7 days of progestogen, is further reduced to 2% with 10 days, and is 0 when progestogens are added for 12 days each month.

Since progestogens may have adverse metabolic effects, **Whitehead** made an attempt to determine the minimum dosage of progestogens necessary to suppress endometrial proliferation.

Studies of intracellular mechanisms have shown that progestogens affect epithelium and stroma in similar ways but the mechanisms of action appear dissimilar. In epithelium, progestogens decrease estradiol and progesterone receptor content and reduce DNA synthesis[11]. These actions are classified as antimitotic or antiproliferative. Additionally, progestogens exert a secretory effect and induce the activities of various enzymes, especially estradiol and isocitrate dehydrogenases. Progestogens also induce certain fine structural features observed by transmission electron microscopy, such as giant mitochondria, nucleolar channel systems and subnuclear accumulations of glycogen. The presence or absence of these features can be used to assess progestational activity.

Using conventional light microscopy, transmission electron microscopy and measurements of DNA synthesis, receptor machinery and enzymatic activity, Whitehead and his colleagues have performed doseranging studies of five progestogens currently available for addition to postmenopausal estrogen therapy. With the C19 norderivatives, the currently recommended dosages can be dramatically reduced without loss of protective effect. With the C21 derivatives, adequate doses induced excellent progestational activity. However, with one preparation, variable responses were obtained. Indeed the nuclear estradiol receptor content decreased in the same extent as in the normal luteal phase with the use of 0.7 mg/d norethisterone (NET) or 150 μg of norgestrel (NG), or 300 mg of micronized progesterone (Table W11.2). The decrease in epithelial

Table W11.2 Comparative effects of various progestins on the endometrium

Minimum daily doses	Endometrial protection	Lipids
Norethindrone 0.7 mg	+ + +	?
dl-Norgestrel 150 μg	+ + +	?
MPA ? 10 mg	Variable responses	Minimal effects
Didrogesterone 20 mg	+ + +	?
Oral progesterone 300 mg	+ +	Minimal effects

multiplication exhibited the same pattern with the reported doses. Whitehead concluded that 0.7 mg/d NET was as equipotent as 150 μg DL-NG or 20 mg/d didrogesterone or 300 mg/d micronized progesterone, but 10 mg/d medroxyprogesterone acetate gave inconstant results.

Good antimitotic effect is attractive clinically, he said, because in the absence of endometrial proliferation, amenorrhea will result. Thus it may be possible to develop regimens in which the endometrium is protected against excessive estrogenic stimulation, yet the patient does not have a withdrawal bleed. Therefore the currently recommended daily dosage of progestins can be dramatically reduced to prevent estrogen-induced dependent endometrial hyperplasia. However this proves true as far as the endometrium is concerned but remains to be demonstrated also in other target cells.

ROLE OF PROGESTOGENS ON THE BONE

While it is now well established that estrogens prevent osteoporosis, the role of progestogens is still in doubt. Since in many situations physicians may wish to prescribe progestogens together with, or even instead of, estrogens, it is important to determine whether or not progestogens by themselves can influence skeletal metabolism or interact with the estrogenic effects on bone.

In a preliminary study, **Lindsay** demonstrated that gestronol, a depot synthetic progestogen, could reduce bone loss in postmenopausal women. However, bone turnover appeared not to be reduced, unlike the effects following estrogen administration. He also demonstrated that norethisterone reduces bone loss, again without any effect on urinary hydroxyproline. However, norgestrel (NG) was poorly tolerated by patients and failed to reduce bone loss. Therefore he underlined the fact that compliance was low in this group of therapy and accounted for the lack of effect. When added to estrogens NG did not reverse the beneficial estrogenic effects. Some preliminary evidence suggests that medroxyprogesterone may also reduce bone loss, said Lindsay.

The addition of a progesterone to estrogen appears from his studies not to affect significantly the action of estrogen in prevention of bone loss.

The mechanism of action of progestogens on the skeleton is unclear. Human and animal experiments give conflicting results, some suggesting reduced turnover, others failing to detect this. Progestogens could, theoretically, interact with glucocorticoid receptors in bone, but the interaction is such as not to be meaningful at physiological or pharmacological concentrations of the progestogens, said Lindsay. No evidence is available to indicate whether or not progestogens influence the PTH–vitamin D–calcitonin axis, as has been suggested for estrogens, concluded Lindsay.

The anabolic effect of norsteroids through their binding to androgen receptors could account for their action. From these data it could be concluded that in women with contraindications to estrogens, 19-norsteroids and mainly NET could be a good alternative to decrease bone loss.

EFFECTS OF PROGESTINS ON PLASMA LIPOPROTEINS

Sipinen's contribution discussed the fact that with any active drug drawbacks exist and side-effects occur. The main reason advocated to accuse progestins was the fact that HDL cholesterol (HDLC) decreased and the beneficial effect of estrogens was reversed. Previously, Fahraeus et al.[12] have shown that norgestrel, the most androgenic progestin, reversed the increase in HDL2 cholesterol induced by estradiol while natural micronized progesterone did not. Sipinen showed that the most androgenic progestins leading to a decrease in sex hormone binding globulin (SHBG) and to an increase in free testosterone index (FTI) were able to increase hepatic lipase and therefore decrease HDLC.

Hepatic endothelial lipase (HL), an enzyme of the liver, has a catalyzing function in the degradation of the surface of the HDL particles prior to its catabolism. The effects of progestins with androgenic properties on plasma HDLC are claimed to be mediated by changes in the activity of HL. Minor daily doses of progesterone-derived megestrol acetate (MGA), medroxyprogesterone acetate (MPA) and ST1435, as well as nortestosterone-derived desogestrel (DG) have no significant effects on plasma lipoprotein, whereas even small daily doses of levonorgestrel (NG) and tibolone (ORG OD14) decrease HDLC and increase the LDL/HDLC ratio. This was also observed when MPA was administered in relatively high daily doses. Progesterone and MGA had no effects on plasma lipoprotein even when high doses were used. Decrease in HDLC after NET administration seems to be dose-dependent, said Sipinen.

The method of progestin administration, oral or parenteral, influences SHBG capacity and the free testosterone (T) in plasma. The free testosterone index (FTI), the ratio between the total T and SHBG, characterizes the androgenicity of a progestin. HL and FTI were increased significantly and HDLC was decreased simultaneously in postmenopausal women treated with NG. On the contrary, DG did not significantly influence either HL, FTI or HDLC. A positive correlation has been observed between the changes in FTI and HL; a negative one between the changes in HL and HDLC. In contrast to estrogens, androgenic progestins decrease SHBG capacity. However, no significant interrelationship was observed between the changes if FTI and HDLC, which supports the idea that the effects of progestins on HDLC are mediated by induction of sex steroid-sensitive hepatic endothelial lipase, concluded Sipinen.

PROGESTIN ACTION ON COAGULATION

There is some epidemiologic evidence that progestins, particularly at higher doses, may predispose patients to increased risks for cerebrovascular accident, to pulmonary embolus, or to deep venous thrombosis.

Kitchens studied women on estrogen (Premarin) and progestin (Provera) containing replacement regimens. He studied three groups of women: (a) control; (b) those on 0.625 mg Premarin and 10 mg Provera; (c) those on 1.25 mg Premarin and 10 mg Provera. Estrogenic agents were given on days 1–21 and progestins on days 15–21 of each month. Samples were drawn at baseline and after 6, 12, and 18 months of administration of these preparations. Plasma was coded and studied by technicians unaware of the patients' pharmacologic regimen. Antithrombin III, $\alpha 1$-antitrypsin, and $\alpha 2$-macroglobulin were unaffected. Total plasminogen activity significantly increased in both hormone-treated groups.

Kitchens said that it does not appear from a coagulation laboratory standpoint that there is any *in vitro* evidence for 'hypercoagulability' in studying plasma from patients taking progestins in the manner prescribed. Rather, he concluded, there is slight evidence that total fibrolytic activity may be enhanced by such agents.

PSYCHOLOGICAL EFFECTS OF PROGESTINS

Progesterone itself exerts hypnotic effects through its 3α-reduced metabolites[13], while nortestosterone derivatives can stimulate aggressivity. The difficult and controversial subject of the psychological effects of progestins was reviewed by **Dennerstein**.

She tested the efficacy of natural micronized progesterone on premenstrual symptoms using a menstrual distress questionnaire in a double-blind, controlled, randomized study using either micronized progesterone (300 mg daily from day 17 to day 26 of the cycle) or placebo. She clearly showed that progesterone was highly effective in correcting premenstrual anxiety and psychological disability[15] (see Fig. W11.2).

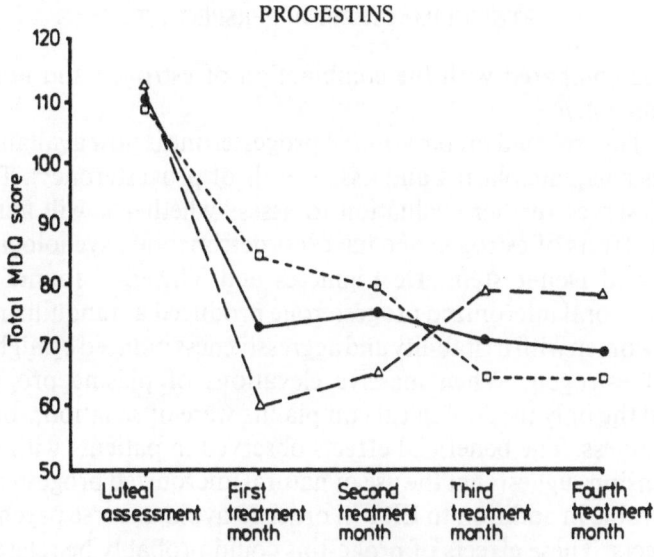

Figure W11.2 Comparison of total scores in menstrual distress questionnaire (MDQ) (transformed) for all subjects (●—●) and subjects grouped according to order of treatment (progesterone followed by placebo: △—△; placebo followed by progesterone: □– – –□).

There has also been some controversy as to the effects of estrogens and progestins on psychological complaints of climacteric women. Once again, discrepancies between studies appear due in part to methodology. The necessity of adequate description of menopausal status; number in sample; psychometric tests for assessing change; length of therapy; crossover design to allow for interpatient variability in response and assessment of change; and reduction of bias by double-blind techniques have been highlighted by Dennerstein et al.[14] When trial methodology has overcome these problems, the beneficial effects of estrogen on psychological complaints have been demonstrated. Few double-blind studies have evaluated the psychological effects of progestins either alone or in combination with estrogen.

In a study of 49 oophorectomized women[14] the effects of an estrogen and a progestin were evaluated alone and in combination, and compared with the effects of placebo. The study was double-blind, crossover and randomized so that each woman received 3 months each of the following medications: ethinyl estradiol 50 μg/d, levonorgestrel 250 μg/d, 'Nordiol', the combination of these two substances; and placebo.

Ethinyl estradiol was found to have beneficial effects on psychological symptoms such as depression, anxiety, irritability and insomnia. The norgestrel when given alone showed less beneficial effects than did estrogen alone, or the combination of norgestrel and estradiol, but was more effective than the placebo. Differences between medications were less obvious by the third therapy month. There were no statistically significant differences in effects on psychological variables when estrogen alone was compared with the combination of estrogen and norgestrel, said Dennerstein.

An oral micronized preparation of progesterone is now available which produces adequate plasma and tissue levels of progesterone[16]. This substance deserves further evaluation to assess whether it will antagonize harmful effects of estrogen and have less detrimental psychological side-effects, said Dennerstein. De Lignières and Vincens[17] found that the addition of oral micronized progesterone produced a tranquilizing effect in those women with irritability and aggressiveness induced by high plasma levels of estrogen. When massive elevations of plasma progesterone occurred the only psychological complaints were of sedation, sometimes with dizziness. The beneficial effects observed in patients with premenstrual tension suggest that the use of natural micronized progesterone will be preferable in addition to ERT in order to avoid adverse psychological side-effects. These effects of progestins could probably be related to the binding of progesterone derivatives to steroid receptors in the central nervous system, as previously reported[18].

To summarize, the value of progestogens in preventing estrogen-stimulated hyperplasia was clearly endorsed during this Workshop. A 13 days/month course should be recommended even in women with hysterectomy.

The potential metabolic side-effects could be avoided by the restriction of progestogen usage to progesterone and its derivatives, or to the prescription of low doses of all progestogens. However the low doses of progestins are active in preventing endometrial hyperplasia but their efficacy at the other target levels remain to be demonstrated.

It must be kept in mind that ERT needs low levels of estrogens to correct symptoms and prevent osteoporosis. Therefore, low doses of progestogens would be sufficient to antagonize estrogen action. Also, as the menopausal women do not need a blockade of the gonadotropins to relieve symptoms, the use of natural progesterone could be more useful in preventing unopposed estrogenic effect, and devoid of side-effects.

REFERENCES

1. Butenandt, A. and Westphal, U. (1974). Isolation of progesterone. Forty years ago. *Am. J. Obstet. Gynecol.*, **120**, 137–41
2. Wambach, G., Higgins, J. R., Kem, D. C. I. (1979). Interaction of synthetic progestogens with renal mineralo-corticoid receptors. *Acta Endocrinol.*, **92**, 560–7
3. Edgren, R. A. and Sturtevant, F. M. (1976). Potencies of oral contraceptives. *Am. J. Obstet. Gynecol.*, **125**, 1029–38
4. Bardin, C. W. (1983). The androgenic, antiandrogenic and synandrogenic actions of progestins. In Bardin, C. W. *et al.* (eds.) *Progesterone and Progestins.* pp. 135–61. (New York: Raven Press)
5. Kuttenn, F., Fournier, S., Durand, J. C. and Mauvais-Jarvis, P. (1981). Estradiol and progesterone receptors in human breast fibroadenomas. *J. Clin. Endocrinol. Metab.*, **52**, 1225–9

6. Fournier, S., Kuttenn, F., De Cicco, N., Baudot, N., Malet, C. and Mauvais-Jarvis, P. (1982). Estradiol 17β-hydroxysteroid dehydrogenase activity in human breast. *J. Clin. Endocrinol. Metab.*, **55**, 428-33

7. Vignon, F., Bardon, S., Chalbos, D. and Rochefort, H. (1983). Anti-estrogenic effect of R5020, a synthetic progestin in human breast cells in culture. *J. Clin. Endocrinol. Metab.*, **56**, 1124-30

8. Malet, C., Gompel, A., Spritzer, P., Kuttenn, F. and Mauvais-Jarvis, P. (1984). Effect of estradiol and the synthetic progestin promegestone (R5020) on the proliferation of human mammary cells in culture. *Ann. NY Acad. Sci.* (In press)

9. Gambrell, R. D. (1984). Proposal to decrease the risk and improve the prognosis of breast cancer. *Am. J. Obstet. Gynecol.*, **150**, 119-32

10. Sitruk-Ware, R., Seradour, B. and Lafaye, C. (1980). Treatment of benign breast diseases by progesterone applied topically. In Mauvais-Jarvis, P. *et al.* (eds.) *Percutaneous Absorption of Steroids.* pp. 219-29. (London: Academic Press)

11. Whitehead, M. I., Townsend, P. T., Pryse-Davies, J., Ryder, T. A. and King, R. J. B. (1981). Effects of estrogens and progestins on the biochemistry and morphology of the post-menopausal endometrium. *N. Engl. J. Med.*, **305**, 1599-604

12. Fahraeus, L., Larsson-Cohn, U. and Wallentin, L. (1983). Norgestrel and progesterone as different influences on plasma lipoproteins. *Eur. J. Clin. Invest.*, **13**, 447-53

13. Gyermek, L., Iriarte, J. and Crabbe, P. (1968). Structure–activity relationship of some steroidal hypnotic agents. *Steroids*, **11**, 117-25

14. Dennerstein, L., Burrows, G. D., Hyman, G. and Sharpe, K. (1979). Hormone therapy and affect. *Maturitas*, **1**, 77-92

15. Dennerstein, L., Spencer-Gardner, C., Gotts, G., Brown, J. B., Smith, M. A. and Burrows, G. D. (1985). Progesterone and the premenstrual syndrome: a double blind crossover trial. *Br. Med. J.*, **290**, 1617-21

16. Whitehead, M. I., Townsend, P. T., Gill, D. K., Collins, W. P. and Campbell, S. (1980). Absorption and metabolism of oral progesterone. *Br. Med. J.*, **280**, 825-7

17. De Lignières, B. and Vincens, M. (1982). Differential effects of exogenous estradiol and progesterone in mood in postmenopausal women: individual dose–effect relationship. *Maturitas*, **4**, 67-72

18. MacLusky, N. J. and McEwen, B. S. (1980). Progestin receptors in the brain and pituitary of the bonnet monkey: differences between the monkey and the rat in the distribution of progestin receptors. *Endocrinology*, **106**, 185-91

Workshop 13

Pharmacology of estrogens

Chairman: **T. E. Shellenberger** (USA)
Co-chairman: **C. Lauritzen** (West Germany)

C. Longcope (USA)
J. Fishman (USA)
B. von Schoultz (Sweden)
B. Düsterberg (West Germany)
R. A. Lobo (USA)
H. Wotiz (USA)

ALTERNATIVE ROUTES OF ESTROGEN ADMINISTRATION

Von Schoultz: Oral *substitution* with estrogen tablets is by far the most common therapy in clinical practice. It is simple, convenient and has a well-documented effect against various postmenopausal symptoms, but cannot be regarded as a physiologic substitution. Following oral treatment, an initial inactivation of steroids commences first in the gut where a considerable part of given estradiol is converted to estrone. The intestinal absorption is rapid and yields extremely high concentrations of hormone in the portal circulation to be further converted in the liver. Within 30–60 min after ingestion of a tablet, rapidly increasing concentrations occur also in the peripheral circulation. Most of the circulating hormone is estrone and during oral treatment the ratio between estrone and estradiol is temporarily highly increased[1]. This pattern contrasts sharply with the physiological situation in women of fertile age (Fig. W13.1).

Hypertension, venous thromboembolism and gall bladder disease are potential side-effects of estrogen treatment and may reflect an estrogenic influence on protein synthesis in the liver. Liver protein synthesis is

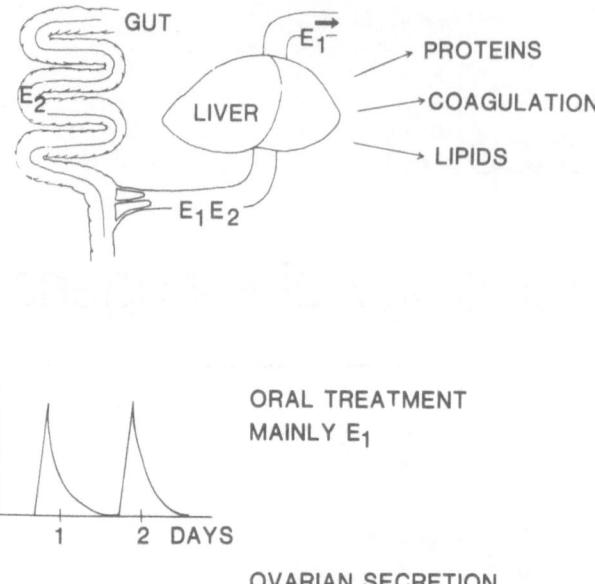

Figure W13.1 Following oral administration the rapid intestinal absorption and conversion of estradiol (E_2) into estrone (E_1) yields high concentrations of hormone in the portal circulation and unphysiological fluctuations of peripheral E_1 levels

extremely sensitive to estrogenic influence and oral therapy increases the serum concentrations of several proteins. The effect is clearly dose-dependent. Sex hormone binding globulin (SHBG), corticosteroid binding globulin (CBG), pregnancy zone protein (PZP) and ceruloplasmin are four highly estrogen-inducible proteins which have been used for dose response comparisons as regards the liver effects of oral therapy[2, 3]. The similar dose-dependent increase in proteins such as renin substrate and coagulation factors may be related to side-effects during oral therapy[4], while the same dose-dependent increase of HDL cholesterol at present is regarded as favorable[5]. Although specific estrogen receptors have been demonstrated in hepatic cells, the liver differs from other target organs in that the hormone is rapidly metabolized and processed. Most active steroids including progestogens are excreted as sulfo- and glucuro-conjugates and hence metabolized in the liver. The interaction between steroids and other substances which are normally metabolized in the liver contributes a further stress to hepatic cells. Some estrogen effects upon the liver are summarized in Table W13.1.

Table W13.1 Estrogen effects on liver metabolism

Affected function	Possible consequences
Plasma protein synthesis	Increase of transport proteins
	Hypertension
Blood coagulation	Increase of clotting factors
	Thromboembolism
Lipid metabolism	Increase of HDL fraction
	Reduced risk of ischemic heart disease
Secretory function	Bile secretion reduced
	Gall bladder disease
	Cholestasis of pregnancy
Glucose metabolism	Reduced glucose tolerance
	Diabetes
Enzymatic metabolism	Sex differences
	Altered drug tolerance
Phagocytic function	Increased phagocytosis
	Immunological effects?

The most important problem during clinical estrogen treatment is not to achieve therapeutic efficacy but rather to avoid overtreatment. While all estrogenic compounds when given at sufficient doses are effective in that they cure menopausal flushing and reverse atrophic changes, they differ considerably with respect to structure, pharmacology and metabolism. *Ethinyl estradiol* is a synthetic and comparatively potent estrogen. As a result of the alkylation in 17-C position it is not a substrate for 17β-dehydrogenase, an enzyme which transforms natural estradiol-17β to the less potent estrone in target organs. Ethinyl estradiol has a half-life of 7 h and is not bound to sex hormone binding globulin (SHBG). Ethinyl estradiol in doses of 30–50 μg is most frequently used in oral contraceptives, and doses around 10 μg daily are often effective in the treatment of menopausal flushing. However, the marked interference with hepatic metabolism should make less potent estrogens the first choice. Treatment with *conjugated estrogens* is the most common regimen in England and the United States. Estrone sulfate is the main component of this preparation but it also contains about 30% of equilin and equilenin. These equine estrogens are very potent when administered in the human species, and like ethinyl estradiol they are not subject to enzymatic metabolism in the liver and other target organs. During postmenopausal replacement doses exceeding 0.625 mg should mostly be considered as overtreatment and a lower dose such as 0.3 mg often has a quite satisfactory effect. *Estradiol-17β* is the terminal biologically active natural estrogen and the pharmacologically active part of estradiol valerate, which is at present the most common compound for postmenopausal therapy in Scandinavia. As compared to ethinyl estradiol it has a half-life of 90 min and is extensively bound to SHBG. Doses of 1–3 mg have well-documented effects on climacteric symptoms and relatively modest effects on metabolic parameters.

Estriol, another naturally occurring estrogen, is often prescribed in doses of 1–3 mg daily for the treatment of local symptoms of urogenital atrophy. As a 'weak' estrogen with a short retention time in the nucleus of target cells it has been proposed also to have anti-estrogenic properties. However, when given at higher doses and repeated intervals estriol is also capable of inducing a complete estrogenic response such as endometrial proliferation. With any kind of therapy, benefits and relief of symptoms have to be carefully weighed against adverse side-effects and possible complications. The route of administration certainly has an effect on the metabolic fate of estrogens. In terms of liver protein induction a single oral dose of 10 μg of ethinyl estradiol roughly equals 1 mg of conjugated estrogens, 4–5 mg of estrone sulfate and 5–7 mg of estradiol preparations.

Alternative routes for estrogen administration have been studied in attempts to reduce the theoretical disadvantages of oral treatment. *Vaginal application* has been found to give a rapid and very efficient absorption of both estrone and estradiol[6]. Estradiol, and in particular estriol, are much more effectively absorbed by the vaginal than by the oral route. Plasma estradiol peak levels after vaginal application of 0.25 mg of estradiol were about 5 times higher than when 2 mg estradiol was given orally. Although there is some conversion into estrone estradiol levels clearly predominate in plasma. The vaginal absorption varies considerably between individuals. The vehicle and the maturation of the vaginal epithelium are important factors in this respect. Compared with oral and vaginal treatment the absorption following *percutaneous application* is slower and less effective, but still allows a satisfactory substitution. Estrogen serum levels are more stable during therapy[1]. When the first liver pass is avoided the conversion of estradiol into estrone, which is a consequence of the oral administration, will be less pronounced and the estrone/estradiol ratio in the circulation will more closely resemble the physiological situation in fertile women. There is no change in estrogen-sensitive liver proteins[4, 7]. Percutaneous application may also allow a flexible therapy. A satisfactory effect on vasomotor symptoms has been reported with a daily dose of 1.5 mg of estradiol-17β, which can be adjusted by ±50%. Treatment with estradiol 2 mg orally and 3 mg percutaneously seem quite equipotent as regards therapeutic effect, FSH inhibition and serum levels of total and free estradiol. There is no evidence that the percutaneous route *per se* would carry an increased risk of overtreatment[8].

PHARMACOLOGICAL AND PHARMACOKINETIC ASPECTS CONCERNING THE THERAPEUTIC USE OF ESTRADIOL IN THE CLIMACTERIC FEMALE

Düsterberg: About 50–80% of all women in the age group between 45 and 65 years show various symptoms accompanying the climacteric.

According to Kuppermann[9] about 40% of all climacteric disorders respond well to placebos. The clinical results obtained with sympatholytic and psychotropic drugs are not much better. While the symptomatic drug therapy eliminates only some of the climacteric symptoms, hormonal substitution, being a causal therapy, influences most of the various climacteric changes[10]. In so far as menopausal treatment is aimed at replacing lost ovarian secretion, it is logical to use 17β-estradiol, the principal circulating estrogen of the women of reproductive age. With the loss of follicular aromatase activity and a decline in ovarian precursors following the menopause, circulating estradiol levels decrease from a premenopausal mean of 120 pg/ml to only 13 pg/ml[11]. Substitution therapy should result in plasma concentrations of 17β-estradiol, estrone and estriol comparable to those observed in the major part of the normal ovulatory cycle. Such a therapy would lead to optimum effect with a desired minimum of side-effects and risks. Some preparations are in use by the medical practitioner which contain 17β-estradiol or estradiol valerate alone or in combination with progestogenic compounds or weak androgens like dehydroepiandrosterone (Table W13.2). Approved preparations for oral and parenteral administration permit individual treatment of women who ask for medication. Special galenic systems in development are noted in Table W13.2.

Estradiol valerate is effective by both the intramuscular and the oral routes of administration and is well suited for the treatment of the characteristic symptoms accompanying the menopause in women. Both routes

Table W13.2

	Dosage forms	Ingredients	
Commercial products	Coated tablets	Estradiol valerate	2 mg
		Estradiol valerate	1 mg
		Estradiol valerate	2 mg + norgestrel 0.5 mg
		Estradiol valerate	1 mg + estriol 2 mg
	Tablets	Estradiol	1 mg
		Estradiol	2 mg
		Estradiol	2 mg + estriol 1 mg
		Estradiol	4 mg + estriol 2 mg + norethisteronacetat 1 mg[a]
		Estradiol	2 mg + estriol 1 mg + norethisteronacetat 1 mg[a]
	Oily solutions	Estradiol valerate	4 mg + dehydroepiandrosterone enanthate 200 mg
		Estradiol valerate	4 mg + testosterone enanthate 90.3 mg
		Estradiol valerate	10 mg
In development		Implants, vaginal rings, transdermal systems	

[a] For sequential regimen

of administration give rise to some major differences in pharmacokinetic behavior and pharmacological efficacy of the drug.

While 1-4 mg of estradiol valerate has to be taken daily by mouth for about 21 days, 4 mg of the same estrogen can be sufficient for 2-4 weeks following a single intramuscular injection as an oily solution. It has been shown in laboratory animals and in humans that, following intramuscular administration, estradiol valerate is completely released from the oily depot at the site of administration[12]. Release of the ester takes place slowly because of increased lipophilia caused by the valeric acid, so that a depot effect is achieved.

The steroid ester released is split by enzymatic hydrolysis into 17β-estradiol and the fatty acid (Fig. W13.2). Estradiol valerate is also split after oral administration during the absorption process and the first liver passage.

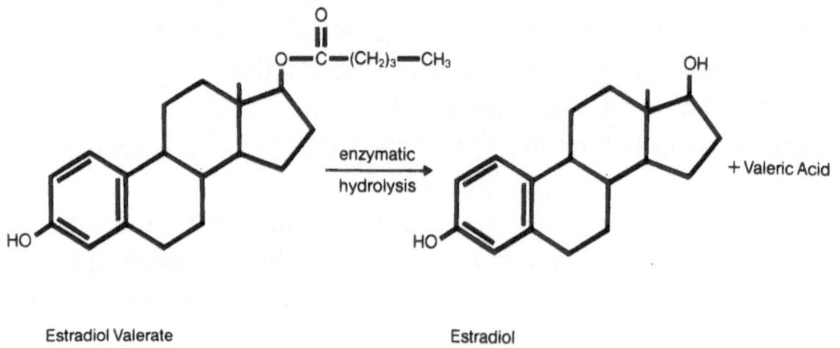

Figure W13.2

As is apparant from comparison of the areas under the curves representing the β-estradiol levels in plasma following intravenous and intramuscular administration of estradiol valerate, 17β-estradiol becomes completely bioavailable in humans when administered intramuscularly as estradiol valerate[12].

Because of the delayed release of the steroid ester from the intramuscular depot referred to earlier the blood level does not reach its maximum before 3-5 days, after which it falls slowly with a half-life of 4-5 days[13]. A distinct increase in the estradiol level can be achieved over a period of about 14 days, with one intramuscular injection of 4 mg estradiol valerate (Fig. W13.3). The systemic availability of estradiol after oral administration of the steroid ester is greatly limited.

As a result of the metabolic process in the gastrointestinal tract, the intestinal wall and the liver, not only does cleavage take place very rapidly, but the free estradiol is subject to further metabolic changes (Fig. W13.4).

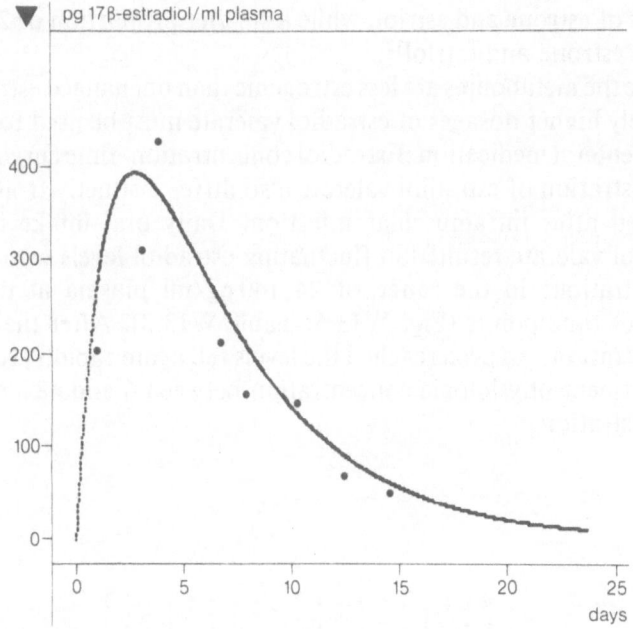

Figure W13.3 Plasma level of 17β-estradiol following a single intramuscular injection of 4 mg estradiol valerate in the human. The curve is the result of an adaptation of measured values produced with the aid of a single compartment model (●, mean values, $n = 2$)

A comparison of the areas under the curve representing estradiol levels following intravenous and oral administration of estradiol valerate in humans made it possible to estimate the system availability. An average of about 3% of the orally administered dose of 2 mg becomes bioavailable as metabolically unchanged estradiol and can exert its effects. About 30%

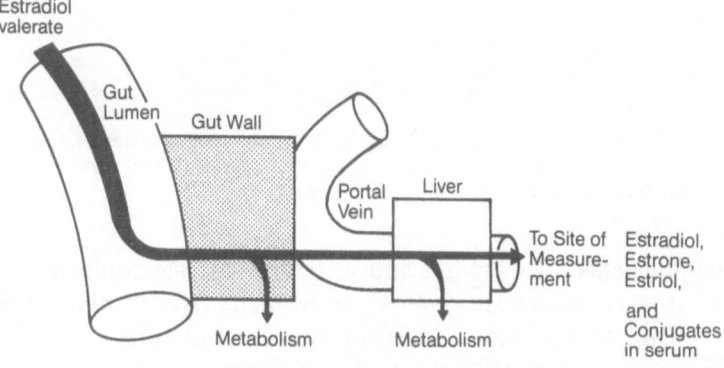

Figure W13.4

of the resulting metabolites are sulfuric acid and glucuronic acid conjugates of estrone and estriol, while a smaller proportion of 2% is made of free estrone and estriol[12].

Since the metabolites are less estrogenic than unchanged estradiol, considerably higher dosages of estradiol valerate must be used for oral than for parenteral medication. Estradiol concentration–time curves after oral administration of estradiol valerate also differ distinctly from the curve obtained after intramuscular injection. Daily oral intake of 2 mg of estradiol valerate resulted in fluctuating estradiol levels with maximum concentrations in the range of 24–140 pg/ml plasma at individually different time points (Fig. W13.5; Table W13.3). After the maximum concentration had been reached the levels fell again rapidly, reaching the pretreatment physiologic concentration between 6 and 48 h after single administration.

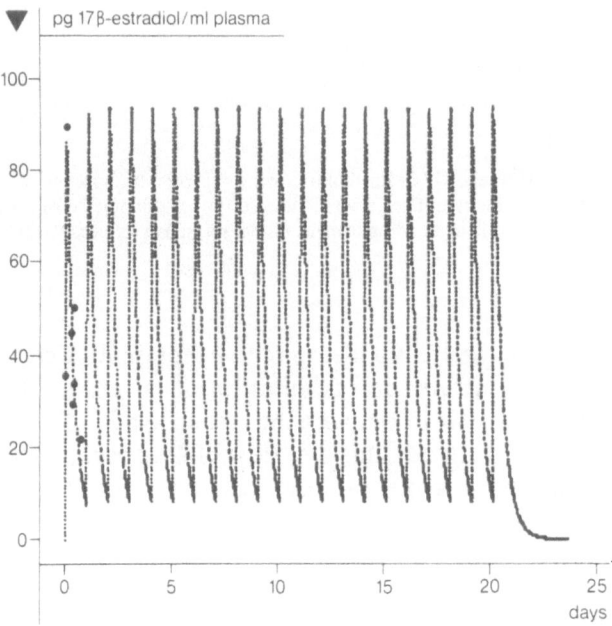

Figure W13.5 Plasma level of 17β-estradiol on daily oral administration of 2 mg estradiol valerate in the human. Computer simulation based on the mean 17β-estradiol level measured after a single oral dose in 2 postmenopausal women

Bioequivalence of estradiol and estradiol valerate could be demonstrated in a crossover study on three women. Oral administration of either 10 mg of estradiol and 10 mg of estradiol valerate resulted in nearly equal concentration–time curves, indicating that there are no major differences in the systemic availability of estradiol between both

Table W13.3 Maximum 17β-estradiol concentrations (c_{max}) and their times of occurrence (t_{max}) after administration of 2 mg estradiol valerate

c_{max} (pg/ml plasma)	t_{max} (hours after administration)	No. of women	Data from reference
90–140	1–3	1 + 1 P	14
24–120[a]	2–12	3	13
50–65	3–6	7 P	15
90–100	6	10 P	16
30–50	6–12	3	17

[a] Adapted to a dose of 2 mg
P = post-menopausal women

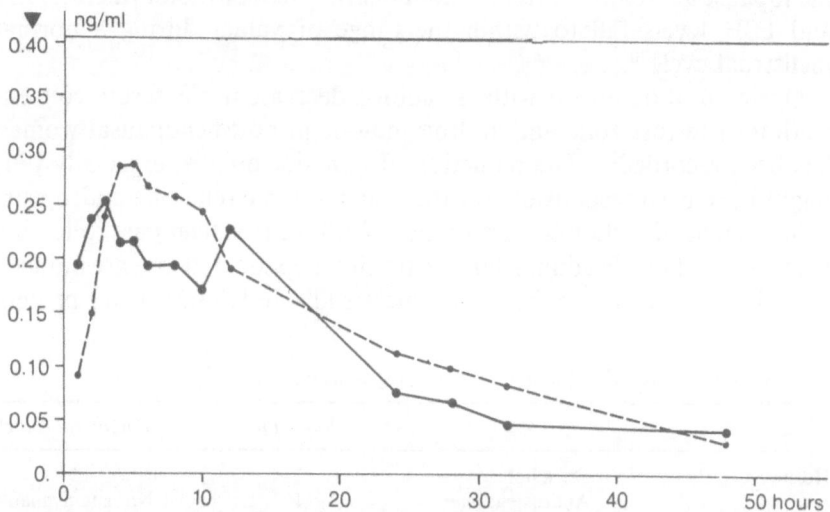

Figure W13.6 Mean plasma levels of 17β-estradiol following single administration of 10 mg of estradiol valerate ●——● and 10 mg of 17β-estradiol ●--● in a crossover study in 3 postmenopausal women

preparations in man (Fig. W13.6). Biodynamic effects of estradiol and estradiol valerate could be recognized at the endometrium. About 4 mg estradiol valerate must be administered orally every day for 14 days to achieve complete endometrial proliferation[18]. Climacteric complaints can be successfully treated with a daily replacement dose of 1–2 mg estradiol valerate, a regimen which leads to only slight changes in the endometrium (Table W13.4). The same effect can be achieved with about the same amount of micronized 17β-estradiol, which is also an indication of the qualitative and quantitative equivalence of estradiol valerate and 17β-estradiol. The estrogenic activity of estradiol valerate can likewise be recognized by the production of cervical mucus and at the vaginal epithelium. In postmenopausal women, estradiol valerate treatment leads to

Table W13.4 Daily replacement dosages and endometrial proliferation dosages in the human

	Daily replacement dose (mg/d)	Full endometrial proliferation dose (mg/14 d)
Estradiol valerate	1.0–2.0	60
17β-Estradiol micronized	2.0	60

From ref. 18

a vaginal cell index which corresponds to that of childbearing age[19]. Moreover elevated gonadotrophin levels observed in most cases after the menopause are reduced after the administration of estradiol valerate. LH and FSH levels fall to within the range of values during a normal menstrual cycle[20].

During oral treatment with estradiol a decrease in the serum concentration of testosterone and androstendione in postmenopausal women has been recorded[21]. The reduction of gonadotrophins, especially LH, might have been responsible for the reduction in circulating androgens, which can be of metabolic importance. With the first liver pass following absorption of orally administered estradiol, hepatic enzymes are induced that alter various biochemical parameters (Table W13.5). Liver protein

Table W13.5 Effects of estradiol on some endogenous parameters

		Oral route	Parenteral route[a]
Hormone levels	Estradiol	↑	↑
	Androstendione	↓	No data available
	Testosterone	↓	No data available
	FSH	↓	↓
	LH	↓	↓
Proteins	SHBG	↑	↔
	CBG	↑	↔
	Ceruloplasmin	↑	↔
Lipids	Triglycerides	↔	↔
	LDL	↓	↔
	HDL	↑	↔

[a] Implants, vaginal rings, percutaneous administration
↑ = Increase; ↔ = unchanged; ↓ = decrease

synthesis is increased, inducing plasma proteins such as sex-hormone-binding globulin, corticosteroid-binding globulin and ceruloplasmin in a dose-dependent fashion[22-25]. The different molecular weight estradiol and estradiol valerate are dose-equivalent in their protein-inducing properties when administered orally[26].

More significant than the changes in protein metabolism is the observed lipoprotein and fatty acid metabolism resulting from treatment with estrogens.

Neither estradiol valerate nor estradiol cause any increase in serum triglycerides and β-lipoproteins when administered by the oral route. Increased concentrations of blood triglycerides may even be reduced by the treatment in individual cases. Low-density lipoproteins (LDL) are reduced, high-density lipoproteins (HDL) are increased – a situation which must be regarded as desirable[18, 27]. High levels of LDL are associated with coronary artery disease, while HDL seem to have some protective effect[22]. However, the increase in HDL may be lost by parenteral administration of estradiol. Apparently the first liver passage is necessary to induce this antiatherogenic lipoprotein[28]. Different therapeutic systems for estradiol avoid the hepatic portal system, by direct absorption of the drug into the peripheral circulation. Percutaneous treatment with estradiol produced no or only minor lipid changes in postmenopausal women[29]. Similar results concerning the protein-inducing hepatotrophic effects of estradiol were obtained from studies with other dosage forms for parenteral administration. Vaginal rings and subcutaneous implants gave stable estradiol levels in plasma, depressed FSH and LH while the sex-hormone-binding-protein levels did not change[30–32].

Regardless of the route of administration, not only estradiol but also estrone and estriol, appears in human plasma following administration of estradiol valerate or estradiol. The formation of estrone and estriol corresponds to the familiar conversion of estradiol. However, the plasma concentration of the three steroids, with their differing estrogenic potency, is low in comparison with the concentration of their conjugates (Fig. W13.7). In contrast to oral estradiol, percutaneous replacement therapy is achieved without elevated estrone levels. The conversion of percutaneous administered estradiol (formulated as a hydroalcoholic gel) into estrone was far less pronounced in comparison to oral therapy[24, 25, 33]. Estradiol may circulate in three forms: free, conjugated and protein-bound. Free estradiol is lipophilic, freely traverses cell membranes, and is then biologically active. Sulfates and conjugates of estradiol are water-soluble, biologically inactive, and can be excreted easily into the urine or bile. Enzymatic cleavage of estradiol conjugates can rapidly convert the inactive form to a potentially active form. Unconjugated estradiol circulates primarily bound to albumin of SHBG. Protein-bound estrogens are presumably biologically inactive.

The contribution of the conjugated estrogens to the formation of active unconjugated estradiol is still unknown. The enzyme estrone sulfotransferase rapidly converts estradiol into estrone sulfate. The reverse reaction is catalyzed by arylsulfatases. Therefore estrone sulfate may be a potential source of active estradiol.

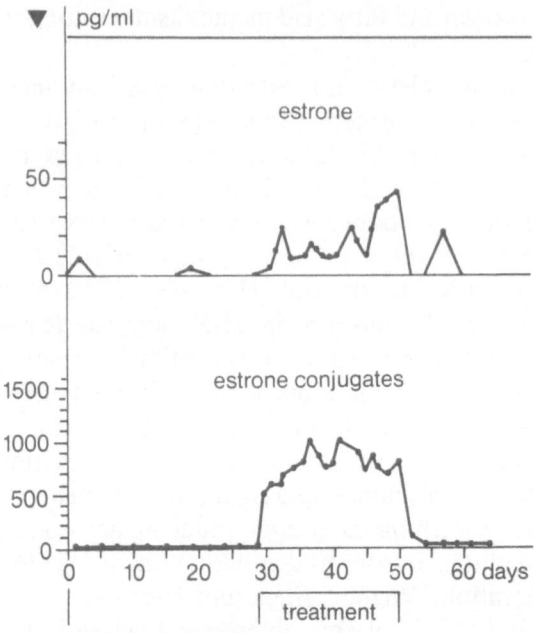

Figure W13.7   Daily oral dose: 2 mg of estradiol valerate in combination with 1 mg of estriol

THE PRODUCTION AND METABOLISM OF ESTROGENS

Longcope: In this review of the production and metabolism of the estrogens, I shall restrict my comments to estrone, estrone sulfate, estradiol and estriol. The catechol estrogens and 16α-hydroxyestrone may have certain properties beyond those mediated by receptor mechanisms[34, 35], but data concerning their production and excretion are relatively scant, and I shall not discuss them further.

When estradiol, as 6,7-[^{3}H]estradiol, is administered to women as an i.v. pulse, the radiolabeled estradiol disappears rather rapidly from the blood with a metabolic clearance rate of about 1200 liters per day. Although some 20% will reappear in the blood as estrone, the major radiolabeled estrogen which is measurable in the blood is estrone sulfate[36]. The disappearance of [^{3}H]estradiol can be described as a function which is the sum of three exponentials. A somewhat similar pattern is also noted when [^{3}H]estrone is administered, with some of the radioactivity measureable as estradiol[36]. However, the conversion ($[\rho]\underset{BB}{E_2},E_1$) of [^{3}H]estradiol to [^{3}H]estrone is less than the conversion of [^{3}H]estrone to [^{3}H]estradiol ($[\rho]\underset{BB}{E_1},E_2$) after the administration of [^{3}H]estrone, findings compatible with the report of Fishman and Bradlow[37] that the equilibrium between

Table W13.6 Intercept (A, B, and C), slopes (α, β and λ) and metabolic clearance rates (MCR) following i.v. pulse of ³H-labeled estrogens

Estrogen administered[a]	A[b]	B	C	α[c]	β (units/ day)	λ	MCR (liters/ day)
[³H]Estradiol	0.076[d]	0.023	0.0029	384.8	64.6	9.40	1170
[³H]Estrone	0.029	0.0079	0.0019	356.2	30.9	4.87	1870
[³H]Estrone sulfate	0.121	0.025	–	324.5	5.1	–	170
[³H]Estriol	0.063	0.0075	–	392.2	17.0	–	2000

[a] Each estrogen administered as an i.v. pulse
[b] A, B and C are the intercepts of each exponential extrapolated to '0' time
[c] α, β and λ are the respective slopes of each exponential
[d] Mean data from refs 35, 39, 40

estrone and estradiol in the blood favors estrone. The metabolic clearance rate of estrone is about 2000 liters per day.

The slopes (λ) of the terminal phases of the disappearance from the blood of [³H]estradiol or [³H]estrone are similar to the terminal slope (β) for the disappearance of [³H]estrone sulfate (Table W13.6). This similarity of the slopes is compatible with estrone sulfate's role as a slowly turning-over reservoir for estrone and estradiol[38, 39]. After the administration of [³H]estrone sulfate as an i.v. pulse, [³H]estrone sulfate disappears slowly from the blood with a metabolic clearance rate of about 150 liters per day. Both [³H]estrone and [³H]estradiol appear in the blood, but the conversions, 15% and 3%, are far less than the formation of [³H]estrone sulfate, about 45%, after either [³H]estrone or [³H]estradiol administration.

When [³H]estriol is administered as an i.v. pulse, its disappearance is relatively rapid with a metabolic clearance rate of about 2000 liters per day[40]. The disappearance can be described as a function which is the sum of two exponentials, suggesting that there is no slowly turning-over sulfate pool as noted for estrone and estradiol.

When [³H]estradiol is administered orally, the pattern of radioactivity in the blood is very different than after i.v. administration. Less than 10% of the [³H]estradiol so administered is measured in the blood as [³H]-estradiol[41, 42]. About the same amount can be measured in the blood as [³H]estrone with most of the radioactivity appearing as estradiol

Table W13.7 Transfer constants ($[\rho]_{BB}$ = percentage of precursor administered into blood and measured in blood as product) of estrogens

Administered estrogen	Estradiol	Estrone	Estrone sulfate
[³H]Estradiol	–	17[a]	42
[³H]Estrone	5	–	41
[³H]Estrone sulfate	3	15	–

[a] Mean data from refs 35, 38

glucuronide and estrone sulfate. Much of the conversion of estradiol to estrone and to estradiol glucuronide may take place in the intestinal wall.

Much of these data were obtained in reproductive-aged women in whom the ovary produces most of the estrone and estradiol. However, in postmenopausal women there is a marked decrease in the production rate of these estrogens and a marked shift in their sources. The ovaries in about 90% of postmenopausal women do not secrete estrogens, although in some 10% of such women the ovaries secrete small but significant amounts of estradiol[43].

The decline in the production rate of estradiol is most marked at the time of the menopause[44], although there is a slight further decrease paralleling a decrease in the metabolic clearance rate with age[45]. The menopausal decline in estrone production does not appear to be followed by any further decrease.

Estrogen production rates are, in part, a function of weight, and heavier women have greater production rates of estrogens (Fig. W13.8)[44]. This would explain, to some extent, why heavier women are at lesser risk for osteoporosis[46] but at greater risk for endometrial carcinoma[47] than lighter women. There is also a direct correlation between weight and androgen production. As androgen production, particularly androstenedione, increases there is a correlated increase in estrogen production in postmenopausal women.

Androstenedione is the major precursor of estrone in postmenopausal women, and as noted by Hemsell et al.[48] and us[49] peripheral aromatization is greater in old as compared to young women. However, there does not appear to be a correlation, in postmenopausal women, between peripheral aromatization and either age or the time since the last menstrual period.

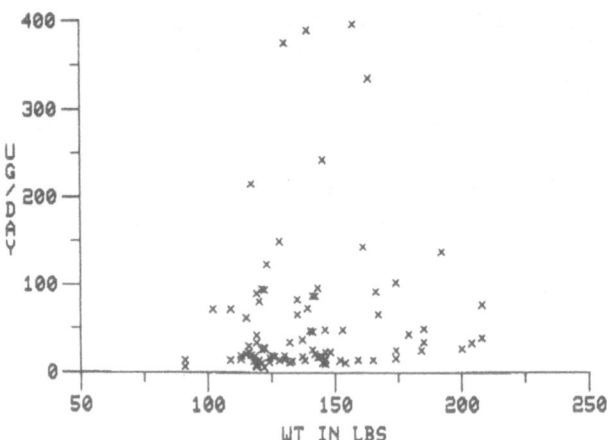

Figure W13.8 Production rates of estradiol (μg/day) related to weight in lb of a group of peri- and postmenopausal women

There is a correlation between aromatization and weight which could be expected, since the stromal cells of adipose tissue are a major site for aromatization[50]. There is a positive correlation between peripheral aromatization normalized for weight and time since the last menses for perimenopausal women who are within 3 months of their last menses (Fig. W13.9). This correlation is not significant for women more than 3 months from their last menses. It would appear, therefore, that the increase in aromatization occurs in association with the climacteric. It is unlikely that changes in gonadotropins or estrogens[51] are the cause for this increase in aromatization, and the exact mechanism remains uncertain.

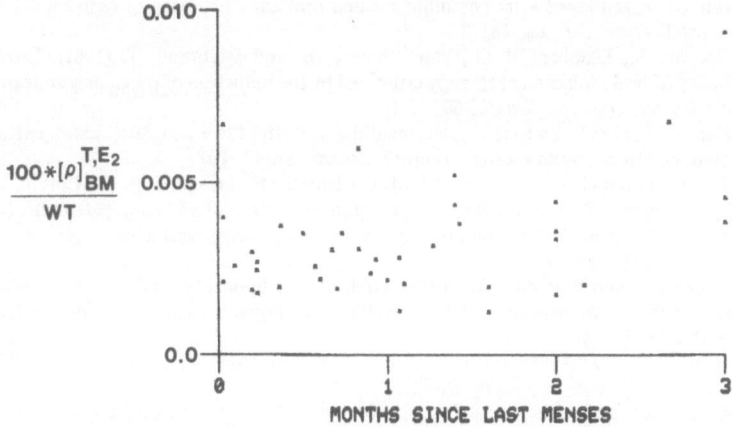

Figure W13.9 Peripheral aromatization normalized for weight ($100 \times [\rho]^{T}_{BM},E_2$/weight in lb) related to time in months since the last menses in a group of perimenopausal women

In most women who are perimenopausal there is a gradual decline in estrogen levels as time from the last menses increases up to about 12 months[52]. After that time, however, there would appear to be little further decline although in certain women, even after a prolonged interval of amenorrhea, a rise in estrone and estradiol can occur and be followed by an isolated episode of vaginal bleeding. Neither our data nor those of others[53] are helpful in predicting which women may have such episodes of bleeding.

As estradiol levels fall FSH concentrations rise, and there is a significant correlation between estradiol and estrone levels and FSH concentrations in women who are perimenopausal (i.e. within 12 months of their last menses) or postmenopausal (i.e. greater than 12 months since their last menses)[52]. The correlation between luteinizing hormone and steroid hormones in these same groups of women is not nearly so strong as those for FSH.

While there are major changes in estrogen production at the time of the menopause, these are primarily due to changes in secretion and source and not to changes in metabolism.

Acknowledgement

Portions of this work were supported by Grants HD-15443, AG-02927 and AG-00058.

REFERENCES

1. Lyrenäs, S., Carlström, K., Bäckström, T. and von Schoultz, B. (1981). A comparison of serum oestrogen levels after percutaneous and oral administration of oestrodiol-17β. *Br. J. Obstet. Gynaecol.*, **88**, 181–7
2. Helgason, S., Damber, M.-G., von Schoultz, B. and Stigbrand, T. (1981). Estrogenic potency of oral replacement therapy estimated by the induction of pregnancy zone protein. *Acta Obstet. Gynecol. Scand.*, **60**, 75–9
3. Helgason, S. (1982). Estrogen replacement therapy after the menopause. Estrogenicity and metabolic effects. *Acta Obstet. Gynecol. Scand.*, Suppl. 107
4. Elkik, F., Gompel, A., Mercier-Bodard, C., Kutten, F., Guyenne, P. N., Corvol, P. and Mauvais-Jarvis, P. (1982). Effects of percutaneous estradiol and conjugated estrogens on the level of plasma proteins and triglycerides in post-menopausal women. *Am. J. Obstet. Gynecol.*, **143**, 888–92
5. Fåhraeus, L. and Wallentin, L. (1983). High density lipoprotein subfractions during oral and cutaneous administration of 17β-estradiol to menopausal women. *J. Clin. Endocrinol. Metab.*, **56**, 797–801
6. Englund, D. (1979). Oestrogen treatment in the menopause. *Doctoral thesis*, Medical Faculty of Uppsala University, Sweden
7. Holst, J., Cajander, S., Carlström, K., Damber, M.-G. and von Schoultz, B. (1983). A comparison of liver protein induction in postmenopausal women during oral and percutaneous oestrogen replacement therapy. *Br. J. Obstet. Gynaecol.*, **90**, 355–60 ·
8. Nilsson, B., Holst, J. and von Schoultz, B. (1984). Serum levels of unbound 17β-oestradiol during oral and percutaneous postmenopausal replacement therapy. *Br. J. Obstet. Gynaecol.*, **91**, 1031–6
9. Kuppermann, H. S. (1963). Clinical management of the climacteric syndrome. *Human Endocrinology*, vol.2, p. 426. (Philadelphia: F. A. Davis)
10. Dapunt, O. (1971). The hormonal therapy of the climacteric syndrome. *Therapie d. Gegenw.*, **110**(1), 34
11. Judd, H. L., Judd, G. E., Lucas, W. E. and Yen, S. S. C. (1974). Endocrine function of the postmenopausal ovary: concentration of androgens and estrogens in ovarian and peripheral vein blood. *J. Clin. Endocrinol. Metab.*, **39**, 1020
12. Düsterberg, B., Schmidt-Gollwitzer, M. and Hümpel, M. (1985). Pharmacokinetics and biotransformation of estradiol valerate in ovariectomized women. *Hormone Res.*, **21**, 145
13. Kolb, K. H. and Schulze, P. E. (1967). Zum Stoffwechsel von Östradiol-valerianat. *Med. Mitteilungen*, **28**, 16–17
14. Kolb, K. H. (1969). Pharmacokinetics of several steroids in man. *Simposio Esteroides Sexuales*, Bogota
15. Vermeulen, A. (1975). Long-acting steroid preparations. *Acta Clin. Belg.*, **30**, 48–55
16. Anderson, A. B. M., Sklovsky, E., Sayers, L., Steele, P. A. and Turnball, A. C. (1978). Comparison of serum oestrogen concentrations in post-menopausal women taking oestrone sulphate and oestradiol. *Br. Med. J.*, **1**, 140–2
17. Staland, B. (1975). Estradiol in climacteric complaints; corresponding doses by different routes of application. *Acta Obstet. Gynecol. Scand.*, Suppl., **47**, 42
18. Lauritzen, C. (1982). *Das Klimakterium der Frau.* (Berlin, Schering and Paris: PIL)

19. Dapunt, O. (1967). Behandlung klimakterischer Beschwerden mit Östradiol-valerianat (Progynova). *Med. Klin.*, **62**, 1356–61
20. Leyendecker, G., Geppert, G., Nocke, W. and Ufer, Y. (1975). Untersuchungen zur Pharmakokinetik von Östradio-17β, Estradiol-Benzoat, Östradiol-Valerianat und Östradiol-Undezylat bei der Frau: Der Verlauf der Konzentration von Östradio-17β, Östron, LH und FSH im Serum. *Geburts. Frauenheilk.*, **35**, 370–4
21. Mattsson, L. A., Abrahamsson, L., Cullberg, G. and Samsioe, G. (1983). Effects of a continuous estrogen-progestogen therapy for climacteric symptoms on circulating sex steroids and gonadotrophins. *Arch. Gynecol.*, **233**(2), 101–7
22. Larsson-Cohn, U. (1976). Lipids and estrogens. In van Keep, P. A. *et al.* (eds.) *Consensus on Menopause Research.* (Lancaster: MTP Press)
23. Schwartz, U., Volger, H., Schneller, E., Moltz, L. and Hammerstein, J. (1983). Effects of various replacement oestrogens on hepatic transcortin synthesis in climacteric women. *Acta Endocrinol. (Copenh.)*, **102**(1), 103–6
24. Holst, J., Cajander, S., Carlstrom, K., Damber, M. G. and von Schoultz, B. (1983). A comparison of liver protein induction in postmenopausal women during oral and percutaneous oestrogen replacement therapy. *Br. J. Obstet. Gynaecol.*, **90**(4), 355–60
25. Holst, J. (1983). Percutaneous estrogen therapy. Endometrial response and metabolic effects. *Acta Obstet. Gynecol. Scand.* (Suppl.), **115**, 1–30
26. Schoultz, B. von, Carlström, K., Damber, M. G., Helgasson, S. and Stigbrand, T. (1980). Estrogenic potency assayed by protein induction. *Acta Obstet. Gynecol. Scand.*, Suppl. **93**, 59–60
27. Lauritzen, C. (1975). Ertahrungen in der Behandlung klimakterischer Beschwerden mit Depot-Injektionen von Östradiolralerianat-Dehydroepiandrosteron-Önanthat. *Therapiewoche*, **30**, 1736–42
28. Tikkanen, M. J., Kunsi, T., Vartiainen, E. and Nikkia, E. A. (1979). Treatment of postmenopausal hypercholesterolaemia with estradiol. *Acta Obstet. Gynecol. Scand.*, Suppl., **88**, 83–8
29. Fahraeus, L. and Wallentin, L. (1983). High density lipoprotein subfractions during oral and cutaneous administration of 17β-estradiol to menopausal women. *J. Endocrinol. Metab.*, **56**(4), 797–801
30. Englund, D. E., Victor, A. D. and Johannsson, E. D. (1981). Pharmacokinetics of pharmacodynamic effects of vaginal oestradiol administration from silastic rings in postmenopausal women. *Maturitas*, **3**(2), 125–33
31. Nichols, K. C., Schenkel, L. and Benson, H. (1984). 17 beta-estradiol for postmenopausal estrogen replacement therapy. *Obstet. Gynecol. Surv.*, **39**(4), 230–45
32. Thom, M. H., Collins, W. P. and Studd, J. W. (1981). Hormonal profiles in postmenopausal women after therapy with subcutaneous implants. *Br. J. Obstet. Gynecol.*, **88**(4), 426–33
33. Holst, J., Cajander, S., Carstrom, K., Damber, M. G. and von Schoultz, B. (1983). Percutaneous estrogen replacement therapy. Effects on circulating estrogens, gonadotropins and prolactin. *Acta Obstet. Gynecol. Scand.*, **62**(1), 49–53
34. Fishman, J. (1981). Biological action of catechol oestrogens. *J. Endocrinol.*, **89**, 59P
35. Fishman, J., Schneider, J., Herschopf, R. J. and Bradlow, H. L. (1984). Increased estrogen-16α-hydroxylase activity in women with breast and endometrial cancer. *J. Steroid Biochem.*, **20**, 1077
36. Longcope, C. and Williams, K. I. H. (1974). The metabolism of estrogens in normal women after pulse injections of ³H-estradiol and ³H-estrone. *J. Clin. Endocrinol. Metab.*, **38**, 602
37. Fishman, J., Bradlow, H. L. and Gallagher, T. F. (1960). Oxidative metabolism of estradiol. *J. Biol. Chem.*, **235**, 3104
38. Longcope, C. (1972). The metabolism of estrone sulfate in normal males. *J. Clin. Endocrinol. Metab.*, **34**, 113
39. Ruder, H. J., Loriaux, L. and Lipsett, M. B. (1972). Estrone sulfate: production rate and metabolism in man. *J. Clin. Invest.*, **51**, 1020
40. Flood, C., Pratt, J. H. and Longcope, C. (1976). The metabolic clearance and blood production rates of estriol in normal, non-pregnant women. *J. Clin. Endocrinol. Metab.*, **42**, 1
41. Longcope, C., Yesair, D. W., Williams, K. I. H., Callahan, M. M., Bourget, C., Brown,

S. K., Carraher, M. S., Flood, C. and Rachwall, P. C. (1980). Comparison of the metabolism in dogs of estradiol 17β-following its intravenous and oral administration. *J. Steroid Biochem.*, **13**, 1047

42. Longcope, C., Gorbach, S., Goldin, B., Woods, M., Dwyer, J. and Warram, J. (1985). The metabolism of estradiol: oral compared to intravenous administration. *J. Steroid Biochem.* (Submitted)

43. Longcope, C., Hunter, R. and Franz, C. (1980). Steroid secretion by the postmenopausal ovary. *Am. J. Obstet. Gynecol.*, **138**, 564

44. Longcope, C., Jaffee, W. and Griffing, G. (1981). Production rates of androgens and oestrogens in post-menopausal women. *Maturitas*, **3**, 215

45. Longcope, C., Jaffee, W. and Griffing, G. (1980). Metabolic clearance rates of androgens and oestrogens in aging women. *Maturitas*, **2**, 283

46. Saville, P. D. and Bilsson, B. E. R. (1966). Height and weight in symptomatic postmenopausal osteoporosis. *Clin. Orthop.*, **45**, 49

47. Corscaden, J. A. and Gusberg, S. B. (1947). The background of cancer of the corpus. *Am. J. Obstet. Gynecol.*, **53**, 419

48. Hemsell, D. L., Groden, J. M., Brenner, P. F., Siiteri, P. K. and MacDonald, P. C. (1974). Plasma precursors of estrogen. II. Correlation of the extent of conversion of plasma androstenedione to estrone with age. *J. Clin. Endocrinol. Metab.*, **38**, 476

49. Longcope, C. (1978). The significance of steroid production of peripheral tissue. In Scholler, R. (ed.) *Endocrinology of the Ovary.* p. 23. (Paris: Editions SEPE)

50. Mendelson, C. R., Cleland, W. H., Smith, M. E. and Simpson, E. R. (1982). Regulation of aromatase activity of stromal cells derived from human adipose tissue. *Endocrinology*, **111**, 1077

51. Franz, C. and Longcope, C. (1979). Androgen and estrogen metabolism in male rhesus monkeys. *Endocrinology*, **105**, 869

52. Longcope, C., Franz, C., Morello, C., Baker, R. and Johnston, C. C. Jr (1985). Steroid and gonadotropin levels in women during the perimenopausal years. (Submitted)

53. Metcalf, M. G., Donald, R. A. and Livesey, J. H. (1981). Pituitary–ovarian function in normal women during the menopausal transition. *Clin. Endocrinol.*, **14**, 245

Workshop 14

Anthropology

Chairman: **P. Kaufert** (Canada)
Co-chairman: **B. Du Toit** (USA)

P. Van Keep (Belgium)
M. Lock (Canada)
J. Wilbush (Canada)
J. Brown (USA)

This Workshop explored the unique contribution which anthropology may make towards an understanding of the menopausal experience. At the same time it examined some of the methodological and conceptual problems with which that discipline is concerned, and which are relevant to menopause research. The Workshop brought together anthropologists and others who, while not necessarily anthropologists, shared with them a similar concern with the importance of collecting crosscultural data. The key questions were how to ensure that these data satisfied the demands for scientific rigour (whether anthropological or epidemiological) yet at the same time adequately represented what was happening in the lives of women at midlife, in terms of their physical and psychosocial well-being.

Wilbush re-examined the debate over whether or not a menopausal syndrome (in the sense of a cluster of symptoms expressing discomfort and associated with menopause) is to be found outside Western, middle-class society. Wilbush himself believed that the syndrome was the product of this society and was restricted to that setting. With customary verve he attacked the use of mail surveys, symptom checklists and structured interview formats by all researchers – regardless of whether they were clinicians, epidemiologists, sociologists or anthropologists – as methodologically wrong and conceptually ill-considered. His contention is that the debate over the existence of a menopausal syndrome was an artefact of differences in the way researchers have elicited symptom data rather than a product of differences in the physiological experiences which accompany a woman's final menses.

Wilbush concentrated his argument in two areas. First he proposed that a distinction should be made between symptoms and semeions. In an earlier paper, Wilbush[1] defined symptoms as the 'spontaneous complaints of patients' and semeions as 'the evidentiary data discovered by the doctor when he questions the patient'. A particular semeion, such as the physiological sensation of the hot flush, may be common to women in two separate societies, yet be reported as a symptom by women in one society, but not in another. In any particular society, while the number of women with hot flushes remains constant, researchers will produce different counts depending on whether their methods produce data on symptoms or semeions. It follows from the same argument that a comparison of results is meaningless if one study is reporting semeions and the other symptoms.

The second point in the argument is that response to physical sensation is mediated through culture, in the sense that people have a tendency to interpret what they feel by what they expect to feel. In Western society, women anticipate a series of menopausal symptoms – a syndrome of discomforts – and cannot distinguish between actual feelings and what they believe that they should feel. This led Wilbush into the deduction that:

> The only women who can tell us about sensations associated with physiological changes of the menopause in their pristine, overlay-free, form are the naive members of other cultures.

Other anthropologists within the Workshop were inclined to dispute Wilbush's characterization of other cultures and peoples as 'pristine' and 'naive', while recognizing the importance of the distinction between semeions and symptoms.

Lock was also looking at issues in the collection of symptom data, but her paper was written from a different perspective. As a medical anthropologist, Lock was concerned with the proper balance between producing data which will permit comparison between studies and which will yet reflect the menopausal experience particular to women in a given society. The material she used as illustration was taken from her recently completed study on the menopause among Japanese women. In the first section of the paper Lock discussed the problems which must be faced when translating words and medical concepts between languages. In her own research, it was not simply a question of finding a literal translation of medical terms: the words used had to be recognisable by Japanese women as meaningful and representative of their own experience. At the same time, Lock wanted to compare the experience of Japanese women at menopause with the experience of Canadian and US women.

(The project is linked with studies in Canada (Kaufert, 1984)[2] and in Massachusetts (McKinlay, 1984).)[3]

Historically, there was, for example, no common Japanese word equivalent to menopause. The term used today for a woman's last menses is a technical one and is rarely used even when a physician is discussing menopause with a patient. Lock traced the commonly used term for menopause to German influence on Japanese medicine towards the end of the nineteenth century. She discussed other words which have an older and Japanese origin, but said that these are rarely used today except by a few of the rural women whom she interviewed.

The Japanese project included a series of in-depth interviews plus a cross-sectional survey in which the questionnaire was a translation and adaptation of ones used in Manitoba by Kaufert and in Massachusetts by McKinlay (Kaufert, 1984). Each study adopted the same checklist approach to eliciting symptom data. A set of symptoms associated with menopause was embedded in a more general list of somatic complaints. There was no reference to menopause and women were asked to report on their current symptom experience.

The list used in the Japanese study included both symptoms particular to the Japanese context plus a translation into Japanese of symptoms which are recognised in both Japanese and North American medicine. While Lock was reporting on a preliminary exploration of these data, there was a marked difference, as compared with the Canadian data, between the overall number of symptoms reported by Japanese women and the frequency of symptoms particular to menopause (such as the hot flush).

The in-depth interviews were used to probe into women's experience at menopause, including their symptom experience. Lock found that few women volunteered hot flushes as a symptom and, when questioned, not many more reported it as a physical sensation. To use Wilbush's terms, hot flushes did not appear to be widespread among Japanese women either as symptom or semeion.

According to the initial plan, the third and fourth papers in the workshop were to focus on the social context of midlife and the extent to which this context might modify the menopausal experience. Brown's paper was to be a general discussion of the structure of family relationships surrounding women at menopause, while McKinlay was to focus on issues of social support and the relationship between social support and psychological well being among menopausal women. Unfortunately, McKinlay was unable to attend the Congress. His place was taken by van Keep who, at very short notice, agreed to discuss menopause and the future.

Brown's paper argued that in many societies the status of women improves rather than declines after menopause[4]. Elaborating on this theme she provided a theoretical rationale out of sociobiology for the survival of women into the postmenopause. Reviewing the available crosscultural evidence, she suggested that middle age appears to bring three types of changes into the lives of women in non-industrialized society. First, they are freed from numerous restrictions and they acquire a greater freedom of movement. Second, special statuses outside their domestic household become available to women, who may serve as mid-wives, curers or priestesses. Third, their position within the family structure changes as do their relationships with other kin. Brown focused her paper on the change in family relationships.

Brown suggests that the marital relationship becomes more tranquil and more equitable as a woman and her husband acquire common interests in property and in the marriages of their children. Furthermore, given that many women were married to husbands much older than themselves, as these men decline into old age, they face wives in vigorous middle age who have the support of adult sons. Even if the husband retains formal authority, there is a shift in the relationships of power within the household. Yet, it is not only through their relationship with their husbands and sons that women in midlife have access to power but also through their relationship with younger women, particularly their daughters and daughters-in-law.

Brown explored differences in authority and 'managerial style', between women living in matrilocal societies and patrilocal societies. In matrilocal societies, married daughters and their children remain with the household of their mother's family. Women have a major role in the productivity of the group and their activities are administered and co-ordinated by women in midlife whose exercise of authority tends to be subtle and benign.

In patrilocal societies, women move into the household of their husband and under the control of their mother-in-law. Women are valued less for their domestic productivity than for their reproductive role. The power of a woman in midlife lies in her ability to subjugate and control her daughters-in-law and to ensure that only her sons have reproductive access to their wives.

Using arguments from sociobiology, Brown suggests that differences in the role of postmenopausal women in patrilocal and matrilocal societies, must be understood as 'the product of an interplay between [sic] biological, sociological and sociocultural conditions'[5]. She uses the concept of 'inclusive fitness', defined by sociobiologists as a measure of the genetic representation of an individual in future generations. In societies in which a daughter's children belong to her husband's kin group, women can guarantee their own 'inclusive fitness' only by ensuring that their genes pass through their son to his descendants. Hence, the need to control access to the daughter-in-law. The more benevolent authority of the mother in matrilocal society reflects the fact that in these societies, her 'inclusive fitness' depends on her daughters' and not on her sons' children. Brown concluded by suggesting that:

> A better understanding of these relationships in other societies will help to illuminate the role of older women in our own, and perhaps rehabilitate that much maligned figure, the American mother-in-law.

While not directly concerned with the menopause, Brown demonstrated how the different perspective of the anthropologist can correct the too facile conclusion that women lose position as they lose their fertility.

Van Keep used the opportunity provided by the Workshop to make a survey of the future. He started by reviewing the different social and demographic factors which have an impact on the symptoms of the climacteric, its timing, its character and its clinical management. He then examined what changes in these factors might be predicted over the next twenty years. He argued that many of these trends will have consequences for the climacteric both as an experience and as a research area. For example, as women marry at younger ages, have smaller families which they complete earlier, the 'empty nest' phase in the family life cycle will occur earlier in their lives and will not coincide with menopause. Furthermore, the idea of 'menopause' as the closure of a woman's fertility must be re-interpreted as more women have hysterectomies or use sterilization as a means of birth control once their family is complete.

Van Keep also predicted change as a result of better information becoming available on the menopause. As women and as their physicians become more aware of what to expect, the medical management of the climacteric and of the climacteric patient will change. Van Keep predicted a growth over the next twenty years in non-sex hormonal treatment for climacteric complaints because he believed that neurohormones might be found to be involved – and be effective – in climacteric complaints. He also suggested that there might be a move towards some form of self-medication. In general, his view of menopause in the year 2000 was an optimistic one. Knowing more about the menopause, women will fear it less. Furthermore, as methods of managing its symptoms and consequences improve, the menopause will become a less traumatic event, whether physically or psychologically, for women.

These four papers made up the formal core of the Workshop presentations, but there was an additional statement by du Toit on his current fieldwork with Black and White, urban and rural women, plus urban Indian women in South Africa. This project is still in process, but promises exciting results which will extend understanding of menopause in crosscultural context.

The remainder of the Workshop was used, not only to question the presenters, but to discuss broader issues arising from the Congress as a whole. Some of the questions revealed the gap between disciplines in terms of what they rank as most important in the methodology of crosscultural research. Epidemiologists see the task as one of charting with maximum accuracy the distribution of such characteristics as age at menopause or the incidence of hot flashes. They are preoccupied with such methodological questions as response rates, sample size and whether the sample is representative. Anthropologists – and in this Lock and Wilbush were in agreement – are concerned with questions of meaning and language. Like Brown, they are anxious that Western concepts – such as those relating to family structure – do not impede understanding of what happens at midlife in the lives of women in other than Western societies. Yet, differences in disciplinary perspectives are not irreconcilable. It is possible for a biostatistician–epidemiologist, a medical anthropologist and a sociologist to collaborate as the link between the Massachusetts, the Japanese and the Manitoba studies show.

The Workshop also turned into a forum for the discussion of issues of particular concern to some women participating in the Congress. For example, there was a strong feeling that the occasional overly negative or disease-focused assumptions about the menopause and the menopausal woman which had occasionally surfaced in earlier sessions required correction. Another concern of women in the workshop was expressed by Voda who queried whether the male researcher could produce results which were both sensitive to women's experience and accurate in their ability to represent what happened at menopause. Both du Toit and Good showed they were conscious of the importance of the issues raised by Voda and by others who supported her position. In reply, they argued both that men were capable of such research and also that the sex of the interviewer was not the only consideration. Du Toit quoted from his own experience in which women preferred an older male interviewer to a younger female one.

Other women argued that conclusions about menopause and its impact on women have been derived from work narrowly based on the characteristics of the middle-class patient. Donna Davis made an eloquent plea that the views should be heard of women, who are non-patient and non-middle class. Citing her own work in Newfoundland, she argued that the role of the anthropologist is to give a voice to such women. It might be added, that it is also the role of the anthropologist to give a voice to the unheard women of the Third World and to the concerns and problems which they face as they enter menopause.

REFERENCES

1. Wilbush, J. (1984). Clinical information – signs, semeions and symptoms: discussion paper. *J. R. Soc. Med.*, **77**
2. Kaufert, P. (1984). Research note: women and their health in the middle years: a Manitoba project. *Soc. Sci. Med.*, **18**(3), 279–81

3. McKinlay, S. M. and McKinlay, J. B. (1986), Health status and health care utilization by menopausal women. In Noteloritz M., and van Keep P. *The Climacteric in Perspective*, pp. 59–75. (Lancaster: MTP)

4. Brown, J. K. (1982). Cross-cultural perspectives on middle-aged women. *Curr. Anthropol.*, **23**, 143–56

5. Van den Berghe, P. and Barash, D. (1977). Inclusive fitness and human family structure. *Am. Anthropol.*, **79**, 809–23

FURTHER READING

Brown, J. K. and Kerns, V. (eds.) (1985). *In Her Prime: A New View of Middle-Aged Women*. (South Hadley, Mass.: Bergin and Garvey)

Kaufert, P. (1985). Midlife in the Midwest: Canadian women in Manitoba. In Brown, J. K. and Kerns, V. (eds.) *In Her Prime: A View of Middle-Aged Women*. pp. 181–97. (South Hadley, Mass.: Bergin and Garvey)

Workshop 15

Joint and musculoskeletal problems

Chairman: J. Dequeker (Belgium)
Co-chairman: C. Christiansen (Denmark)

J. Dequeker (Belgium)
C. C. Johnston (USA)
R. R. Recker (USA)
R. B. Mazess (USA)
R. Lindsay (USA)
C. H. Chesnut (USA)

Osteoporosis is clinically defined as the loss of bone (osteopenia), sufficient to result in fractures with minimal trauma, generally of the spine, but also of the hip and wrist, and does not affect everyone in the older age groups. One out of four women will develop osteoporosis after the menopause.

In order to have a better insight in the problem of osteoporosis, it is necessary (a) to know the relationship between osteoporosis and joint and bone aging; (b) to detect the people at risk for postmenopausal osteoporosis; and (c) to evaluate the possible way to prevent and treat osteoporosis.

Joint and bone aging

Dequeker reviewed the clinical experience and the epidemiological evidence that primary osteoporosis and primary osteoarthrosis, although very common in postmenopausal women, are rarely seen together.

When postmenopausal osteoporosis and osteoarthrosis cases are compared with normal controls matched for age, it is found that these disease states, although both occur frequently in the older age groups, represent

419

two extreme groups. At an individual level it is often difficult to differentiate between cases of osteoporosis and osteoarthrosis and normal controls, but as groups they represent two different populations: osteoporosis with osteopenia, slender body status, and little degenerative joint changes; and osteoarthrosis with above-normal bone mass, more fat, more muscle strength and less fractures.

The pathophysiology causing this phenomenon is not clear. Cases with clinical osteoporosis have a rate of bone loss greater than normal, but may also have a lower bone mass from youth onwards. Primary osteoarthrosis cases, on the other hand, have little or no bone loss with age, or may have started adult life with more bone. No significant differences in serum PTH, 24 OH and 1.25 OH vitamin D metabolite levels between osteoporosis and osteoarthrosis could be established.

Important and significant alterations in the protein profile of bone matrix was found in osteoarthrosis and in osteoporosis, which might explain the opposite biomechanical behavior of bone and cartilage in the two conditions. In osteoarthrosis the change to a lower collagen/non-collagenous ratio can be responsible for an abnormal shock-absorbing capacity of subchondral bone with cartilage destruction as a consequence. Conversely for osteoporosis the higher ratio might explain the inability of osteoporotic bone to withstand abnormal stress, and the sparing effect on cartilage in osteoporosis.

Furthermore, the bone metabolism data indicate that patients who develop osteoarthrosis at the small hand joints are not at risk for fracture and do not need preventive therapy for osteoporosis, while those who do not develop these nodes, are more likely to be candidates for osteoporosis and could benefit from a preventive therapy.

Estrogen treatment started within 1 year after cessation of menstruation prevents bone loss but does not prevent the development of osteoarthrosis at the hand joints. Growth hormone, on the other hand, may be involved in the pathogenesis of osteoarthrosis since above-normal fasting growth hormone levels have been found in women suffering from osteoarthrosis and not in women suffering from osteoporosis.

These data support the idea that postmenopausal osteoporosis and osteoarthrosis are two different disease entities, and not simply the end-result of normal aging, aggravated by wear-and-tear phenomena.

DETECTION OF PATIENTS AT RISK FOR POSTMENOPAUSAL OSTEOPOROSIS: GENETIC, CLINICAL AND ENDOCRINOLOGICAL SCREENING

Johnston first stressed the importance of excluding causes of secondary osteoporosis, such as hyperparathyroidism, multiple myeloma, metastatic disease, infection and osteomalacia when evaluating patients for postmenopausal osteoporosis. The simple screening tests for exclusion of secondary osteoporosis include serum calcium, phosphorus and alkaline phosphatase concentrations, and serum protein electrophoresis. In the unusual case, cortisol, thyroxine, and PTH determinations are helpful, and bone biopsy may be necessary, especially to exclude osteomalacia.

Although osteoporosis is characterized by a decrease in bone mass, leading to structural failure of the skeleton and an increased frequency of atraumatic fractures, the pathogenesis may be more complex than the simple loss of bone substance. Thus, low bone mass is only one factor in the pathogenesis of fracture. There also may be a heterogeneity of the fracture syndromes, some fractures due to cortical bone loss, and others to trabecular bone loss.

The amount of bone which remains in old age is a result of the inter-action between the amount present at maturity and subsequent rates of loss. Different environmental and genetic factors may influence each of the determinants to produce the end-result: low bone mass. Johnston and collaborators have attempted to evaluate some of the factors important in the development of adult bone mass and subsequent loss. In a study of twins they found that there is a strong genetic component responsible for determining bone mass, but environmental factors may also play a role, including possibly calcium intake and exercise.

The prevailing view that loss of bone mass with age is a linear function beginning in the fourth and fifth decade in women, and that different individuals lose bone at the same rate, is at present not substantiated. Accelerated bone loss has been observed with estrogen deficiency, a sedentary lifestyle, calcium deficiency, with alcohol and tobacco abuse, and in disease states such as hyperparathyroidism, hyperthyroidism, and with corticosteroid excess.

Screening tests to detect accelerated bone loss associated with increased bone turnover include bone Gla protein (osteocalcin) measurements, serum alkaline phosphatase activity, and hydroxyproline : creatinine and calcium : creatinine ratios in a morning fasting urine sample.

The principal risk factors for osteoporosis are, at present: female sex, Caucasian race, low bone mass at maturity, early menopause, a family history of osteoporosis, calcium deficiency, alcohol and tobacco abuse, and perhaps a sedentary lifestyle.

RELEVANT BONE MEASUREMENTS

Mazess reviewed the non-invasive quantitation of bone mass and density *in vivo*. Bone can currently be measured by diagnostic radiology methods (radiogrammetry, photodensitometry and X-ray computed tomography) and by nuclear medicine techniques (single and dual photon absorpti-ometry and ^{125}I computed tomography). In an experimental phase are Compton-scattering, neutron activation and $99^{m}Tc$ diphosphonate scanning.

In a normal population there is a moderate correlation between different skeletal sites of the appendicular skeleton and the axial measurements compared to the high ($r = 0.9$) intercorrelation measurements at different peripheral sites. In patient groups, however, the correlations are lowered, and measurements at the site of involvement have to be made in order to reach valid conclusions. For predicting osteoporosis of the spine or proximal femoral, none of the present techniques is perfect. Some overlap is seen between patients with vertebral crush and femoral fractures and age–sex matched controls, particularly in older (> 80 years) patients. This is also true for the invasive iliac crest biopsy measurement of trabecular bone volume.

Problems involved with computed tomography (QCT) were discussed in comparison with dual photon absorptiometry of the spine. The rates of menopausal bone loss reported in the literature are considerably different according to the techniques used to evaluate the bone changes. QCT of the spine showed an annual loss rate of 10% in oophorectomized women and 6% in menopausal women, while with dual photon absorptiometry of the spine the annual loss rate at menopause was half this. At the radius, using single photon absorptiometry, the annual loss rate in oophorectomized as well as in menopausal women was also 2–3%.

According to Mazess the sites for screening, diagnosis and monitoring of osteoporosis shown in Table W15.1 are recommended. Not everyone at the workshop agreed with these proposals. The radius has been used in the past as a reliable site of measurement for monitoring treatment and longitudinal evaluation.

Table W15.1 Screening, diagnosis and monitoring sites for osteoporosis

	Radius	Spine	Femur	Total skeleton
Screening	Yes	±	No	No
Diagnosis	±	Yes	±	Yes
Monitoring	No	Yes	±	Yes

TREATMENT OF POSTMENOPAUSAL OSTEOPOROSIS

Dietary calcium and bone health

Recker from Omaha reviewed the present value of dietary calcium for the prevention of postmenopausal bone loss.

Early attempts at demonstrating a relationship between low dietary calcium and fractures due to osteoporosis late in life were largely unsuccessful. In fact there is still little direct evidence to support this relationship.

Nevertheless, a substantial amount of data has been accumulated which demonstrates that nutrition, and perhaps nutrient interactions, may influence calcium balance in healthy postmenopausal women. In a group of nearly 200 women carefully studied on their own self-selected intakes, calcium balance was positively correlated with calcium intake, i.e. higher intake resulted in more positive balance[1]. Long-term studies of the effect of self-selected calcium intake on balance in this cohort of 200 women continue to demonstrate a positive effect of diet calcium on calcium balance. In two separate studies, in which calcium intakes were consciously increased by giving calcium as carbonate[2] in one case and as milk[3] in the other, calcium balance became more positive. These data support the notion that maintenance of bone mass in healthy women past menopause requires a calcium intake of about 1.5 g/d; however, longer studies are necessary to document that this will help prevent bone loss and fractures late in life. A survey of two communities in Yugoslavia[4] suggests that early nutrition may prevent later fractures. Nutrient interactions with calcium may be important in maintenance of bone health, and increases in protein, fiber and, perhaps, oxalate intakes are examples that may cause deterioration in calcium balance. Alcohol and caffeine ingestion may also[5]. These negative influences of diet on calcium balance must be viewed along with others, such as the effect of achlorhydria and independent effects that are attributable to the anion which accompanies dietary calcium. An example of the former is supplied by studies of 11 patients with achlorhydria[6] who absorbed calcium from carbonate poorly but hyperabsorbed calcium from a pH-adjusted citrate; and the latter, by studies in 28 healthy women showing that bone remodeling rates were significantly less suppressed by milk supplements than by calcium carbonate supplements[2,3]. Finally the interactions between diet calcium and hormone status and their combined effects on calcium balance are important. At any given self-selected intake, calcium balance is more positive in estrogen-replete women than in estrogen-deprived. Intakes required for average zero balance in the former are nearly 1 g/d and in the latter nearly 1.5 g/d. Conclusions from these data are: (1) bone health is favorably affected by higher calcium intakes in free-living healthy women; (2) optimum intake is about 1.5 g/d in women past menopause and about 1 g/d prior to menopause; (3) nutrient interactions may play a significant role in calcium balance; (4) long-term data on the antifracture efficacy of increased calcium intakes are needed.

Recker also stressed the fact that there is an exponential decline of bone mass after the menopause and that therefore this exponential pattern has an impact for timing of studies. Studies started early after the menopause will show more important changes than those started 10 or 15 years after the menopause when the rate of loss is almost nil.

PREVENTION OF OSTEOPOROSIS: ESTROGENS AND PROGESTOGENS

Lindsay discussed the use of estrogens as a preventive therapy for osteo-porosis. In asymptomatic younger women several well-designed clinical studies have now demonstrated that estrogens prevent the increased bone loss which occurs after oophorectomy or menopause. Such studies have been conducted using single photon absorptiometry and radiological techniques. One recent study has been conducted using computerized axial tomographic measurements of vertebral trabecular bone, but as yet no studies are available using dual photon absorptiometry. The effects of estrogens persist for as long as treatment is continued (now 10–12 years) and in some studies when estrogen therapy is terminated there is an acceleration of bone loss equivalent to that following oophorectomy or a natural menopause. The most acceptable theory for mechanism of action of estrogens requires for the direct stimulation of calcitonin. Increased production of calcitonin, and the subsequent biochemical changes, could explain many of the calcium kinetics and the bone effects which follow estrogen treatment.

The fact that women appear relatively calcitonin-deficient, in com-parison to men, might then explain the sexual dichotomy of osteoporosis. Certain facts currently do not fit this hypothesis and the possibility of a non-genome-dependent (i.e. receptor-independent) effect of estrogens on bone cells must not be overlooked. That estrogen renders the organism a more efficient utilizer of available calcium (using calcitonin as the first intermediary) is an attractive hypothesis. If that were so, calcium loss should be preventable by the supply of excessive calcium in the diet. This has been suggested by two controlled studies but has not been found sub-sequently. Certainly, bone loss in the early postmenopause appears more estrogen-dependent than dietary calcium-dependent and bone mass in younger women is equally more dependent on ovarian status than dietary lifestyle. The effect of estrogen in reducing bone turnover is, however, not specific, and certain progestogens and anabolic agents may also be effective therapeutic agents for prevention of bone loss. While such anti-resorptive agents play a key role in prevention of bone loss, the role by themselves in therapy of established disease is less obvious, although combination therapies have shown a reduction in fracture incidence.

CURATIVE TREATMENT: CALCITONIN, ANABOLIC STEROIDS AND SODIUM FLUORIDE

Chesnut reported results on curative treatment in osteoporosis. Salmon calcitonin in a daily dosage of 100 MRC units transiently but significantly increased total bone mass (+2%) through 18 months in 24 treated patients with postmenopausal osteoporosis and spinal compression fractures. In the osteoporotic patient with fractures and a reduced bone mass, calcitonin does appear to slow bone mass loss, but presumably such therapy is of limited value in replacing bone previously lost; possibly greater benefit in the osteoporotic patient could be achieved with a lesser calcitonin dosage administered intermittently, or through utilization of calcitonin in combination with other therapeutic agents known to stimulate bone formation.

In osteoporotic patients who have already developed fractures, the aim of therapy must be not only the prevention of further bone loss but, more importantly, the restoration of bone mass previously lost. In these individuals treatment should be directed at increasing bone mass above the hypothetical fracture threshold. In this clinical situation the use of anti-resorptive agents as the sole therapy is questionable; agents which stimulate bone formation ('positive bone-formers') are necessary to persistently increase bone mass. Fluoride is accepted as an agent capable of stimulating bone formation; in addition, data from a number of laboratories, including our own, suggest that anabolic steroids stimulate bone formation, rather than inhibiting bone resorption as was originally thought.

A double-blind controlled study with stanozolol in 23 treated and 21 control postmenopausal osteoporotic females with spinal compression fractures revealed a significant 4.4% ($+25.6$ g) increase in total bone mass (TBC-NAA) in the treated group through 29 months. An increase in the rate of bone formation as assessed by iliac crest bone biopsy was noted in the treated group ($p = 0.06$), and no new spinal compression fractures were noted in this group through 29 months. It would appear, therefore, that stanozolol, and presumably other anabolic steroids, will persistently increase bone mass and may prevent compression fractures, and therefore would be of value as 'positive bone-formers'.

Sodium fluoride is the other proven 'positive bone-former'; it is of value in increasing bone mass and conceivably in preventing fractures. Concern has arisen, however, regarding the structural integrity and possibly greater fracture potential of bone produced during fluoride therapy. Such bone is of greater crystallinity due to the substitution in the hydroxyapatite crystal of fluoride ions for hydroxyl ions, producing fluorapatite. Current data do suggest satisfactory skeletal strength in patients treated with fluoride. Side-effects to fluoride include gastric upset, tendonitis/fasciitis, and possibly exacerbation of arthritic symptoms. In addition, about 25% of osteoporotic patients show a limited response to fluoride therapy.

The individual patient response to these various medications will obviously vary; since osteoporosis is a heterogeneous disease, therapeutic responses would also presumably be heterogeneous. Nevertheless, the mean response of bone mass to these therapeutic perturbations would indicate potential value for the prevention of osteoporosis (calcitonin), and for the treatment of osteoporosis after the disease occurs (stanozolol and the anabolic steroids, and sodium fluoride). In the future there will undoubtedly be further utilization of these individual agents in combination therapies, and as part of sequential therapeutic programs.

REFERENCES

1. Heaney, R. P., Recker, R. R. and Saville, P. D. (1978). Menopausal changes in calcium balance performance. *J. Lab. Clin. Med.*, **92**, 953–63
2. Recker, R. R., Saville, P. D. and Heaney, R. P. (1977). Effect of estrogens and calcium carbonate on bone loss in postmenopausal women. *Ann. Int. Med.*, **87**, 649–55
3. Recker, R. R. and Heaney, R. P. (1985). The effect of milk supplements on calcium metabolism, bone metabolism and calcium balance. *Am. J. Clin. Nutr.*, **41**, 254–63
4. Matkovic, V., Kostial, K., Simonovic, I., Buzina, R., Brodarec, A. and Nordin, B. E. C. (1979). Bone status and fracture rates in two regions of Yugoslavia. *Am. J. Clin. Nutr.*, **32**, 540–9
5. Heaney, R. P. and Recker, R. R. (1982). Effects of nitrogen, phosphorus, and caffeine on calcium balance in women. *J. Lab. Clin. Med.*, **99**, 46–55
6. Recker, R. R. (1985). Calcium absorption and achlorhydria. *N. Engl. J. Med.* (In press)

FURTHER READING

Avioli, L. V. (ed.) (1983). *The Osteoporotic Syndrome: Detection, Prevention, and Treatment.* (New York: Grune & Stratton)

Chesnut, C. H. (1984). Treatment of postmenopausal osteoporosis. *Comprehen. Ther.*, **10**, 41–7

Dequeker, J. (1985). The relationship between osteoporosis and osteoarthritis. *Clin. Rheum. Dis.*, **11**, 271–96

Epstein, S., McClintock, R., Bryce, G., Poser, J., Johnston, C. C. and Hui, S. (1984). Differences in serum bone Gla protein with age and sex. *Lancet*, **1**, 1307–10

Johnston, C. C. Jr, Hui, S. L. and Christian, J. C. (1985). Some determinants of peak bone mass and subsequent rates of bone loss. In Christiansen, C. *et al.* (eds.) *Osteoporosis.* pp. 263–8. Glostrup Hospital, Glostrup. Proceedings of Copenhagen International Symposium on Osteoporosis, 3–8 June, 1984

Johnston, C. C. Jr, Norton, J. A. Jr, Khairi, R. A. and Longcope, C. (1979). Age-related bone loss. In Barzel, U. S. (ed.) *Osteoporosis II.* pp. 91–100. (New York: Grune & Stratton)

Kruse, H. P., Kuhlencordt, F. and Ringe, J. D. (1976). Correlation of clinical, densitometric and histomorphometric data in osteoporosis. In Pors Nielsen, S. and Hjorting-Hansen, E. (eds.) *Calcified Tissues.* pp. 437–61. (Copenhagen: FADL)

Lindsay, R., Hart, D. M. and Clark, D. M. (1984). The minimum effective dose of estrogen for prevention of postmenopausal bone loss. *Obstet. Gynecol.*, **63**, 759–63

Mazess, R. B. (1982). On aging bone loss. *Clin. Orthop. Rel. Res.*, **165**, 239–52

Mazess, R. B. (1983). Noninvasive methods for quantitating trabecular bone. In Avioli, L. (ed.) *The Osteoporotic Syndrome.* pp. 85–114. (New York: Grune & Stratton)

Mazess, R. B., Peppler, W. W., Chesney, R. W., Lange, T. A., Lindgren, U. and Smith, E. Jr (1984). Does bone measurement on the radius indicate skeletal status? *J. Nucl. Med.*, **25**, 281–8

Recker, R. R. and Heaney, R. P. (1985). The effect of milk supplements on calcium metabolism, bone metabolism and calcium balance. *Am. J. Clin. Nutr.*, **41**, 254–63

Riggs, B. L. (1983). Evidence for two distinct syndromes of involutional osteoporosis (editorial). *Am. J. Med.*, **75**, 899–901

Riggs, B. L., Seeman, E., Hodgson, S. F., Taves, D. R. and O'Fallon, W. M. (1982). Effect of the fluoride/calcium regimen on vertebral fracture occurrence in postmenopausal osteoporosis. *N. Engl. J. Med.*, **306**, 446-50

Smith, D. M., Nance, W. E., Kang, K. W., Christian, J. C. and Johnston, C. C. Jr (1973). Genetic factors in determining bone mass. *J. Clin. Invest.*, **52**, 2800-8

Wahner, H. W., Dunn, W. L. and Riggs, B. L. (1983). Noninvasive bone mineral measurements. *Sem. Nucl. Med.*, **13**, 282-9

Wahner, H., Dunn, W., Mazess, R. B., Towsley, M., Lindway, R., Markhardt, L. and Dempster, D. (1984). Dual-photon (153-Gd) absorptiometry of bone. *Radiology*, **156**, 203-6

Workshop 16

Psychoneuroendocrinology

Chairman: **L. Speroff** (USA)
Co-chairman: **L. Zichella** (Italy)

           J. Simpkins (USA)
           J. Fishman (USA)
           S. Zeisel (USA)
           I. Schiff (USA)
           L. Zichella (Italy)

Simpkins, from the Department of Pharmaceutical Biology at the University of Florida, reviewed his work on CNS neurotransmitters and aging. Age-related changes in Long Evans rats are characterized by a loss of LH surges in the development of constant estrus. The amplitude of estrogen-induced LH surges is also reduced, and prolactin levels are increased. GnRH concentrations in rat brains, however, are not changed in old rats. The concentration and turnover of norepinephrine is decreased in the preoptic, suprachiasmatic and median eminence areas.

The change in LH secretion is characterized by decreased amplitude and pulse frequency. In view of the GnRH and norepinephrine changes, this appears to be due to catecholamine CNS changes with age. This is supported by the fact that the administration of clonidine to old rats increased LH responses to a more youthful pattern.

In Fischer 344 rats, old age is associated with elevated prolactin levels which produce a pseudopregnant state. The administration of bromocriptine restores estrus cycles. No differences in GnRH concentration were found in areas of the brain, but as in previous studies norepinephrine concentration and turnover were decreased.

Dr Simpkins concluded that the hyperprolactinemia of aging in rats is the cause of a defect in the dopamine tuberoinfundibular tract.

Fishman, of the Rockefeller University, reviewed catecholestrogens, which have a clearance rate of 50–100 times that of estradiol, and this may explain the lack of activity in peripheral target tissues such as the uterus. However, catecholestrogens may function *in situ*.

Rat brain formation of catecholestrogens changes dramatically with the estrus cycle in rats. This activity is influenced by endogenous opiates. The action of catecholestrogens is inhibitory, but inhibitory only of the positive feedback action of estradiol on LH with no effect upon negative feedback. This inhibitory action operates only during the initial period of rising estradiol levels. The catecholestrogens of estrone, estradiol and estradiol-17α were all effective, but 2-hydroxyestrone was more effective at a later period while 2-hydroxyestradiol was more effective at the beginning of the estradiol rise. Thus, 2-hydroxyestrone and 2-hydroxyestradiol-17α are antagonists, while 2-hydroxyestrone has antagonist and agonist properties depending on the timing. The antagonistic action is avoided by the administration of GnRH, suggesting a hypothalamic site of action.

2-hydroxyestrone has no effect on postmenopausal LH levels in women. If LH is first reduced by estrogen priming, then 2-hydroxyestrone has an inhibitory action on LH levels.

Is there a physiologic role? Are catecholestrogens a mechanism for preventing repetitive LH surges? What do catecholestrogens have to do with aging? At the present time Dr Fishman does not have the foggiest idea.

Zichella, Chairman of the first clinic of obstetrics and gynecology in Rome, reported his studies of dopamine agonists and antagonists in the treatment of hot flushes. Bromocriptine treatment was studied in postmenopausal and ovariectomized women. Bromocriptine was superior to placebo in the reduction of hot flushes. This was associated with a decrease in the frequency of LH pulsatile peaks, as well as a decrease in the amplitude of the LH peaks. This reduction was greater with time; whether this effect is a primary dopamine effect or a secondary effect is, of course, unknown.

Bromocriptine was compared to veralipride, a drug which is a dopamine antagonist and crosses the blood–brain barrier. The effects of the two drugs in a crossover study were similar. Why were the end-results the same with two opposite-acting drugs? The administration of two other drugs, one a dopamine agonist and the other a dopamine antagonist, also inhibited hot flushes. At least we learned that dopamine is involved in hot flushes but why both agonist and antagonist work is unclear. The answer is lost in speculation on hypothalamic pathways.

Zeisel, from the Boston University School of Medicine, discussed nutrition and neurotransmitters. Some brain neurotransmitters clearly require blood amino acids for their synthesis. The blood amino acids are in turn dependent upon dietary intake. There exists a transport carrier system across the blood–brain barrier, to move these substances into the brain. Entry is dependent upon blood concentration of all substances which bind to the carrier as all must compete for the available carrier-binding sites.

There is a rhythm to blood levels of amino acids determined in part by diet. After a meal, insulin promotion of uptake of branched-chain amino acids by muscles results in decreased competition with tyrosine, and tryptophan for entry into brain. The result is an increase in serotonin, dopamine, and norepinephrine formation in the brain. Choline uptake by the brain is also increased after ingestion of meals supplemented with choline, leading to increased acetylcholine synthesis.

The clinical consequence of these principles include the following: (1) Because serotonin influences carbohydrate selection during eating, carbohydrate-induced insulin secretion and the secondary consequence of increased tryptophan entry into the brain, leads to serotonin-induced avoidance of carbohydrates. (2) Hyperalimentation alteration in amino acids can be expected to alter brain catecholamines and perhaps behavior. (3) Abnormal liver function leads to decreased blood levels of branched amino acids, which allows increased brain uptake of tryptophan and phenylalanine. The resulting increase in brain serotonin can contribute to sleepiness or coma while inhibition of dopamine and norepinephrine synthesis by the phenylalanine can also decrease alertness.

Food can be designed, therefore, so that it can be used as a drug. Lecithin-rich food can increase brain choline levels, for example to decrease movement in patients with tardive dyskinesia. Choline-enriched diets improve short-term memory in rats. Besides a potential use in older people, a sure-fire market exists during examination weeks on every campus. Tryptophan-enriched feedings make babies fall asleep sooner and sleep better, while valine, because it competes for transport, lowers tryptophan levels and hence serotonin, and produces the opposite effect. The same results can be seen in adults with insomnia. Manipulation of neurotransmitters in aging people can therefore be aided by dietary changes.

Schiff, from Harvard, told of his studies of sleep in postmenopausal women. The time it takes to fall asleep increases with aging. The time spent asleep, however, declines with aging. Although there is no major overall change at the time of menopause, individual patients do report sleep difficulties at and immediately after menopause.

In a crossover study on a sleep study unit, women on estrogen fell asleep faster and slept better compared to women on placebo medication (Table W16.1 and Fig. W16.1). A variety of mood and psychological tests showed improvement on estrogen (Fig. W16.2). Is the improvement a direct effect of estrogen, or does it reflect the loss of hot flushing either clinical or subclinical? Greater spikes of GnRH have been measured by

Table W16.1 Effects of placebo and estrogen treatment on various sleep factors in 27 patients[a]

	Placebo	Drug
Sleep latency* (min)	19.1 ± 6.1	12.2 ± 8.6
Total sleep time (min)	426.2 ± 55.6	438.3 ± 43.2
Total REM sleep** (min)	70.4 ± 9.7	$95.4 - 14.8$
Percentage REM time*	16.5 ± 1.1	21.7 ± 2.1
Percentage awake time	13.7 ± 2.2	10.4 ± 1.9
Sleep stage (percentage of time)		
I	10.2 ± 1.3	10.9 ± 1.7
II	40.3 ± 2.1	38.3 ± 2.1
III	11.0 ± 1.0	10.4 ± 1.2
IV	8.3 ± 1.3	8.3 ± 1.1

[a] All values given as means and standard errors of the mean
*$p < 0.05$
**$p < 0.005$

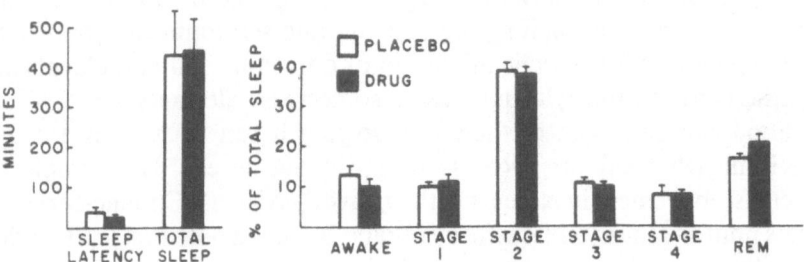

Figure W16.1 Mean sleep measurements during placebo and during drug conditions

Table W16.2 Comparisons between mean symptom scores

Symptom	Last drug week vs. first drug week	Last drug week vs. last placebo week	First placebo week vs. last placebo week	First placebo week v. first drug week
Hot flashes	Less[b]	Less[a]	Less[b]	Less[b]
Sweating		Less[a]	Less[b]	Less[a]
Depression			Less[b]	Less[a]
Breast pain			More[b]	More[a]
Discharge	More[a]	More[b]		

[a] $p < 0.05$
[b] $p < 0.005$

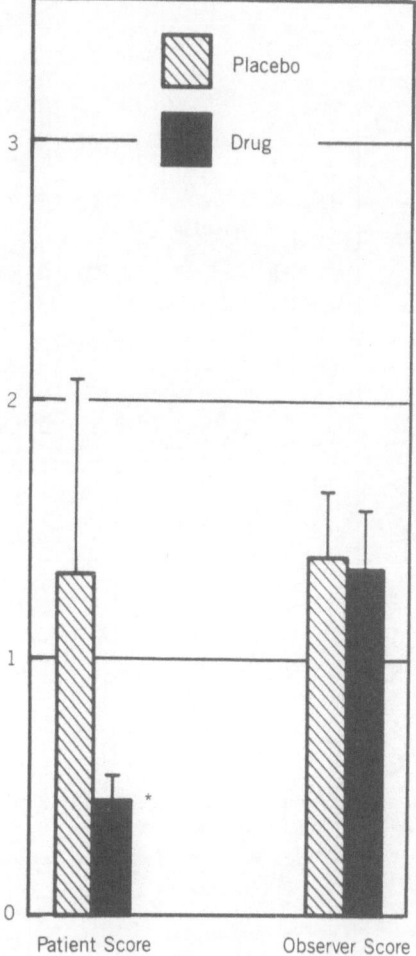

Figure W16.2 Clyde mood scores for aggression, on scale of 0 (least) to 3 (maximal). Asterisk indicates $p < 0.001$

this group in women who are symptomatic with hot flushes suggesting greater catecholamine changes (Figs. W16.3 and W16.4). The role of hot flushes therefore is a good bet. This study emphasizes the importance of the hot flush, extending its significance beyond the physical manifestations to a psychological and behavioral impact. Regardless of the mechanism, a good night's sleep helps individuals to meet the stresses and problems of life. This applies to all of us, and I assure you, to a greater and greater extent as we get older.

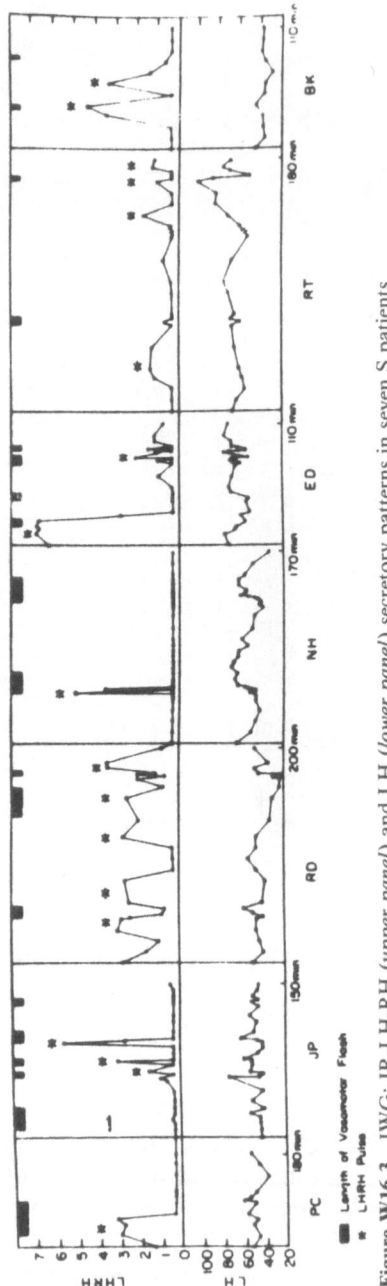

Figure W16.3 IWG: IR-LH-RH (*upper panel*) and LH (*lower panel*) secretory patterns in seven S patients

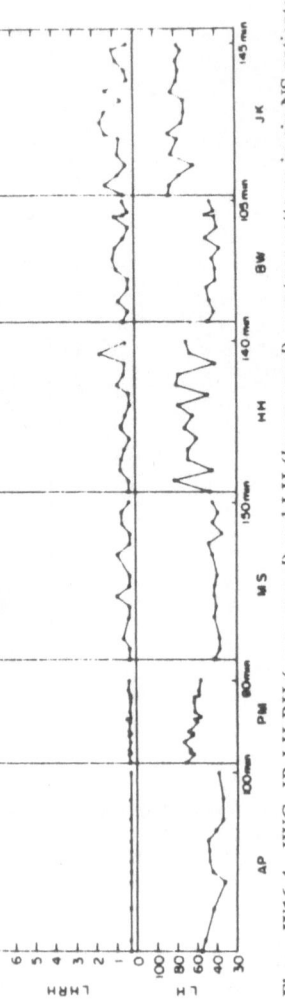

Figure W16.4 IWG: IR-LH-RH (*upper panel*) and LH (*lower panel*) secretory patterns in six NS patients

FURTHER READING

Erlik, Y., Tataryn, I., Meldrum, D. *et al.* (1981). Association of waking episodes with meno-pausal hot flashes. *J. Am. Med. Assoc.*, **245**, 1741

Fernstrom, J. D. and Wurtmann, B. J. (1972). Brain serotonin content: physiological regulation by plasma amino acids. *Science*, **178**, 414–16

Ravnikar, V., Elkind-Hirsch, K., Schiff, I., Ryan, K. J. and Tulchinsky, D. (1984). Vasomotor flushes and the release of peripheral immunoreactive luteinizing hormone-releasing hormone in postmenopausal women. *Fertil. Steril.*, **41**, 881–997

Regestein, Q. R., Schiff, I., Tulchinsky, D. and Ryan, K. J. (1981). Relationships among estrogen-induced psychological changes in hypogonadal women. *Psychosom. Med.*, **43**, 147–55

Schiff, I., Regestein, Q., Schinfeld, J. S. and Ryan, K. J. (1980). Interactions of oestrogens and hours of sleep on cortisol, FSH, LH, and prolactin in hypogonadal women. *Maturitas*, **2**, 179–83

Schiff, I., Regestein, Q., Tulchinsky, D. and Ryan, K. J. (1979). Effects of estrogens on sleep and psychological state of the hypogonadal women. *J. Am. Med. Assoc.*, **242**, 2405–7

Yogman, M. W. and Zeisel, S. H. (1983). Diet and sleep patterns in newborn infants. *N. Engl. J. Med.*, **309**, 1147–9

Zeisel, S. H. (1981). Dietary choline: biochemistry, physiology and pharmacology. *Ann. Rev. Nutr.*, **1**, 95–211

FURTHER READING

Other scientific contributions

Special Lectures

1. SOCIAL SCIENCE (Chairman: S. Ballinger;
Co-chairman: A. Holte)

A study of the climacteric as experienced by Glasgow women.
  K. Honigman, D. M. Barlow, H. M. Hart and D. M. Hart

The zero explanatory effect: sociological parameters and climacteric symptoms.
  A. Mikkelsen and A. Holte

A longitudinal study of sexuality through the menopause.
  N. McCoy and J. Davidson

Relationships between psychological symptoms, somatic complaints and menopausal status.
  M. Hunter, R. Battersby and M. I. Whitehead

Epidemiology of the climacteric syndrome in Linkoping, Sweden.
  G. Berg, M. Hammar, L. Fahraeus and U. Larsson-Cohn

Psychological and sexual adjustment to hysterectomy; a prospective study.
  M. Ryan, L. Dennerstein and R. Pepperell

Management of the menopause in British general practice.
  J. Coope

Natural history of the human menopause: a comparative approach.
  J. F. Donaldson

2. BASIC SCIENCE (Chairman: V. H. T. James;
Co-chairman: J. H. Thijssen)

In vitro observation of impaired testicular endocrine function in elderly men.
  M. Hammar, C. Ahlstrand and A. Berg

Oestrogens and immune reactivity.
  B. von Schoultz, B. Nilsson, A. Bergovist, E. Sodergard and M. G. Damber

Biosynthesis of oestriol in man: biological properties of intermediate and end products.
  J. Fishman and R. J. Herschcopf

Endogenous concentration of oestrone and oestradiol in atrophic and pathological human post-menopausal endometrium.
  C. Vermeulen-Meiners, J. Poortman, A. A. Haspels and J. H. Thijssen

Progesterone receptors in human vaginal tissue.
  S. Batra and S. Iosif

Peripheral androgen metabolism in post-menopausal women and in women with hirsutism.
  R. A. Lobo and P. C. Serafini

Oestradiol binding in endometrial cancer tissues.
  T. Csermely, G. Keller, J. Szekely and M. Vertes

Pharmacokinetic properties of oral oestrone sulphate piperazine and oestradiol valerate in post-menopausal women.
  A. R. Aedo, B. M. Landgren and E. Diczfalusy

3. OSTEOPOROSIS: RECENT RESEARCH (Chairman: D. Hart; Co-chairman: J. Dequeker)

Menopausal bone loss: effects of conjugated oestrogen and/or high calcium diet.
  B. Ettinger, C. Cann and H. K. Genant

Effect of oestrogen: progestogen treatment on bone turnover in early post-menopausal women.
  B. J. Riis, L. Nilas, C. Christiansen, P. Rodbro, B. D. Catherwood and L. J. Deftos

Regional variations in bone density in relation to total body calcium in the early post-menopausal period.
  J. C. Stevenson, L. M. Banks, C. Freemantle, T. Spinks, I. MacIntyre, R. Hesp, M. Padwick and M. Whitehead

Effect of castration on calcium regulating hormones.
  M. I. Whitehead, G. Lane, J. Morsman, J. Endacott, C. H. Myers and J. C. Stevenson

Relationship between calcium absorption, serum dehydroepiandrosterone and bone density in normal and osteoporotic post-menopausal women.
  B. C. Nordin, A. Robertson, T. Steurer, A. Bridges, B. E. Chatterton, R. F. Seamark and T. F. Hartley

Determinants of bone mass and bone loss response to oestrogen therapy in oophorectomized women.
  H. I. Abdalla, D. M. Hart, R. Lindsay and M. Aitken

Osteoporosis in menopausal women related to level of physical activity.
  L. D. Lutter and J. M. Lutter

Short communications

1. Basic investigation: physiology; pharmacology
(Chairman: D. Barlow; Co-chairman: R. Lobo)

Growth hormone, oestrogens and liver-protein synthesis.
B. von Schoultz and M.-G. Damber

Comparison of calcium-regulating hormones and calcitonin gene-related peptide levels in osteoporotic and non-osteoporotic women.
J. C. Stevenson, G. Abeyasekera, C. H. Myers, S. I. Girgis, C. Self and P. P. Allen

Role of melatonin in the regulation of the hypothalamic pituitary axis during the menopause.
F. A. Aleem, U. Weinberg and E. Weitzman

A primate model of human menopausal hot flushes.
J. Jelinek, E. Schonbaum and P. Lomax

Pharmacokinetics of orally administered oestriol in elderly women.
G. Samsioe, P. Eneroth and A. Jarnfelt-Samsioe

Effect of long-term oestrogen replacement therapy on plasma prolactin.
D. H. Barlow, C. Conaghan, F. A. Al-Azzawi and D. M. Hart

Effects of exogenous oestrogens on the prostacyclin/thromboxane balance in oophorectomized women.
G. Silfverstolpe, E. Enk, B. Kallfelt, G. Samsioe and N. Crona

Hormonal regulation of regional fat distribution in women.
L. Enk, N. Crona, M. Rebuffe-Scrive and P. Bjorntorp

Pharmacodynamic effects of orally active oestrogen formulations in peri-menopausal women.
E. Johannisson, B.-M. Landgren, M. le Donne and E. Diczfalusy

Changes in vaginal physiology during the menopause and the effect of exogenous oestrogen therapy.
J. P. Semmens, C. C. Tsai, E. C. Semmens, C. B. Loadholt and G. Wagner

Correlation between skin collagen content, skin thickness and an index of bone density: effect of years since menopause on these indices.
M. Brincat, C. Moniz, A. L. Magos, E. Versi and J. W. Studd

In-vivo induction of progesterone receptors (PR) in normal post-menopausal endometrium – evidence of lack of inhibitory control of PR synthesis.
I. G. Gorodeski, A. Geier, R. Beery, B. Lunenfeld and C. M. Bahary

2. Clincial: endometrium: progestin/estrogen therapy
(Chairman: B. Wren; Co-chairman: L. Rauromo)

Amenorrhoea and endometrial atrophy following continuous oral oestrogen and progestogen therapy in post-menopausal women.
A. L. Magos, M. Brincat, T. O'Dowd, P. Schlesinger, P. Wardle and J. W. Studd

Continuous combined treatment with conjugated oestrogens and either medroxyprogesterone acetate or norethisterone.
N. Siddle, M. Padwick, J. Endacott, H. Cooper and M. Whitehead

Effects of dydrogesterone, medroxyprogesterone acetate and oral progesterone on the oestrogenized post-menopausal endometrium.
M. Padwick, G. Lane, N. Siddle, J. Pryse-Davies, T. Ryder, R. J. King, P. Townsend and M. I. Whitehead

Effect of oestriol addition to oestradiol to protect the post-menopausal endometrium.
M. Padwick, N. Siddle, J. Endacott, H. Cooper, J. Pryse-Davies and M. Whitehead

Effects of high-dose treatment with oestriol in post-menopausal women.
O. Frankman, G. Valldor, K. G. Tillinger and B. von Schoultz

Controversies over estrogen replacement therapy; are progestogens necessary?
A. Haspels

Effect of oral medroxyprogesterone acetate on climacteric symptoms, plasma gonadotrophins and oestradiol levels.
F. A. Aleem

Treatment of menopausal symptoms with oral medroxyprogesterone acetate.
N. O. Siseles, A. Selzer, H. Benencia and R. Nicholson

Clinical and lipid metabolic effects of a new combination of conjugated esterified oestrogens and medroxyprogesterone acetate for the treatment of post-menopausal climacteric complaints.
G. Cullberg and G. Rybo

Plasma lipid and serum androgen levels in post-menopausal women treated with depomedroxyprogesterone acetate.
R. B. Barnes, S. Roy and R. A. Lobo

Continuous combined oral oestradiol and norethisterone acetate in post-menopausal women: effect on vasomotor symptoms, plasma lipids and lipoproteins.
D. A. Davey, G. M. Berger, D. Yon and F. E. Hardie

Progesterone is an antihypertensive!
M. Brincat, P. Rylance, V. P. Parsons and J. W. Studd

3. Clinical: pellet implants: general topics (Chairman: J. Studd; Co-chairman: W. Utian)

Endometrial and menstrual response to subcutaneous oestradiol and testosterone implants and continuous oral progestogen therapy in post-menopausal women.
A. L. Magos, M. Brincat, T. O'Dowd, P. Schlesinger, P. Wardle and J. W. Studd

Effect of long-term hormone replacement by implantation on plasma hormone levels and other parameters.
D. H. Barlow, A. D. Roberts, C. Conaghan and D. M. Hart

Problems of postmenopausal oestradiol implant therapy and their prevention: comparison of 25, 50 and 75 mg doses.
N. Siddle, M. Padwick, J. Endacott, H. Cooper and M. Whitehead

Subcutaneous hormone implants for the control of climacteric symptoms - a prospective study.
J. W. Studd, M. Brincat, A. L. Magos, E. Versi, L. D. Cardozo, T. O'Dowd and P. J. Wardle

Treatment of premenstrual syndrome with subcutaneous estradiol implants - a double-blind, placebo-controlled study.
A. L. Magos, M. Brincat and J. W. Studd

Psychological and physical side effects of cyclical norethisterone in post-menopausal women on pellet implants.
A. L. Magos, M. Brincat and J. W. Studd

Thermal entrainment testing - a new way of looking at menopausal flushing.
M. Brincat, K. Lafferty, J. de Trafford and J. W. Studd

Effects of topical oestrogen therapy in post-menopausal climacteric patients.
C. G. Netto, A. M. Fonseca, R. Hegg, N. R. Mello, J. R. Rilassi, M. M. Okada, S. B. Zynnier and C. A. Salvatore

Lower urinary tract symptoms, urodynamic findings and skin collagen in normal postmenopausal women.
E. Versi, L. Cardozo, M. Brincat and J. Studd

Oestrogen implants in the management of the menopausal urethra.
C. Richards

4. General: lipids and lipoproteins (Chairman: C. Lauritzen; Co-chairman: D. Davey)

Effect of hysterectomy on time of ovarian failure.
N. Siddle and P. Sarrell

Non-hormonal treatment of peri-menopausal women.
T. M. C. M. Schellen

Contraception in the middle-aged woman.
J. C. Stryker

Post-menopausal oestrogen replacement: prevention of osteoporosis and systemic effects.
F. W. Lafferty and D. O. Helmuth

Endometrial hyperplasia in women receiving oestrogen therapy.
C. Nezhat and A. Karpus

Breast tissue alterations – diagnosis by ultrasound.
D. Mulz

Cardiovascular risk factors: plasma lipids in the climacteric.
O. Blašková

Lipoprotein lipids and Apolipoprotein A1 – effects of Org OD 14.
N. Crona, G. Samsioe and G. Silfverstolpe

Hormonal and fibrinolytic effects of the synthetic steroid Org OD 14 in menopausal women.
R. W. Yates, A. Richards, H. P. McEwan, J. R. Coutts, I. D. Walker and J. F. Davidson

Effects on serum lipoproteins of 2 mg and 4 mg doses of oestradiol valerate.
G. Silfverstolpe, L. Enk, U. Lindberg, G. Samsioe and N. Crona

Effects of equine oestrogens alone and in combination with a progestogen on mineral and lipoprotein metabolism in post-menopausal women.
E. Farish, C. D. Fletcher, D. M. Hart and B. F. Allam

Hormonal therapy in the climacteric.
L. Rauramo

5. Clinical: psycho-social aspects: general (Chairman: A. Haspels; Co-chairman: J. Hailes)

Tryptophan studies in depressed post-menopausal women.
A. Teran, J. S. Chaddha, R. A. Roesel and R. B. Greenblatt

Biopsychological and sociological aspects of 'climacteric complaints'.
A. Mikkelsen and A. Holte

Work patterns and personal circumstances of midlife female nurses.
J. Nolan

Vasomotor and psychic climacteric symptoms according to age at menopause.
C. Campagnoli, F. D. Tetto, A. Sandri, P. Belforte and T. Maraschiello

Who speaks for women.
  D. Birnbaum

Menopausal stress, menopausal status and personality: a study of climacteric lifestyles among Indian women.
  V. K. Sharma

Characteristics of peri-menopausal women seeking assistance.
  R. W. Rebar, E. Anderson, S. Hamburger and J. Liu

Living in a post-menopausal body.
  B. T. Parker

Effects of regular exercise on self-perception of health and well-being in older women.
  J. M. Lutter

Exercise patterns of women aged 46–76: current physical activity compared with youthful patterns.
  J. M. Lutter and L. D. Lutter

Psychological effects of progestogens on oestrogen-treated post-menopausal women.
  N. Siddle, V. Williams, O. Young and M. Whitehead

Poster session

PARTICIPANTS (Chairman: R. Tesar; Co-chairman: R. Abrams)

Effects of the aging process and ovarian function on calcium metabolism in women.
J. C. Stevenson, G. Abeyasekera, C. H. Myers, G. Lane, M. Padwick, J. A. Endacott and M. I. Whitehead

Naturally occurring sex-related changes in lipoprotein metabolism.
W. F. Riesen and R. Mordasini

Comprehensive breast self-examination training.
G. H. Stein, H. S. Pennypacker and M. K. Goldstein

Anticarcinogenic effects of oestriol in DMBA-induced rat mammary cancer.
H. H. Wotiz, R. E. Muller, L. A. Cupples and M. Bennett

Urinary incontinence in post-menopausal women.
E. Versi, L. Cardozo and S. Williams

Changing profiles of FSH, LH, oestrone, oestradiol, progesterone and androstenedione from pre-menopause to post-menopause.
G. Rannevik, K. Carlstrom, S. Jeppsson, B. Bjerre and L. Svanberg

Salivary and plasma steroid levels in aging men following oral testosterone undecanoate administration.
M. Luisi, F. Franchi, P. M. Kicovic, G. F. Argenio, D. Barletta and A. D'Acunto

Assessment of patient and physician knowledge about osteoporosis.
C. Rector, B. Cook, J. Krischer and M. Notelovitz

Salivary testosterone in males at different ages.
G. Sorcini, M. Genderini, M. Palermo, M. Iozzo, M. Verri, M. Pepe, R. Sperone and M. Sperone

Development and testing of an instrument to evaluate the dynamic characteristics of the circumvaginal musculature.
M. C. Dougherty and R. Abrams

Transdermal administration of dihydrotestosterone for 3 months. Effects on hormone levels and lipids.
J. P. Deslypere and A. Vermeulen

Pharmacokinetics of oral micronized progesterone.
M. Padwick, J. Endacott and M. Whitehead

Effects of load bearing during treadmill walking in women aged 57 to 67 years.
K. E. Caramelli and M. Notelovitz

A plea for a uniform menopausal index.
L. J. Benedek Jaszmann

Provocation and objective assessment of menopausal hot flushes.
L. M. Germaine and R. R. Freedman

Conjugated oestrogens and clonidine: a new regimen for the treatment of post-menopausal women.
A. E. Schindler, D. Heners, T. Pater and U. Wendel

Clinical and laboratory trial of non-oestrogenic drugs in climacteric syndrome.
R. Hegg, A. M. Fonseca, C. G. Netto, J. R. Filassi, N. R. Mello, A. Z. Souza and C. A. Salvatore

Testosterone binding globulin levels in peri-menopausal women with benign and malignant breast disease.
A. Gorins, H. Rozenbaum, I. Husson, I. Loiseau, A. Barbey, M. Egloff and H. Degrelle

Oestriol treatment of urinary discomforts in elderly women.
A. Jarnfelt-Samsioe, A. Brandberg, S.-M. Samuelson, J. Ursing and G. Samsioe

Incompetent bladder neck in post-menopausal patients.
L. Cardozo, E. Versi, M. Brincat and J. Studd

Plasma β-endorphin in post-menopausal women.
F. A. Aleem and T. K. McIntosh

Oral discomfort during the menopause.
R. W. Wardrop, P. C. Reade, J. Hailes and H. G. Burger

An absorption study and clinical evaluation of two oestriol formulations for vaginal application.
L.-A. Mattsson and G. Cullberg

Long-term implant therapy and the prevention of post-menopausal osteoporosis.
D. H. Barlow, A. D. Roberts, F. A. Al-Azzawi and D. M. Hart

Management of persistent menopausal symptoms with oestradiol-testosterone implants: clinical, biochemical and hormonal results.
J. Hailes and H. Burger

Subcutaneous implantation of pure crystalline 17β-oestradiol and its effect on blood lipids and lipoproteins.
M. Oettinger, D. Yeshurun, A. Lanir, L. Kahana, S. Degani and M. Sharf

Detection of endometrial hyperplasia and endometrial cancer.
R. Erny, M. Garcia and F. Serradimigni

Hormonal profiles in women at risk for endometrial carcinoma.
T. von Holst, D. Klinga and B. Runnebaum

Use of conjugated oestrogen and progesterone in the treatment of climacteric complaints.
R. S. Samil, I. A. Rachman, T. Z. Jacoeb, E. J. Surjana and S. Soebijanto

Menopausal oestrogen therapy and the risk of endometrial, ovarian and breast cancer.
H. B. Peterson, N. C. Lee, P. A. Wingo, R. W. Sattin and G. L. Rubin

Premarin and low-dose sequential norethisterone and norgestrel treatment for climacteric women.
N. Siddle, M. Padwick and M. Whitehead

Enterohepatic recirculation of orally administered oestriol in menopausal women.
G. Heimer and D. Englund

Distinct actions of progesterone on human endometrial epithelial glands and stromal cells.
L. Tseng

Evaluation of skeletal metabolism before and after oophorectomy.
M. L. Smith, I. Fogelman, D. M. Hart, W. McIntosh, J. Bevan, J. Poser, I. Leggat and R. Cowan

Use of X-ray phalangeal mineral density to identify fast and slow bone losers.
R. S. Bachtell and C. Colbert

Prophylactic treatment for age-related bone loss in women.
C. Christiansen

Prolonged oestrogen substitution in post-menopausal women – a prospective study.
M. Furuhjelm

Treatment of vaginal mucosa in postmenopausal women before and after vaginal surgery.
S. Milojevic and P. M. Kicovic

Non-hormonal treatment of the post-menopausal syndrome.
N. E. Siseles, M. Diaz, H. Benencia and A. Foix

Randomized comparative trial of a sequential oestradiol/progestogen combination and oestradiol alone in the treatment of climacteric complaints.
U. J. Gaspard, J. Doyen, D. Gillian and R. Lambotte

Clinical, haematochemical and cytohormonal assessment of menopausal women treated with oestriol.
L. Zichella and G. C. Urbinati

An endocrine, metabolic and psychological study of the climacteric.
L. Zichella

Calendar-oriented compliance.
D. A. Leonard and W. G. Leonard

Medroxyprogesterone acetate in the treatment of post-menopausal syndrome.
J. Andor, R. Goldberg, T. Modly and W. Obolensky

Absorption of oral progesterone and its conversion into deoxycorti-costerone during oestrogen replacement therapy.
U. B. Ottosson, K. Carlstrom, J. E. Damber, B. Nilsson and B. von Schoultz

Effects of bilateral oophorectomy on lipoprotein metabolism.
C. D. Fletcher, E. Farish, D. M. Hart and L. Smith

Lipoprotein studies in climacteric men treated with pure testosterone.
J. S. Chaddha, A.-Z. Teran, E. B. Feldman and R. B. Greenblatt

Effects on two apolipoproteins of four different oestrogen-progestogen preparations administered continuously to post-menopausal women.
T. Sporrone, L.-A. Mattson and G. Samsioe

Effects of physiological sex steroids on haemostasis during menopause.
P. Fenichel, J. Y. Gillet, J. Bayle and M. Harter

Cyproterone acetate as a progestogen in post-menopausal oestrogen replacement therapy.
M. L. Padwick, J. Endacott, T. Ryder, J. Pryse-Davies, R. J. King and M. I. Whitehead

Consideration for calcium balance: a dietary calcium intervention pro-gramme for post-menopausal women.
R. Tesar, E. Shim and M. Notelovitz

Single photon absorptiometry – a valid method for detecting osteopenia.
R. Tesar, M. Notelovitz and W. Harris

Endocrine and clinical effects of veralipride and cyclophenyl in post-menopausal women.
M. Gambacciani, G. B. Melis, A. M. Paoletti, A. Cagnacci, F. Beneventi and P. Fioretti

Pharmacological manipulation of dopaminergic system in the control of post-menopausal hot flushes.
G. B. Melis, A. M. Paoletti, M. Gambacciani, A. Cagnacci, F. Fruzzitti, and V. Mais

Use of osteocalcin and a short infusion of calcium to predict post-menopausal women at risk to lose vertebral spongiosa rapidly.
B. S. Roof, D. Frey, C. Hudson, P. Ross and A. Gross

Hysteroscopy and the postmenopausal female.
H. Michlewitz

Effect of vaginal oestriol (E3) applications on receptor kinetics in oestrogen target tissues of postmenopausal women.
M. van Haaften, J. Poortman, G. H. Donker, M. A. H. M. Wiegerinck, A. A. Haspels and J. H. H. Thijssen

The effect of premarin on coagulation, fibrinolysis, and platelet function in perimenopausal Asian women.
F. H. M. Tsakok, S. Koh, S. E. Chua, R. Yuen and B. L. Ng

Oestrogen implants in the management of the menopausal urethra.
C. J. Richards

Some metabolic effects of trisequens, a combined hormone preparation.
C. D. Fletcher, E. Farish and D. M. Hart

Histological-hormonal profile in the pre-menopausal and post-menopausal phases.
R. Trevoux, J. Brux, M. Castanie and R. Scholler

Oestrogen (mestranol) in postmenopausal oophrectomized women: its effect on free thyroxine concentration and on TSH response to TRH.
H. I. Abdalla, D. M. Hart and G. H. Beastall

Effect on bone loss of long-term estrogen therapy commenced at different times after oophrectomy.
H. I. Abdalla, D. M. Hart and R. Lindsay

A holistic health management approach for menopause disorders.
C. Morse, L. Dennerstein, B. Cook and J. Krischer

A mobile unit for osteoporosis screening.
M. Notelovitz, C. Rector, B. Cook and J. Krischer

Comparison of single photon absorptiometry of the radius with radiographic absorptiometry of the phalanges.
L. McKenzie, R. Bachtell, R. Tesar, C. Colbert, J. Pendergast and M. Notelovitz

The metabolic effects of 50 mg and 25 mg 17β-estradiol pellet therapy in surgically menopausal women.
M. Johnston, S. Smith, Y. Suggs, S. Devine, I. Levenson and M. Notelovitz

A five year study prospective of oral oestriol succinate therapy.
C. Lauritzen

Change in plasma lipid fractions with menopause and the response to different hormonal treatments.
D. W. Thomas and B. E. Nordin

A male–female coalescence model of communicative change with aging.
H. Hollien and K. Massey

Response of a liver protein, sex hormone binding globulin (SHBG), to modulations of circulating oestradiol.
P. Stumpf and T. Lloyd

Skeletal alterations in ovariectomized rats.
T. J. Wronski, P. L. Lowry and C. C. Walsh

Tibolone (Org OD 14) in the control of the climacteric.
P. Fioretti, E. P. Grimaldi, G. B. Melis, M. Gambacciani, F. Stringini, and F. D. Petacchi

Self-limiting forearm bone loss in normal post-menopausal women.
B. E. C. Nordin, T. Huber, T. Steurer, C. Walker and B. Chatterton

The effect of three exercise treatments on the cardiovascular fitness of sedentary post-menopausal women.
C. Fields, K. Caramelli, Y. Suggs, W. Harris, K. Dunn and M. Notelovitz

Selective luteinizing hormone hypergonadoreophiam – pre-menopausal, peri-menopausal and post-menopausal forms.
S. Geller

Index

aging, and inactivity 43–5
alcohol use 37
  effects on nutrients 344, 345
  excess, link with cancer 347
  influence on osteoporosis 83
  vitamin deficiency 344, 349
androgen therapy 341
andropause, *see* male menopause
androstenedione, conversion to estrone
    193–7
animal experimentation, and pharmacologic
    evaluation of hot flushes 213–51
aromatase activity 194,196
atherosclerosis 55–6
Australia, population age structure 51

bereavement, effect on climacteric
    symptoms 309–10, 311
black women
  incidence of depression 185
  see also Nigeria: study of symptoms
blood coagulation 323–5
  action of progestins 388
blood pressure, age- and race-related
    differences 31
bone
  calcium blance 105
  cellular mechanisms 87–8
  decline in trabecular bone mass 89
  effect of progestogens 386–7
  factors determining mass 88–9
  fracture threshold 356–7
  loss, following oophorectomy 89
  mass and density measurement 421–2
  peak mass and calcium intake 356
  performance of collagen with age 332
  see also osteoarthrosis, osteoporosis
bone mineral analysis 95
  clinical applications 102–4
  neutron activation 98
  photodensitometry 97

  photon absorptiometry 97–8, 109
  quantification techniques 329
  quantitative computed tomography
    99–101
  radiogrammetry 97
  radiography 96
brain
  effect of reduced ovarian hormones
    207–9
  mediation of response to naloxone, in rat
    model of hot flushes 229–36
breast
  action of progestins 384
  atypical hyperplasia (atypia) 289, 290
  benign non-proliferative lesions 289,
    290
  changes 164
  fibrocystic mastopathy 286–7, 289
  see also Xeromammography
breast cancer
  comparison of estrogen, estrogen and
    progestogen therapies, and non-users
    of hormones 289
  diet 32, 347
  estrogen therapy involvement 12, 287–8
  free estradiol fraction 199–200
  hormone sensitivity 287
  incidence 285
    related to age 285
    related to age of first birth 291
  mortality 285
  risk factors 289–91
  screening criteria 288, 289, 291, 292
  temperature abnormalities 293

caffeine, influence on osteoporosis 83
calcitonin levels 89–90
calcium
  malabsorption 90, 104, 357–8
  metabolism 105–6
  and peak bone mass 356
  plasma levels 90

calcium intake   31, 34, 82, 343–5
  before and after menopause   357
  and bone fracture threshold   356–7
  nutritional factors   355
  and osteoporosis   422–3
  and skeletal mass   88–9
calcium therapy
  effectiveness   358
  estrogen-sparing action   358–9
caloric intake
  excess, linked with cancer   347
  reduction   27–8, 343
cancers
  dietary considerations   343, 345–8
  see also breast cancer, endometrial
    cancer, ovarian tumors
cardiovascular disease   10–11
  related to age at menopause   321
childbearing
  age, related to breast cancer incidence
    291
  completion, related to menopause   180
  cultural differences in attitude   141
  dietary influences   144–5
  influence on status of Indian women   186
children, effect on climacteric complaints
  134
cholesterol levels
  age-related   29, 30–1, 351–2
  during hormone replacement therapy   115
climacteric
  as research field   128
  attitudes and therapies
    during French Revolution   125–6
    18th century   124–5
    19th century   126–7
    20th century   127–8
    'poisonous menstrual blood' theory
      123–4
    prior to 18th century   123
    Tilt's influence   126–7
  attitudes of hetero- and homosexual
    women compared   303
  characteristics   19, 20, 177
  duration   19
  epidemiology   131–2
  historical sources   121–2
  lifestyles influencing   299–300
  medical model, challenged by
    anthropological and social research
    299
  medical requirements   20–1
  Newfoundland village study   149–59
  role of scientist in devising therapies
    23–6
  studies in non-Western cultures   135–6
  studies in the West   133–4
  see also menopause, perimenopause

clonidine   241–4, 246
  in treatment of hot flushes   236, 255,
    256, 273
collagen
  bone, performance with age   332
  skin thickness related to   316–17, 318,
    332
computed tomography (CT), see quantitative
    computed tomography (QCT)
contraception
  choice   369
  evaluation   367–8
  guidelines on requirement   368–9
  hormonal   83
    for women over 40 years   369–72
    risks   324, 325, 373–5
  increasing availability   127
  intrauterine devices   375–6
  side effects   368
  sterilization   376–8
  triphasic   370–1
  vasectomy   378
coping skills   302–3
cortisol, and aromatase activity   194, 196
cultural influences   177
  in Japanese women   412–13
  in Mayan Indian and Greek women
    compared   140–6
  in non-Western societies   135–6
  increasing prestige with age   179–80
  on attitudes to menopause   139–40
  on variety of women's roles   186
  study of Newfoundland village   149–59
  variations   133
cystadenomas, ovarian   315

danazol therapy   272
dehydroepiandrosterone sulfate (DHA-S)
  198
depression
  Nigerian women   171, 173
  pre-menopausal, related to coping skills
    307
  reporting, related to life stress   307
  situational causes   185
destrusor instability (DI)   317
developing countries
  expenditure on health and on defence   13
  increase in menopausal women   7
  life expectancy   5
  osteoporosis   8–10
  population growth   2–4
diabetes mellitus   31
diet
  Greek and Mayan Indians compared
    143, 144–5
  influences on menstruation and
    childbearing   144–5

dizziness, reported by Nigerian women
171, 172
dopamine
metabolism, in morphine-dependent rats,
after withdrawal 236–40
role of agonists and antagonists in hot
flushes 430
dual photon absorptiometry 98, 330
diagnosis of crush fracture osteoporosis
331
precision 330
spine 422
technical requirements 331–2
dyspareunia 165, 174, 339

endogenous opioid peptide (EOP) activity
217
endometrial cancer
and diet 32
preventive measures 383
protective dosages of progestin 318
endometrial hyperplasia
effect of progestins with estrogen therapy
385
estrogen risk 12–13
epidemiology of the climacteric 131–2
methodology 132–3
estradiol
availability 199–200
conversion of estrone to 197–9
levels, and symptoms of menopause 216
receptor sites in brain 208, 209
sex differences in reaction 209
estradiol therapy
pharmacological and pharmacokinetic
aspects 396–403
vaginal rings 334
estrogen
action on bone 89
carcinoma-inhibiting and -promotion
roles 288
decreased production 193
effect on lipids 353
effect on nerve cell function 208
fibrocystic breast disease 287
presentation to target tissues 193–200
production and metabolism 404–8
regulating calitonin secretion 89
synthesis and reabsorption, related to fat
intake 33
estrogen therapy 8
alternative routes of administration 27,
325–6, 334, 393–6
benefits after withdrawing therapy 112,
114
blood clotting 324
breast cancer 286
correlation with sexual activity 339–40

early forms 272
effect on atherosclerosis 56
effect on brain 209
effect on hot flushes 254, 255, 266
effect on osteoporosis 424
effect on sexuality 55
effect on sleep 431–3
effect on stress incontinence 317–18
length of treatment 277
modes of administration 334
opposed by progestogen 287–8, 382
dosage levels 25–6, 318
following hysterectomy 288–9
regimens 277
risks 12–13
studies of efficacy 275, 277
with calcium supplement 358–9
see also hormone replacement therapy
estrone
conversion to estradiol 197–9
from androstenedione 193–7
ethamsylate, in therapy for hot flushes
273
exercise 35
adverse considerations 88
and aging 43–5
changes following physical conditioning
44
effect on fitness decline in men 296
effect on osteoporosis 83, 88
for postmenopausal women 41–7
influence on physiological age 41, 42
measuring activity 42–3
medical screening 45–6
planning 45
program design 46–7

fats, dietary 31
and cancers 32–3, 347
fertility
decrease with age 368
premenopausal, monitoring 333
fiber, dietary 33–4, 347–8
fibrocystic mastopathy 286
prolactin and estrogen involvement 287
related to incidence of breast cancer 289
flexibility of joints 45
folk knowledge 150, 151–2, 157–8
see also cultural influences
fractures
hip: age distribution 96
osteomalacia as cause 354
prevalence 106–7
risk period 89
factors affecting 79–80
vertebral 96, 331
diagnosis 331

genetic factors 145
Greek study 140-6

hand, thermoregulatory role 254
see also metacarpal index
headaches, reported by Nigerian women
171, 172
see also symptoms
health care, uptake by women 52-3
hormone replacement therapy (HRT)
blood clotting 323-5
cardiovascular disease 321-2
cost-benefit considerations 114-15, 117
improvements 56-7
limitations 272
monitoring 333-4
possible misunderstandings 260
risks 12-13, 57
time span 266
see also estrogen therapy
hormones
changes with age, animal studies 429-30
effect on lipids 353
polypeptides in women with multiple
breast cysts 292-3
hot flushes (flashes)
action of clonidine 236
age at first onset 262-3
animal model for pharmacologic
evaluation 213-51
areas for research 267
blood flow measurements 316
characteristics 215
decrease over time 265, 267
degrees of intensity 263-4
duration 134, 214-15, 256, 266
early treatments 271-2
frequency 264-5
Greek women 143
in men 254, 279
in Nigerian women 169
incidence 261
and duration 214-15, 256
measurement methods 253
morphine-dependent rat model 218-25
brain mediation of response to
naloxone 229-36
effect of withdrawal on norepinephrine
and dopamine metabolism 236-40
narcotic antagonist studies 226-9
role of α-adrenergic neurons in skin
temperature response to naloxone
240-6
role of dopamine agonists and
antagonists 430
self-reporting methods 262
severity, comparison of clinic patients
and non-patients 305

skin temperature increase 260
study design and methodology 261-3
therapies 271-81
non-estrogenic 272-4
triggers 254-5
vascular response pattern 253-4, 256
compared with non-flushing women
256
viewed as disease symptom 260-1
women's views on 263
hysterectomy 378

incontinence, stress-related 317
insomnia, reported by Nigerian women
171, 172
see also symptoms
intrauterine devices 375-6
iron deficiency 343, 349
irritability, reported by Nigerian women
169
see also symptoms

Japanese study 412-13
joints, flexibility of 45

life events
as source of stress 300-2
comparison of clinic patients and
non-patients 304-7
coping skills 302-3
perimenopausal symptoms 307-11
vulnerability model 310
life expectancy 4-5
sex ratios 6
lipid levels
effect of estrogen 353
effect of progesterone 353
factors influencing 351-3
lipoproteins
effect of progestins 383, 387-8
hormone replacement therapy 322
liver response, in estrogen therapy 325-6

male menopause 341
hot flushes 254, 279
social context 295-6
males
changes in sexual parameters 296-7
fertility levels 296
physical fitness related to age 296
mammography, *see* xeromammography
Mayan Indian study 140-6
medical aid, factors influencing desire for
133
menopause
age: factors influencing 7
Greek and Mayan Indian women 142
Indonesian women 135
Nigerian women 162, 173

artificial 63, 64, 65-6, 69, 72-3
attitudes among Nigerian women 162-3, 173
celebratory ritual 183
common perceptions 59, 60
consultations with relatives or friends 72
definition 7, 63
duration, in Indonesia 136
and end of childbearing 180
epidemiological research needs 73
future factors 415
lack of information from developing countries 7
local understanding of term 154
related to population growth 6-7
sources of information, in small communities 156-7
stereotypes 259-60
studies of health status 60-3, 72
variety of experience 266, 267
women's attitudes to 71-2
see also climacteric, perimenopause, postmenopause, premenopause
menstruation
coping style, related to climacteric coping style 303
cultural differences in attitudes 141
cultural restrictions on activity during 180, 181
dietary influences 144-5
Islamic restrictions 184
related to childbearing, Mayan Indian and Greek women compared 143, 145
metacarpal index (MI), in osteoporosis screening technique 332-3
methyldopa therapy, for hot flushes 274
mood changes, related to estradiol and progesterone levels 208-9
see also symptoms
muscular strength 45
musculoskeletal disorders 11

naproxen therapy, for hot flushes 274
neutron activation analysis, for bone mineral assessment 98
Newfoundland village study 149-59
Nigeria, study of symptoms 161-75
demographic data 162, 163
norepinephrine, action of clonidine 236
numbness, reported by Nigerian women 171
see also symptoms
nutrition 27-39
additives and contaminants 348
and cancer 343, 345-8
current recommendations 37-8
deficiencies 33-5

dietary fiber 347-8
and calcium intake 355
effect of medication 35
effect on neurotransmitters 430-1
excesses 27-33
factors in osteoporosis 355-9
influence on middle life health 343
need for variety 343, 344, 345
and osteoporosis 82-3, 423
recommendations 344-5
sources of information 37

obesity
and conversion of androstenedione to estrone 193-4
correlation with cancers 347
determinants 27-8
and protection of skeletal mass 355
related disease risks 30
opiate withdrawal, similarity to menopause symptoms 217, 218
opipramol therapy, for hot flushes 274
osteoarthrosis, characteristics 420
osteomalacia 106
and vitamin D deficiency 354
osteopenia 34, 106
osteoporosis
bone collagen loss 317
change in cellular activity 88
characteristics 420
counseling 95-6
cultural and dietary influences 145
definition 419
diagnostic methods 8
and endocrine status 83
etiology 87-91
in developing countries 8-10
incidence 34
and cost 79
related to weight 356
influence of exercise 83, 88
nutritional factors 82-3, 343, 355-9
pathogenesis 79-84
postmenopausal and senile 96
preventive measures 424
risk assessment 84
risk factors 8, 81-2, 83-4, 96, 421
savings effected by estrogen therapy 56
screening 332-3, 420-1
structural changes 80
treatment 422-3
curative 424-6
optimal dose of optimal prophylaxis (study) 108, 111-14
optimal preventive treatment (study) 108, 109-11
therapeutic agents 8-9
vitamin D therapy 355

with calcium malabsorption 357-8
see also estrogen therapy, hormone
  replacement therapy
ovarian cystadenomas 315
ovarian hormones
  effect on brain 207-9
  relationship between decline and hot
    flushes 215-16
  withdrawal phenomena 217
  see also estradiol, progesterone
ovarian tumors
  detection by non-invasive means 23-4
  study 315-16
ovaries, volume, correlation with
  menopausal age 316

parathyroid hormone 90, 105
perimenopause
  definition 7, 63
  in Mayan Indian and Greek women
    compared 140-6
  symptoms: Nigerian study 161-75
    related to life events 307-11
  see also climacteric
phentolamine 245-6
phosphate intake 355
phosphorus intake, effect on calcium
  homeostasis 82-3
photodensitometry, for bone mineral
  assessment 97
photon absorptiometry, *see* dual photon
  absorptiometry, single photon
  absorptiometry
population, sex ratios in Australia 51
population growth 1-2
  environmental effects 3-4
  in developing countries 2-4
  and urbanization 4
postmenopause
  cultural differences in attitude 136
  definition 7
  dominant western view 139
  exercise requirements 41-7
  Mayan Indian and Greek women
    compared 140-6
  problems 53-5
  summary of requirements 57
potassium intake 31
pregnancy
  complications related to age 368
  cultural attitudes to late pregnancies
    180-1
  patterns among Greek and Mayan Indian
    women compared 143-4, 145
premenopause
  loss of fine skin microcirculation 316
  Mayan Indian and Greek women
    compared 140-6

risk of pregnancy 368
progesterone
  effect on lipids 353
  mechanism of action 203-5
  natural 381
  receptors 204-5, 208-9, 384-5
  salivary, immunoassay 333
  stimulating E_2DH 198
  synthesis of progestins 381
  vaginal rings 334
progestins
  action on blood coagulation 388
  characteristics 381-2
  counteracting estrogen therapy 25-6
  dosage levels 318
  effects on lipoproteins 387-8
  prevention of endometrial cancer 383
  psychological effects 388-90
progestogens
  effect on bone 386-7
  therapy of hot flushes 274-5, 277
  with estrogen therapy 56-7, 277
prolactin, and fibrocystic breast disease
  287
propranolol therapy, for hot flushes 273-4
prostaglandins 325
pulse rate, during hot flushes 257

quantitative computed tomography (QCT)
  330
  for bone mineral assessment 99-101
  minimum radiation exposure 330
  precision 330
  vertebral 422

radiogrammetry, for bone mineral
  assessment 97
radiography, for bone mineral assessment
  96
rituals, to celebrate menopause 183

saliva, steroids in 333-4
salt intake 31
  excess, link with cancer 347
sedatives 272
sedentary lifestyles 43
self-help groups 362-4
  aims 362
  Climacteric Outreach 362
  for men 364
  philosophy 361-2
  post-mastectomy 362
  Swedish summer camps 363
senility, prevention of 13
sexual activity
  cultural restrictions 180-1
sexual desire, loss of 167-8, 173
sexuality after menopause 55

sexuality at menopause   173-4
  decline in interest   337, 339
  etiology of changes   339-40
  following surgical menopause   340
  management of problems   340-1
  of aging males   296-7, 341
  study   338
  touch impairment   339, 340
  types of changes   338-9
single-photon absorptiometry (SPA)   332
  for bone mineral assessment   97, 109
skin thickness
  related to bone collagen   316-17
  related to skin collagen   318, 332
sleep, differences with age   431-3
socioeconomic factors   134-5
status of older women
  as mother   184-5
  close-knit societies   182-3
  cultural variations   182
  effect of menopause   125, 133, 139
  Greek and Mayan Indian societies   141-2
  Newfoundland village   155
  non-industrialized societies   414-15
  sociocultural factors   178-9
  Western societies   185-6
sterilization   376-8
steroid receptor assays   286
steroids, in saliva   333-4
stilboestrol   272
stress
  definition   300
  factors   310-11
   study of perceptions   300-2
  genuine stress incontinence (GSI)   317
  incidence   300-1
  provoking hot flushes   255
  related to seeking medical help   304-7
  related to symptom reporting   307
  response based on past behaviour   303
symptoms   214
  among Japanese women   136
  anthropological study   411-13
  comparison between clinic patients and non-patients   304-7
  incidence   133-4
  influence on attitudes to menopause   163, 173
  Mayan Indian women   142
  Nigerian study   161-75
  perimenopausal, related to life events   307-11
  postemenopausal   134
  premenopausal   134
  problems for research   149-50
  reported by Greek women   142-3
  serum estradiol levels   216
  similarity to opiate withdrawal   217, 218

views on hot flushes   260-1
  see also hot flushes (flashes)

tachycardia, preceding hot flush   215
temperature, skin   262
testerone levels   297
testerone therapy   296, 297
thermography, in cancer screening   293
thermoregulation   215
trace elements   350
  history of study   350
  recommended intakes   350-1
tranquilizers   252
triglyceride levels, age relationship   29, 31, 352

ultrasound screening, for ovarian cancer   315, 316
urbanization, related to population growth   4
urethral instability (UI)   317
urological symptoms   317-18
uteroglobin, interaction with progesterone receptors   203-4

vaginal dryness   167, 339
vaginal rings   334
vaginismus   174, 339
vasectomy   378
vasodilatation, peripheral, in hot flushes   256
vegetarian diet   33-4
venous occlusion plethysmography   253
vitamin A deficiency   348
vitamin C deficiency   348
vitamin D   105
  levels, geographical influences   353-4
  metabolism   106
  supplements   353, 354-5
vitamin deficiencies   344, 349
vitamin E therapy   272
vitamin intake   349-50
vitamin supplements   35, 36, 344
  misuse   350, 351
  professional supervision   350

weight
  ideal   35
  reducing diets   36
working women, and experiences of complaints   134-5

xeromammography   291
  radiation dosage   292
  screening criteria   292